NARCOTICS AND THE HYPOTHALAMUS

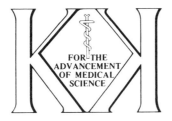

FOR THE
ADVANCEMENT
OF MEDICAL
SCIENCE

Kroc Foundation Symposia
Number 2

Narcotics
and the
Hypothalamus

Editors

Emery Zimmermann
Department of Anatomy
and Brain Research Institute
School of Medicine
University of California at Los Angeles

Robert George
Department of Pharmacology
and Brain Research Institute
School of Medicine
University of California at Los Angeles

Raven Press ▪ New York

Dedication

When Dr. David M. Hume died in a plane crash in May 1973, the many notices of his death in newspapers and medical publications referred extensively to his career in transplant surgery; however, the fact that this remarkable man was also one of the founders of neuroendocrinology was largely ignored. Born in Michigan in 1917, Dr. Hume received his M.D. from the University of Chicago in 1943 and his surgical training at the Peter Bent Brigham Hospital and Harvard. He assumed the chairmanship of the Department of Surgery at the Medical College of Virginia in 1958 and held that position until his death.

He was a man of many interests and great energy. One of his major interests was the body's response to stress. It was in Boston, while carrying out his first experiments on kidney transplantation, that he hit upon the idea that the pituitary-adrenocortical response to stress might be triggered via the hypothalamus. To test this hypothesis, he made hypothalamic lesions in dogs and demonstrated that these lesions abolished the stress response. He published these studies with Wittenstein at the same time that Harris and de Groot published their similar observations on rabbits. However, he went further. Working with Dr. P. H. Forsham and others in the late 1940's, he prepared extracts of beef hypothalamic tissue and showed that these extracts increased ACTH secretion in lesioned dogs. The results of these experiments were published only in abstract form, but they clearly anticipated by several years the subsequent studies demonstrating the existence of corticotropin-releasing factor.

Dr. Hume subsequently devoted more and more of his time to his work on organ transplantation, and dropped out of neuroendocrinology. However, his pioneering work clearly stimulated many others, including myself, to investigate further the concept of neuroendocrine control. Indeed, a remarkably large part of neuroendocrinology in the United States stems from the studies initiated by David Hume. This book, which is concerned with several aspects of hypothalamic function, is therefore dedicated to him.

William F. Ganong
Department of Physiology
University of California, San Francisco

Preface

In the summer of 1972, a highly successful conference entitled "Drug Effects on Neuroendocrine Regulation" was held near Aspen, Colorado, as a satellite symposium of the Fifth International Congress on Pharmacology. That conference reviewed and identified significant advances in the rapidly expanding fields of neuropharmacology and neuroendocrinology and provided for the fruitful interchange of ideas on problems in several areas of common interest in these two disciplines.

Subsequently, a unique opportunity to explore one of these areas in greater depth was made available by the generosity of The Kroc Foundation. Through the support and encouragement of the Foundation, its founder, Ray A. Kroc, and its president, Dr. Robert L. Kroc, another very successful meeting, "Effects of Drugs of Abuse on Hypothalamic Function," took place on February 27 to March 1, 1974, at Foundation headquarters, the J & R Double Arch Ranch in the Santa Ynez Valley near Santa Barbara, California. All participants agreed that the efficient but relaxed exchange of information and ideas at the meeting was due in part to its limited size, excellent facilities, and picturesque setting. More important, however, was the warm and gracious hospitality of Dr. and Mrs. Robert Kroc and of Dr. Peter Amacher, who played a key role in organizing and conducting the meeting and in providing valuable editorial advice.

The scientific sessions of the meeting covered autonomic, neuroendocrine, and developmental aspects of drug actions on hypothalamic activity. I would like to thank Drs. Peter Lomax, Charles Sawyer, and Roger Gorski for moderating the various sessions. Special thanks are given to Dr. Robert George, who helped with advice and with editing the manuscripts, and to Mrs. Barbara Pettley for her secretarial assistance. Finally, I would like to thank each of the participants for taking part and for their prompt submission of manuscripts.

Emery Zimmermann
Los Angeles

Contents

Participants and Contributors

P. Amacher
The Kroc Foundation
Santa Ynez, California

M. Ary
UCLA School of Medicine
Los Angeles, California

B. Branch
UCLA School of Medicine
Los Angeles, California

M. Braude
National Institute of Drug Abuse
Rockville, Maryland

P. Brazeau
Salk Institute
La Jolla, California

H. Brøndsted
University of Utah College of Medicine
Salt Lake City, Utah

P. Cushman, Jr.
Columbia University College of Physicians
    and Surgeons
New York, New York

W. de Jong
University of Utrecht Medical Faculty
Utrecht, The Netherlands

G. A. Deneau
University of California
Davis, California

D. de Wied
University of Utrecht Medical Faculty
Utrecht, The Netherlands

D. H. Ford
Downstate Medical Center, State Uni-
    versity of New York
Brooklyn, New York

W. F. Ganong
University of California
San Francisco, California

J. M. George
The Ohio State University
Columbus, Ohio

R. George
UCLA School of Medicine
Los Angeles, California

A. Goldstein
Stanford University School of Medicine
Palo Alto, California

R. A. Gorski
UCLA School of Medicine
Los Angeles, California

R. Guillemin
Salk Institute
La Jolla, California

P. G. Harms
University of Texas Southwestern Medical
    School
Dallas, Texas

J. Hayward
UCLA School of Medicine
Los Angeles, California

C. Johanson
University of Utah College of Medicine
Salt Lake City, Utah

F. W. L. Kerr
Mayo Graduate School of Medicine
Rochester, Minnesota

A. Koestner
Ohio State University
Columbus, Ohio

N. Kokka
University of California
Irvine, California

M. J. Kreek
Rockefeller University
New York, New York

R. L. Kroc
The Kroc Foundation
Santa Ynez, California

L. Krulich
University of Texas Southwestern Medical
    School
Dallas, Texas

C. Libertun
University of Texas Southwestern Medical
    School
Dallas, Texas

H. H. Loh
University of California
San Francisco, California

P. Lomax
UCLA School of Medicine
Los Angeles, California

B. H. Marks
Wayne State University College of
    Medicine
Detroit, Michigan

S. McCann
University of Texas Southwestern Medical
    School
Dallas, Texas

I. A. Mirsky
Brentwood Veterans Administration
    Hospital
Los Angeles, California

S. R. Ojeda
University of Texas Southwestern Medical
    School
Dallas, Texas

W. H. Oldendorf
UCLA School of Medicine
Los Angeles, California

C. N. Pang
UCLA School of Medicine
Los Angeles, California

R. K. Rhines
Downstate Medical Center, State Uni-
    versity of New York
Brooklyn, New York

K. K. Sakai
Ohio State University
Columbus, Ohio

C. Sawyer
UCLA School of Medicine
Los Angeles, California

U. Scapagnini
University of Naples Faculty of Medicine
Naples, Italy

A. N. Taylor
UCLA School of Medicine
Los Angeles, California

L. F. Tseng
University of California
San Francisco, California

W. Vale
Salk Institute
La Jolla, California

J. M. van Ree
University of Utrecht Medical Faculty
Utrecht, The Netherlands

K. Voeller
Downstate Medical Center, State
    University of New York
Brooklyn, New York

E. L. Way
University of California
San Francisco, California

E. T. Wei
University of California
San Francisco, California

R. Weiner
University of Southern California
Los Angeles, California

A. Wikler
*University of Kentucky College of
    Medicine
Lexington, Kentucky*

D. M. Woodbury
*University of Utah College of Medicine
Salt Lake City, Utah*

J. Young
*UCLA School of Medicine
Los Angeles, California*

E. Zimmermann
*UCLA School of Medicine
Los Angeles, California*

Narcotics and the Hypothalamus, edited by
E. Zimmermann and R. George. Raven Press,
New York © 1974

General Overview of Theories of Opiate Tolerance and Dependence

Gerald A. Deneau

Department of Pharmacology, University of California, Davis, California 95616

This volume is devoted to detailed examinations of some of the factors involved in the development of tolerance to and physiologic dependence on narcotic analgesic drugs. No attempt will be made here to establish the precise mechanisms of these biologic phenomena. Our purpose is merely to outline the possibilities from a pharmacologic viewpoint.

First some limiting definitions are in order. By tolerance we mean that successive doses of a drug produce diminishing biologic responses, thus necessitating ever-increasing doses to achieve responses equal in magnitude to the initial effect. When an organism becomes tolerant to a given chemical agent (drug), it shows cross-tolerance to all other chemicals having similar pharmacologic properties but not to drugs with dissimilar properties.

Physiologic dependence develops in a biologic organism after a prolonged exposure to some foreign chemicals, such as the narcotic analgesics. When such exposure is discontinued, either by removal of the foreign chemical from the environment or, in the case of the narcotic analgesics, by the addition of a specific antagonist, there is a change of responsivity in the biologic organism, usually in the direction opposite to that produced by the foreign chemical. The syndrome of signs resulting from this altered reactivity of the biologic system is the abstinence or withdrawal syndrome. It usually persists for several days in large animal and human subjects, although some elements may be detected for weeks or months.

To understand how a drug might induce tolerance and/or physiologic dependence, it is necessary to have a working concept of how drugs act. The "receptor theory" is now almost universally accepted. Biologic organisms are composed of a multitude of chemical substances which are combined in many forms, some to provide rigid structures such as bone; some to provide cell membranes with a wide variety of specific properties; some to provide intracellular substances with specific functions such as contraction, secretion, and metabolism; and some, such as blood, lymph, and extracellular fluid, to transport oxygen, carbon dioxide, nutrients, waste products, endocrine messenger substances, etc. from one part of the body to another. The receptor theory postulates that drugs react with specific chemicals or "receptors" of some tissues in such a way as to increase or decrease the activity of that tissue.

Such an alteration in activity is the "drug response." The magnitude of the response depends on the number of receptors occupied by, or in combination with, drug molecules at any given moment. Most drug–receptor combinations are readily reversible, being of hydrogen or Van der Waal's bonding. If we assume that the number of receptors is constant at any moment, then the magnitude of the response depends on the number of drug molecules available for such chance reversible drug–receptor combinations and recombinations.

Now let us examine how a drug like morphine can occupy receptors in the human central nervous system.

The drug first has to be administered to the person. This can be by mouth in solid form or in solution, by smoking the volatilized form, by subcutaneous, intramuscular, or intravenous injection of solutions, or by subcutaneous implantation of solid pellets. Next the drug has to be absorbed into the circulating blood by crossing the membranes of the intestinal mucosa or the lung, then traversing the capillary wall into the bloodstream. When the drug is injected parenterally, only the capillary wall has to be traversed. Intravenous injection avoids the transmembrane aspects of absorption. When solid morphine is implanted subcutaneously, it must first be solubilized before it can cross the capillary wall, thus delaying absorption. This delay can be extended by implanting the alkaloid base, which is much less soluble than the commonly employed sulfate and hydrochloride salts. Once into the bloodstream, morphine molecules can be either carried in simple solution or bound to plasma proteins.

Distribution of the drug proceeds after its absorption into the blood. As the blood circulates, that morphine which is in simple solution in the serum passes out through the capillary wall into the extracellular fluid in amounts that depend on the local circulation. Some of this morphine then binds to the local tissue in amounts determined by the composition of that tissue (morphine is less lipophilic than hydrophilic). The brain provides an exception to this general sequence of distribution because of the blood-brain barrier. The nature of this barrier will be described in detail in subsequent chapters (Oldendorf; Woodbury et al.). It is sufficient at this point to say that the blood-brain barrier provides a reduced permeability for some substances, including morphine, into cerebral tissue. Nevertheless, measurable amounts of morphine do enter the central nervous system. The morphine then combines with specific receptors to initiate a cellular chain of events which produces the typical response to morphine.

Termination of drug action is accomplished by processes known as drug metabolism and excretion. Circulating morphine is metabolized in the liver, mainly by conjugation with glucuronic acid and by N-demethylation. These products are then excreted into the bile or via the kidneys. As the concentration of circulating morphine falls, the morphine in the brain diffuses back into the bloodstream and thus drug action is gradually terminated.

On the other hand, drug metabolism or biotransformation may result in the formation of one or more metabolites which also possess narcotic activity. This appears to be the case with L-alpha-acetylmethadol.

POSSIBLE MECHANISMS OF TOLERANCE

One can postulate that tolerance to the narcotic analgesic drugs can develop by an alteration of any of the processes mentioned above—namely, absorption, distribution, drug–receptor interaction, cellular response, metabolism, and excretion. It is also possible that an immune response develops.

Alterations in the process of absorption can fairly well be discounted. Most narcotic abusers of the current era utilize the intravenous route for self-medication, which readily permits tolerance to occur while completely bypassing all barriers to absorption. Moreover, clinical studies of orally effective narcotic analgesics demonstrate that tolerance develops less rapidly by the oral route than by parenteral routes. The mucosal lining of the gastrointestinal tract is apparently not the site in question.

For the past 40 years several groups of investigators have studied the possibility that tolerance to morphine results from an altered distribution between blood and brain. In fact, this postulated effect of an increased selectivity by the blood-brain barrier has been reinvestigated with each new refinement in procedures for the detection of morphine. To date, no significant differences in distribution have been found between tolerant and nontolerant subjects. These findings, however, have not ruled out the possibility of altered distribution within the central nervous system.

There have been an abundance of hypotheses but a paucity of data concerning alterations in drug–receptor interactions as the mechanism of tolerance development. Axelrod (1) noted a marked reduction in the ability of liver microsomal preparations from morphine-tolerant rats to demethylate morphine. He postulated that a reduction in the number of morphine receptors in the brain might parallel the reduction of N-demethylating capacity that he observed in rat liver microsomal preparations.

Other suggestions have been made to the effect that drug responses are proportional not to the total number of receptors occupied, but rather to the rate at which drug–receptor combinations and recombinations occur. While this might explain the development of acute tolerance or tachyphylaxis as the result of tissue saturation by a drug, it is difficult to conceive how it would account for the persistence of tolerance weeks or months after a single administration of a drug.

In recent years, Takemori (2) has developed a body of evidence which he believes indicates the development of qualitatively different receptors to morphine-like drugs. This is an interesting concept and merits further investigation.

Another concept—one that has received repeated attention for nearly a century—postulates the development of an immunologic response. The results of early attempts to demonstrate this were equivocal, but with refined technology more recent studies by Winters and co-workers (3) indicate a clear possibility that the basis of tolerance may be immunologic.

As the methodology for studying the biogenic amines has developed and improved in the past several years, many investigators have studied their possible roles in the development of tolerance and physiologic dependence. The results of these studies have often been contradictory in that opposite effects have been observed between species, between laboratories and, more recently, between strains of the same species.

Similar contradictory results have been reported concerning the role of serotonin in mediating analgesia and in the development of tolerance and physiologic dependence. Rech and Tilson (4), in a recent study of these factors in two strains of rats (Sprague-Dawley and Fisher), used p-chlorophenylalanine to inhibit the synthesis of serotonin. This pretreatment attenuated the analgesic effect of morphine in the Sprague-Dawley but not the Fisher rats. Tolerance to morphine developed equally in both strains and the severity of naloxone-precipitated withdrawal was diminished only in the Sprague-Dawley rats. Norepinephrine and serotonin clearly seem to be involved in the modulation of the actions of morphine, but these interactions have yet to be elucidated.

PHYSIOLOGIC DEPENDENCE

One of the earlier hypotheses concerning morphine dependence was the "dual-action theory," proposed by Tatum, Seevers, and Collins (5) and based on the fact that while morphine depresses some central nervous functions, it stimulates others. They suggested that the stimulant effects outlasted the depressant effects; thus, more and more morphine would be required to counteract the accumulating stimulant effects if analgesia were to be maintained. Tolerance would therefore be accounted for as well as physiologic dependence, since, upon withdrawal of treatment, the longer lasting stimulant effects would manifest themselves as the abstinence syndrome. This hypothesis had to be discarded with the advent of the antagonists, when it was shown that simultaneous administration of antagonists (which block the depressant but not stimulant narcotic effects) and morphine prevented the development of physiologic dependence.

A concept of physiologic adaptation was developed by Himmelsbach (6), who felt that when morphine depressed certain functions of the central nervous system, counteracting processes were activated. This would account for tolerance development during the course of morphine administration and also for physiologic dependence, because, upon withdrawal of morphine treatment, the unchecked adaptive process would give rise to the abstinence syndrome.

Denervation supersensitivity is another attractive hypothesis that would explain both tolerance and physiologic dependence development. It has repeatedly been demonstrated that chronic pharmacologic blockade of the peripheral autonomic nervous system produces supersensitivity of the effector neuron or organ in a manner similar to anatomic denervation. Jaffe and Sharpless (7) have suggested that this phenomenon may be extended to the central nervous system. They postulate that narcotic analgesics suppress certain neurons by some unknown mechanism. It then follows that the next neuron in these affected pathways would become supersensitive to the normal neurotransmitter, causing it to respond normally to less than normal amounts of the transmitter. Thus, larger doses of narcotic would be required to reduce further the release of the neurotransmitter in order to achieve the initial narcotic effect. If narcotic treatment should be abruptly discontinued, normal amounts of the neurotransmitter would reach the supersensitive neurons and would produce exaggerated effects opposite to those produced by the narcotic. These exaggerated effects would constitute the abstinence syndrome. Both tolerance and physiologic dependence are thus explained on the basis of the hypothesis of pharmacologic denervation supersensitivity.

This brief overview is by no means complete nor has any attempt been made to cite all investigators who have contributed to the areas outlined above. The intention rather is to point out those potential mechanisms of tolerance and physiologic dependence that are under active investigation.

The phenomena of tolerance and physiologic dependence are of immense biologic interest, and an understanding of their mechanisms would greatly advance our understanding of biology in general. Neither phenomenon is necessary for drug abuse (chemical dependence, addiction, etc.) to occur. Tolerance to the effects of cocaine does not develop, nor does physiologic dependence occur with chronic use of cocaine or the amphetamines. The only feature shared by all classes of drugs that produce dependence is the creation of a new urge. This urge is often more powerful than such basic urges as hunger, sleep, sex, self-respect, and social responsibility, and sometimes surpasses even the instinct for survival.

REFERENCES

1. Axelrod, J. Possible mechanism of tolerance to narcotic drugs. *Science*, 124:263–265, 1956.
2. Takemori, A. E. The effects of morphine, other opioids and their derivatives on the metabolism of the cerebral cortex. In: *The Addictive States*, edited by A. Wikler, *Res. Publ. Assoc. Res. Nerv. Ment. Dis.*, Vol. 46, p. 53. Williams and Wilkins, Baltimore, 1968.
3. Nakamura, J., and Winters, W. D. Attenuation of the morphine EEG continuum following a repeat dose within 16 days: Delayed tolerance in the rat. *Neuropharmacology*, 12:607–617, 1973.
4. Rech, R. H., and Tilson, H. A. Effects of *p*-chlorophenylalanine (PCPA) on morphine analgesia and development of tolerance and dependence in two strains of rats. *Pharmacologist*, 15:202, 1973.

5. Tatum, A. L., Seevers, M. H., and Collins, K. H. Morphine addiction and its physiological interpretation based on experimental evidence. *J. Pharmacol. Exp. Therap.*, 36:447, 1929.
6. Himmelsbach, C. K. With reference to physical dependence. *Fed. Proc.*, 2:201–203, 1943.
7. Jaffe, J. H., and Sharpless, S. K. Pharmacological denervation supersensitivity in the central nervous system: A theory of physical dependence. In: *The Addictive States,* edited by A. Wikler, *Res. Publ. Assoc. Res. Nerv. Ment. Dis.,* Vol. 46, p. 226. Williams and Wilkins, Baltimore, 1968.

DISCUSSION

Mirsky: Is there any correlation between the rate at which tolerance develops to different drugs of different classes? In other words, is there a common mechanism involved in the development of tolerance to different drugs which are known to produce tolerance?

Deneau: Evidence would suggest that a common mechanism is involved in the development of tolerance to drugs of a given class or structurally related configuration since we know that cross-tolerance between such agents does occur.

Goldstein: There are several published observations regarding tolerance and physical dependence which take us beyond the realm of theory and make several things quite clear. One is that the myenteric plexus of the guinea pig ilium responds to opiates in much the same way as does the brain, namely, that comparable concentrations of opiates are effective, that these effects are stereospecific for one set of the opiate isomers, and that these effects are blocked by naloxone, which is a pure antagonist of the opiates. In the myenteric plexus preparation, the plexus has been stripped off and adheres to the longitudinal muscle of the ilium, thus eliminating any permeability barrier to the plexus neurons. Myenteric plexuses from guinea pigs made tolerant to morphine are tolerant to the drug in the bath. The degree of tolerance is approximately equal to that in whole guinea pigs, in our experience about tenfold. This observation disposes of the idea that the drug in the tolerant animal is unable to reach the site at which it acts to produce its effect. Rather, it reflects a change at the cellular level in the myenteric plexus. Regarding the chemical basis for this tolerance, we have found that the plexus is supersensitive to serotonin, which is a stimulatory neurotransmitter in the plexus which is antagonized by morphine. Again, there is a tenfold supersensitivity to serotonin. We feel that the supersensitivity to serotonin is sufficient explanation for both tolerance and physical dependence in this preparation.

Narcotics and the Hypothalamus, edited by
E. Zimmermann and R. George. Raven Press,
New York © 1974

Behavioral and Neurohormonal Relationships to Thermoregulatory Adaptive Changes in Morphine Abstinence

E. Leong Way, H. H. Loh, L. F. Tseng, and E. T. Wei*

*Department of Pharmacology and Langley Porter Neuropsychiatric Institute, University of California, San Francisco, California 94143, and * School of Public Health, University of California, Berkeley, California 94720*

INTRODUCTION

It is well established that the development of physical dependence on morphine or any of its surrogates is the consequence of repeated and frequent administration of high doses of agents acting on the central nervous system. The morphine-abstinent or withdrawal syndrome is easily identifiable by a number of characteristic signs which reflect central autonomic nervous system hyperreactivity. Himmelsbach et al. (1) postulated that physical dependence on morphine might constitute a part of body defenses to the continued effect of the drug, and that abstinence reflects an exaggeration of normal physiologic effects to maintain homeostasis. Since then, others have attempted to describe physical dependence in general physiologic or biochemical terms without identifying the specific counteradaptive process that might be involved.

The theories more or less agree that the development of physical dependence represents a normal compensatory reaction and that the withdrawal phenomenon involves an exaggerated rebound or overshoot of some function that is overly depressed. Thus the miosis, respiratory depression, decreased body temperature, sedation, and analgesia resulting from acute morphine inhibition become mydriasis, hypernea, hyperexia, excitability, and hypergesia, respectively, during withdrawal. Although none of the explanations of abstinence has been verified experimentally, it is of interest to mention briefly a few examples. It has been suggested that as a compensatory consequence of the blockade of nervous pathways following repeated morphine administration, the innervated effector sites become more sensitive to their exciting neurohormone (2), or hypertrophy of an alternate pathway ensues (3). In either case, exaggerated function seen as abstinent hyperexcitability occurs upon withdrawal of morphine. The biochemical theorists relate drug tolerance and dependence either to overproduction of an endogenous hormone (4, 5) or to an adaptive increase of the target receptor which would manifest in abstinence signs upon morphine withdrawal (6).

In recent studies on the neuroanatomic correlates of morphine withdrawal,

9

we found that brain areas associated with the wet-shake behavior of precipitated abstinence in the rat appeared to be closely adjacent to central pathways of heat dissipation and heat gain (7–9). Since morphine has complex
effects on central thermoregulatory mechanisms (10), the possibility was considered that derangement of central temperature homeostasis may account for
the appearance of some abstinence signs. The findings, discussed below, summarize a series of experiments by Wei and his associates to localize the central nervous system sites and to assess the thermoregulatory processes that
may be involved in abstinence.

BRAIN SITES INVOLVED IN MORPHINE ABSTINENCE

The central sites related to physical dependence have been studied by
localized manipulation of brain tissue. Wikler (11, 12) reported that removal
of the cortex in dogs did not attenuate the abstinence syndrome but that
spinal cord section interfered with some withdrawal signs. This work was
subsequently extended by Martin and Eades (13), who demonstrated in the
spinal dog that morphine dependence had supraspinal and spinal components.
Kerr and Pozuelo (14) have recently reported that the intensity of precipitated withdrawal signs in rats was attenuated after lesions were made in
the ventromedial nucleus of the hypothalamus. That morphine dependence
has a central component is suggested by the studies by Eidelberg and Barstow (15) in the monkey and Watanabe (16) in the rat, showing that withdrawal could be precipitated by administering opioid antagonists into the
ventricular fluids. Herz et al. (17) reported that withdrawal signs were elicited
in morphine-dependent rabbits after administration of opioid antagonists into
the fourth ventricle. Part of this rather confusing information may be due to
the fact that different actions of morphine were assessed in different species.

Our findings (7–9) indicate that the medial mesodiencephalic sites are
more sensitive than neocortical, hippocampal, striatal, lateral thalamic, and
lateral mesencephalic structures to naloxone-precipitated withdrawal. From
what is currently known concerning the physiologic, anatomic, biochemical,
and behavioral aspects of medial mesodiencephalic function, there is considerable attraction in considering these areas to be intimately involved in morphine dependence.

These conclusions are based on studies which were designed to localize the
areas sensitive to naloxone-precipitated withdrawal in the brain of the morphine-dependent rat. Stainless steel guide cannulas were implanted into different brain areas of male albino rats. One to five days after cannula implantation, physical dependence on morphine was induced by subcutaneous
implantation of a pellet containing 75 mg of morphine base (18, 19).
Naloxone hydrochloride crystals were applied via each cannula 70 to 76 hr
after morphine pellet implantation, and observations were made for precipitated abstinence signs of wet shakes and escape behavior occurring

within 10 min. The application of naloxone to various brain regions in morphine-dependent animals selectively precipitated the abstinence syndrome in the medial thalamus and in areas at the junction of the diencephalon and mesencephalon. The lateral thalamus, cortex, hippocampus, subthalamus, and striatum were relatively inactive.

NEUROANATOMIC CORRELATIONS OF WET-SHAKE BEHAVIOR

Wet shakes appear to occur in response to sensory irritation in normal rats (15) and could be a heat gain mechanism similar to shivering. It was of interest, therefore, to determine if the neural elements underlying shaking behavior in normal rats have commonalities with those associated with morphine withdrawal (9).

Rats were anesthetized with sodium pentobarbital, and transverse brain lesions, extending 2 to 4 mm on each side of the midline, were made in brain areas corresponding to areas A–E as shown in Fig. 1. The scalp incision was closed with a wound clip, and 3 to 10 min later the colonic temperature was measured. The rat was then held by the nape of the neck and placed in ice water. The animal was initially completely immersed in the water and then immediately raised so that only the head was above water. The number of shakes was then counted over a 5-min period. Colonic temperature was measured again after removal of the animal from the water.

The repetitive shaking movements elicited in pentobarbital-anesthetized rats

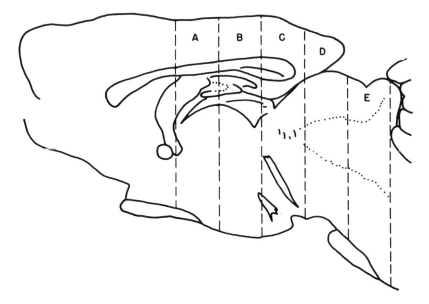

FIG. 1. Brain areas in which transverse lesions were made bilaterally with an iridectomy knife.

after immersion in water resembled those seen in the morphine-dependent rat upon withdrawal. The frequency of shakes was inversely related to the temperature of the water and apparently to the drop in body temperature.

The brain areas influencing the wet-shake response to ice water are shown in Fig. 1. Lesions in the anterior diencephalon, septal area, and striatum (area A and anterior to A) did not significantly affect the frequency of shaking when compared with sham-operated controls. Lesions in the midbrain (areas D and E) blocked the ability of the animals to make the wet-shake response to the cold water stimulus. The transition point for inhibiting wet shakes appeared to be in the posterior diencephalon and rostral midbrain (areas B and C). Morphine sulfate, 10 mg/kg i.p., completely antagonized the wet-shake response to ice water. Tolerance to the 10 mg/kg dose of morphine sulfate could be partially induced by implanting subcutaneously a morphine pellet for 3 days.

The results of this and the previous study strongly indicate that the wet shakes of morphine abstinence and shivering have common neural elements. Wet shakes appear to resemble shivering in that pentobarbital anesthesia does not inhibit these reflexes in the rat. Head shakes and wet shakes apparently are characteristic behavioral responses of the rat to noxious stimuli, since stimuli which provoke this behavior, namely cold water, wetness, and tissue damage to the ear, are generally considered unpleasant. Morphine, which is antinociceptive, also antagonizes the wet-shake response of the rat to ice water. It is of interest to note that the areas where the wet-shake response to ice water- and naloxone-precipitated withdrawal are attenuated bear considerable resemblance to the loci of the shivering center in the cat (20).

EFFECT OF ENVIRONMENTAL TEMPERATURE ON ABSTINENCE

Body temperature fluctuates widely during withdrawal from morphine (21–23) and some of the symptoms and signs of abstinence may reflect disruption of thermoregulation. For example, shivering, gooseflesh, sensations of cold and warmth, profuse sweating, rhinorrhea, and lacrimation are well-known characteristic symptoms and signs of withdrawal in man. Martin (24) has suggested that trembling, a withdrawal sign in the dog, may result from the activation of heat generating mechanisms which have hypertrophied against the hypothermic effects of morphine. In the rat, during precipitated withdrawal at room temperature, teeth chattering, wet shakes, vasoconstriction, ptosis, and a huddled posture may be observed (8). This behavior may reflect activation of heat gain mechanisms. Other withdrawal signs are salivation, the spreading of saliva on the body, and escape behavior. The latter signs may be manifestations of heat loss mechanisms. These conjectures were validated by experiments on morphine-dependent rats designed to assess the effect of environmental temperature on naloxone-precipitated wet shakes and escape behavior.

Rats rendered dependent on morphine by pellet implantation were placed in gallon-sized glass jars and then randomized into three groups. One group was kept at room temperature (22 to 24°C). The other groups were transferred to a hot (34 to 37°C) or cold (6 to 10°C) room. After 1 hr the abstinence syndrome was precipitated by injecting naloxone hydrochloride. Animals placed in jars at the three different temperatures did not manifest any shaking behavior or escape attempts. However, animals in the hot environment exhibited reddening of the ears and tails, extended posture, and salivation after 1 hr of exposure. These signs have been reported as being characteristic behavior of rats acutely exposed to a hot environment (25). Animals kept in the cold, on the other hand, maintained a huddled position and had blanched ears and some degree of ptosis.

The injection of naloxone in morphine-dependent rats kept at room temperature provoked the typical abstinence signs of wet shakes and escape behavior (18) that were dose-dependent, whereas saline provoked no response. Injection of naloxone in animals in cold or hot environments produced dramatic alterations in the withdrawal signs. As can be seen in Fig. 2A, escape behavior, precipitated by naloxone in a hot environment, was markedly enhanced; jumping was elicited in some animals with a dose of naloxone as low as 0.04 mg/kg whereas at room temperature the same dose was ineffective. At 4 mg/kg most animals repeatedly jumped out of the jars as fast as the observer was able to put them back into the container, and the most active rat jumped out of its jar 132 times within a 10-min period. On the other hand, wet-shakes behavior was completely suppressed in the hot environment and even the 4 mg/kg dose was ineffective (Fig. 2B).

In striking contrast, in the cold environment the frequency of wet shakes was enhanced but no change in the escape attempt frequency was noted (Fig. 2B). Thus the results demonstrate that certain withdrawal signs can be markedly influenced by environmental temperature. Since pharmacologic agents frequently affect more than one component of the thermoregulatory system (26, 27, 28), considerable caution should be exercised in the interpretation of drug effects on morphine dependence. To seek meaning regarding the alterations of withdrawal signs through environmental temperature in the morphine-dependent rat, it may be worthwhile to consider the physiologic significance of wet shakes and escape attempts in the behavioral repertoire of the normal rat.

Hainsworth (25) has observed that normal rats placed in a 40°C environment for 2 hr or a 44°C environment for 1 hr will attempt to escape from its cage by trying to push the top off the cage. By contrast, wet shakes in the normal rat appear to occur in response to extreme cold and to sensory irritation (9). For example, cold water wetness, hypothermia, and irritation to tissue around the ears will provoke this behavior. It appears, therefore, that escape attempts and wet shakes, under certain experimental conditions, are forms of adaptive behavior which enable the rat to maintain normal body

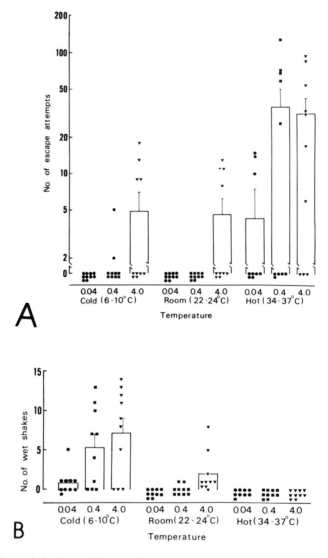

FIG. 2. Abstinence behavior at different ambient temperatures. Two pellets containing 75 mg of morphine base were implanted 48 hr apart in male Sprague-Dawley rats weighing 235 ± 21 (SD) g. Three days after the first pellet, withdrawal was precipitated at different ambient temperatures by injecting naloxone hydrochloride at 0.04, 0.4, or 4.0 mg/kg i.p. Withdrawal behavior was observed for 10 min after naloxone administration. Each point represents the datum from one rat.

temperature. Escape attempts could be a heat loss mechanism: the animal "feels too warm" and attempts to escape from its environment. Wet shakes could be a heat gain mechanism similar to shivering.

Intravenous administration of opioids provokes a sensation of warmth but, during withdrawal in individuals dependent on opioids, a frequent complaint is "feeling cold." During withdrawal marked fluctuations occur in body temperature. The sensation of cold is also intimately associated with emotional affect. The antinociceptive action of morphine on the wet-shake response to ice water to some extent would mimic the inhibitory effect of anterior hypothalamic efferents on the shivering center. It seems possible, therefore, that some of the central actions of morphine may involve hypothalamic efferents to the brainstem.

The data we have presented indicate that naloxone acts principally in medial mesodiencephalic regions of the brain to precipitate the abstinence syndrome. There is considerable attraction in considering nuclei in these regions as primary sites involved with morphine dependence. The medial thalamic nuclei contain rostral components of the diffuse, extralemniscal reticular system which is thought to mediate pain (29, 30) and arousal (31). Electrolytic lesions of these nuclei in different species apparently decrease the affective reaction to noxious stimuli while sparing the ability of the organs to perceive discrete stimuli (32, 33). Electrical stimulation of some medial mesodiencephalic structures can also inhibit avoidance behavior provoked by painful stimuli (34). Anatomically these nuclei receive extensive inputs from the bulbar and midbrain reticular formation (29). The main projection of the medial thalamic nuclei in the rat is to the globus pallidus and neostriatum rather than directly to the cortex, since removal of the cortex does not lead to retrograde degeneration in these nuclei whereas removal of the striatum does (35).

The medial mesodiencephalon has traditionally been considered to be an important brain area for the integration of thermosensory information and for the regulation of body temperature (26). Thus, from an anatomic viewpoint, it would appear plausible that certain precipitated withdrawal signs resemble a derangement of central thermoregulatory mechanisms. Escape behavior and wet shakes may be viewed as behavioral events triggered by the sudden occurrence of an error signal in the thermosensory or thermal control system: compensatory heat gain and heat loss mechanisms are then activated to return the set-point to normality.

From these considerations a tentative generalization may be proposed for interpreting the effects of some drugs which modify the withdrawal signs of wet shakes or escape attempts. It is proposed that drugs which make the animals "feel hot" will increase the frequency of escape behavior and, possibly, suppress wet shakes, whereas drugs which make the animal "feel cold" will enhance the frequency of wet shakes without affecting escape behavior. Such changes are likely to involve the various neurotransmitters which may play a role in temperature regulation. Acetylcholine, dopamine, norepinephrine, and serotonin have all been studied and considered.

Current evidence strongly suggests that the initiating sites for many morphine effects are cholinergic, although gabaminergic sites have not been eliminated from consideration. Our studies on the brain sites of morphine action and abstinence provide increasing evidence that some of the effects of morphine reside in the medial mesodiencephalic area, and that some of these sites may be common to those for initiating antagonist-precipitated withdrawal.

Few of the dopaminergic, serotonergic, or adrenergic pathways mapped by histofluorescence techniques originate, traverse, or terminate to any significant degree in the medial thalamic nuclei (36). On the other hand, high levels of acetylcholinesterase and cholinesterase have been found in these nuclei by Shute and Lewis (37) and by Olivier et al. (38). Behaviorally, electrical (39, 40) or cholinergic (41) stimulation of medial thalamic and hypothalamic regions in the brain elicits avoidance behavior, i.e., as if the stimulation was interpreted as being unpleasant. Stein (41) has suggested a central punishment system in the brain with acetylcholine as the neurotransmitter. Thus, if the biochemical action of morphine were to inhibit acetylcholine release (42–44), an inhibited release of acetylcholine in the rostral portions of ascending reticular system may be expected to result in a decreased cortical reaction to noxious stimuli. It would not be unreasonable then to seek relationships between tolerance and physical dependence and the release of acetylcholine in this area of the brain.

CHOLINERGIC–DOPAMINERGIC ACTIVITY IN MORPHINE ABSTINENCE

In studies initiated to assess cholinergic mechanisms that might influence naloxone-precipitated withdrawal escape or jumping behavior, naloxone-precipitated withdrawal jumping in morphine-dependent mice was markedly attenuated by elevating brain acetylcholine by cholinesterase inhibition. When physostigmine was given immediately prior to naloxone, it greatly increased the amount of naloxone necessary to induce the withdrawal jumping syndrome as evidenced by a striking increase in the naloxone ED_{50} by over 100-fold (45). Conversely, when hemicholinium-3 was injected intracerebrally in the dependent mouse to inhibit acetylcholine synthesis, naloxone-precipitated withdrawal jumping was enhanced. A dose of hemicholinium-3 which reduced brain acetylcholine by 40% reduced the naloxone ED_{50} by 50% (46). Furthermore, cholinergic agonists of both the muscarinic and nicotinic types, including nicotine, tremorine, oxytremorine, arecoline, and physostigmine, significantly reduced naloxone-induced jumping, whereas cholinergic antagonists such as atropine, benztropine, pempidine, and mecamylamine enhanced naloxone effects (47). During naloxone-precipitated withdrawal in dependent mice or rats, brain acetylcholine levels are significantly decreased, suggesting that brain acetylcholine release is enhanced (Bhagarva and Way, *unpublished*). Thus there is considerable evidence indicating that acetylcholine participates in the withdrawal jumping response.

In addition to acetylcholine, dopamine also appears to be important for the manifestation of the escape or jumping in the morphine-dependent animal.

In mice rendered dependent on morphine by pellet implantation, naloxone-precipitated withdrawal jumping was accompanied by a sudden elevation of dopamine. The increase in dopamine was noted to occur within 2 min and to reach a maximum between 5 and 10 min, when the incidence of jumping was at its peak. On the other hand, brain levels of norepinephrine and serotonin were not altered by naloxone at any of the test times. The dopamine increase in dependent mice after naloxone challenge was about 30% at 5 min and the response was over by 30 min. The increase in brain dopamine occurred primarily in the corpus striatum and hardly at all in the other brain areas (48). In rats made dependent on morphine after destruction of the substantia nigra zona compacta to effect unilateral degeneration of the left nigroneostriatal pathway, the injection of naloxone caused turning toward the right or non-lesioned side (49). This contralateral turning behavior corresponds to that produced in other groups of lesioned rats by dopaminergic-receptor blocking agents such as haloperidol and pimozide (50). Thus the contralateral circling behavior observed in dependent rats during naloxone-precipitated withdrawal suggests that a diminution of dopamine in the neostriatum may be occurring (49).

Our studies indicate, therefore, that both cholinergic and dopaminergic neurons participate in the manifestation of morphine withdrawal, and indeed, the two substances appear to be interrelated. Elevation of brain acetylcholine by cholinesterase inhibition in the morphine-dependent mouse, for example, blocks not only naloxone-precipitated withdrawal jumping but also the sudden elevation of brain dopamine which occurs (48). We have presented findings elsewhere that the two neurotransmitters do not appear to be the primary substances involved in dependence development (45, 51), but there can be little argument that both are associated with the acute effects of morphine and in the expression of certain signs of morphine withdrawal.

There is other circumstantial evidence implicating dopamine in narcotic-precipitated withdrawal. Apomorphine, which is known to stimulate the dopamine receptor (52), has recently been reported to inhibit some withdrawal signs in the rat (49) and in man (53). We have also found an inhibition of precipitated and abrupt withdrawal jumping behavior by apomorphine in morphine-dependent mice. On the other hand, the dopamine antagonist haloperidol does not block jumping, but significantly blocks the inhibitory effect of apomorphine. Apparently, the stimulation of dopamine receptors by apomorphine antagonizes the jumping behavior associated with narcotic withdrawal.

From these considerations, a partial explanation for the role of dopamine in morphine withdrawal can be advanced. It is possible that a compensatory inactivation of dopaminergic neurons occurs during precipitated narcotic withdrawal and the sudden increase of dopamine in dopamine neurons may be due to the decrease in the release of dopamine by dopaminergic neurons with a consequent accumulation of newly synthesized dopamine. It has been well established that a single dose of morphine increases dopamine turnover (54–56). Inasmuch as the steady-state levels of dopamine are not affected, any increase in turnover of dopamine must be the consequence of its increased synthesis, release, and/or degradation. In animals made tolerant to the antinociceptive effect of morphine by chronic morphine treatment, no increase in dopamine turnover is observed (56). Thus, it is possible that during tolerance development, the animal has activated some sort of braking system to normalize the effects of morphine on the dopaminergic system. In so doing, however, the animal now requires the presence of morphine for the maintenance of dopamine turnover within the normal range. Upon withdrawal of morphine, therefore, with the braking system still functioning, dopamine turnover decreases and, thus, there is less inhibitory influence of the dopaminergic neurons which, in turn, leads to a hyperexcitable state that is manifested by jumping behavior. Experiments are in progress to further substantiate this operational hypothesis.

ACKNOWLEDGMENTS

The findings summarized here represent collaborative studies supported by research grants DA-00036, 00091, and 000564 from the National Institute on Drug Abuse.

REFERENCES

1. Himmelsbach, C. K., Gerlach, G. H., and Stanton, E. J. A method for testing addiction, tolerance and abstinence in the rat. *J. Pharmacol. Exp. Ther.*, 53:179–188, 1935.
2. Jaffe, J.H., and Sharpless, S. K. Pharmacological denervation supersensitivity in the central nervous system: A theory of physical dependence. *Res. Publ. Assn. Nerv. Ment. Dis.*, 46:226–246, 1968.
3. Martin, W. R. Pharmacological redundancy as an adaptive mechanism in the central nervous system. *Fed. Proc.*, 29:13–27, 1970.
4. Shuster, L. Repression and depression of enzyme synthesis as a possible explanation of some aspects of drug action. *Nature*, 189:314–315, 1961.
5. Goldstein, A., and Goldstein, D. B. Enzyme expansion theory of drug tolerance and physical dependence. *Res. Publ. Assn. Nerv. Ment. Dis.*, 48:265–267, 1968.
6. Collier, H. O. J., Francis, D. L., and Schneider, C. Modification of morphine withdrawal by drugs interacting with humoral mechanisms: Some contradictions and their interpretation. *Nature*, 237:220–223, 1972.
7. Wei, E., Loh, H. H., and Way, E. L. Brain sites of precipitated abstinence in morphine-dependent rats. *J. Pharmacol. Exp. Ther.*, 185:108–115, 1973.
8. Wei, E. Brain lesions attenuating wet shake behavior in morphine abstinent rats. *Life Sci.* (part I), 12:385–392, 1973.
9. Wei, E., Loh, H. H., and Way, E. L. Neuroanatomical correlates of wet shake behavior in the rat. *Life Sci.* (part II), 12:489–496, 1973.
10. Lotti, V. J. Body temperature responses to morphine: Central sites and mechanisms of action. In: *The Pharmacology of Thermoregulation*, edited by E. Schoenbaum and P. Lomax. Karger, Basel, 1973.
11. Wikler, A. Recent progress in research on the neurophysiologic basis of morphine addiction. *Amer. J. Psychiat.*, 105:329–338, 1948.

12. Wikler, A. Sites and mechanisms of action of morphine and related drugs in the central nervous system. *Pharmacol. Rev.,* 2:435–506, 1950.
13. Martin, W. R., and Eades, C. G. A comparison between acute and chronic physical dependence in the chronic spinal dog. *J. Pharmacol. Exp. Ther.,* 146:385–394, 1964.
14. Kerr, F. L., and Pozuelo, J. Suppression of physical dependence and induction of hypersensitivity to morphine by stereotaxic hypothalamic lesions in addicted rats. *Proc. Mayo Clin.,* 46:653–665, 1971.
15. Eidelberg, E., and Barstow, C. A. Morphine tolerance and dependence induced by intraventricular injection. *Science,* 174:74–76, 1971.
16. Watanabe, H. The development of tolerance to and of physical dependence on morphine following intraventricular injection in the rat. *Jap. J. Pharmacol.,* 21:383–391, 1971.
17. Herz, A., Teschemacher, H., Albus,. K., and Ziegelgansberger, S. Morphine abstinence syndrome in rabbits precipitated by injection of morphine antagonists into the ventricular system and restricted parts of it. *Psychopharmacologia,* 26:219–236, 1972.
18. Wei, E., Loh, H. H., and Way, E. L. Quantitative aspects of precipitated abstinence in morphine-dependent rats. *J. Pharmacol. Exp. Ther.,* 184:398–403, 1973.
19. Gibson, R. D. and Tingstad, J. E. Formulation of a morphine implantation pellet suitable for tolerance-physical dependence studies in mice. *J. Pharm. Sci.,* 59:426–427, 1970.
20. Hemingway, A. Shivering. *Physiol. Rev.,* 43:397–422, 1963.
21. Martin, W. R., Wikler, A., Eades, C. G., and Pescor, F. T. Tolerance to and physical dependence on morphine in rats. *Psychopharmacologia,* 4:247–260, 1963.
22. Herz, A., Teschemacher, H., Albus, K., and Ziegelgansberger, S. Morphine abstinence syndrome in rabbits precipitated by injection of morphine antagonists into the ventricular system and restricted parts of it. *Psychopharmacologia,* 26:219–236, 1972.
23. Schwartz, A. S., and Eidelberg, E. Role of biogenic amines in morphine dependence. *Life Sci.* (part I), 9:613–624, 1970.
24. Martin, W. R. Opioid antagonists. *Pharmacol. Rev.,* 19:464–521, 1967.
25. Hainsworth, F. R. Saliva spreading activity and body temperature regulation in the rat. *Am. J. Physiol.,* 212:1288–1292, 1967.
26. Hardy, J. D. Posterior hypothalamus and the regulation of body temperature. *Fed. Proc.,* 32:1564, 1973.
27. Cramer, J. E., and Bligh, J. Body temperature and responses to drugs. *Brit. Med. Bull.,* 25:299–306, 1969.
28. Lomax, P. Drugs and body temperature. *Int. Rev. Neurobiol.* 12:1–43, 1970.
29. Bowsher, D. The anatomophysiological base of somatosensory discrimination. *Int. Rev. Neurobiol.,* 8:35–75, 1965.
30. Casey, K. L., and Melzack, R. Neural mechanism of pain: A conceptual model. In: *New Concepts in Pain and its Clinical Management,* edited by E. L. Way, pp. 13–31. Davis, Philadelphia, 1967.
31. Papez, J. W. Central reticular path to intralaminar and reticular nuclei of thalamus for activating EEG related to consciousness. *Electroencephalogr. Clin. Neurophysiol.,* 8:117–128, 1956.
32. Ervin, F. R. Effects of opioids on electrical activity of deep structures in the human brain. *Res. Publ. Assn. Nerv. Ment. Dis.,* 46:150–155, 1968.
33. Mitchell, C. L., and Kaelber, W. W. Effect of medial thalamic lesions on responses elicited by tooth pulp stimulation. *Amer. J. Physiol.,* 210:263–269, 1966.
34. Mayer, D. J., Wolfle, T. L., Akil, H., Carter, B., and Liebskind, J. C. Analgesia from electrical stimulation in the brainstem of the rat. *Science,* 174:1351–1354, 1971.
35. Powell, T. P. S., and Cowan, W. M. The connections of the midline and intralaminar nuclei of the thalamus of the rat. *J. Anat.,* 88:308–319, 1954.
36. Ungerstedt, U. Stereotaxic mapping of the monoamine pathways in the rat brain. *Acta. Physiol. Scand.,* 82, 1 (Supplement 367), 1971.
37. Shute, C. C. D., and Lewis, P. R. The ascending cholinergic reticular system: Neocortical, olfactory and subcortical projections. *Brain,* 90:497–540, 1967.

38. Olivier, A., Parent, A., and Poirer, L. J. L. Identification of the thalamic nuclei on the basis of their cholinesterase content in the monkey. *J. Anat.*, 106:37–50, 1970.
39. Olds, M. E., and Olds, J. Approach-avoidance analysis of rat diencephalon. *J. Comp. Neurol.*, 120:259–295, 1963.
40. Kaelber, W. W., and Mitchell, C. L. The centrum medianum–central tegmental fasciculus complex. A stimulation, lesion and degeneration study in the cat. *Brain*, 90:83–100, 1967.
41. Stein, L. Chemistry of reward and punishment. In: *Psychopharmacology. A Review of Progress, 1957–1967*. Public Health Service Publication No. 1836, Washington, D.C., 1968, pp. 105–124.
42. Schaumann, W. Inhibition by morphine of the release of acetylcholine from the intestine of the guinea pig. *Brit. J. Pharmacol. Chemother.*, 12:115–116, 1957.
43. Paton, W. D. M. The action of morphine and related substances on contraction and on acetylcholine output of coaxially stimulated guinea pig ileum. *Brit. J. Pharmacol. Chemother.*, 12:119–127, 1957.
44. Jhamandas, K., Phillis, J. W., and Pinsky, C. Effects of narcotic analgesics and antagonists on the *in vivo* release of acetylcholine from the cerebral cortex of the cat. *Brit. J. Pharmacol.*, 43:53–66, 1971.
45. Bhargava, H. N., and Way, E. L. Acetylcholinesterase inhibition and morphine effects in morphine tolerance and dependent mice. *J. Pharmacol. Exp. Ther.*, 183: 31–40, 1972.
46. Bhargava, H. N., Chan, S. L., and Way, E. L. Influence of hemicholinium (HC-3) on morphine analgesia, tolerance, physical dependence and on brain acetylcholine. *Europ. J. Pharmacol.*, 1974 (*in press*).
47. Brase, D. A., Tseng, L. F., Loh, H. H., and Way, E. L. Cholinergic modification of naloxone-induced jumping in morphine-dependent mice. *Europ. J. Pharmacol.*, 26:1–8, 1974.
48. Iwamoto, E. T., Ho, I. K., and Way, E. L. Elevation of brain dopamine during naloxone precipitated withdrawal in morphine-dependent mice and rats. *J. Pharmacol. Exp. Ther.*, 187:558–567, 1974.
49. Iwamoto, E. T. Circling behavior precipitated by naloxone in morphine dependent rats with unilateral lesions of the substantia nigra. *Fed. Proc.*, 33:487, 1974.
50. Costall, B., Naylor, R. J., and Olley, J. E. Catalepsy and circling behavior after intracerebral injections of neuroleptic, cholinergic and anticholinergic agents into the caudate-putamen, globus pallidus and substantia nigra of rat brain. *Neuropharmacol.*, 11:645, 1972.
51. Friedler, G., Bhargava, H. N., Quock, R., and Way, E. L. The effect of 6-hydroxydopamine on morphine tolerance and physical dependence. *J. Pharmacol. Exp. Ther.*, 183:49–55, 1972.
52. Andén, N. E., Rubsnsen, A., Fuxe, K., and Hökfelt, T. Evidence for dopamine receptor stimulation by apomorphine. *J. Pharm. Pharmacol.*, 19:627–629, 1967.
53. Hedri, A. Apomorphi bei Opiat-Entziehungskur. *Schweiz. Rundschau Med.* (*Praxis*) 61:488–489, 1972.
54. Gunne, L. M., Jonsson, J., and Fuxe, K. Effects of morphine intoxication on brain catecholamine neuron. *Europ. J. Pharmacol.* 5:338–343, 1969.
55. Clouet, D. H., and Ratner, M. Catecholamine biosynthesis in brains of rats treated with morphine. *Science* 168:854–856, 1970.
56. Fukui, K., and Takagi, H. Effect of morphine on the cerebral content of metabolites of dopamine in normal and tolerant mice: Its possible relation to analgesic action. *Brit. J. Pharmacol.* 44:45–51, 1972.

DISCUSSION

Kerr: I am interested in your localization of the origin of withdrawal phenomenon by the implantation of naloxone into various brain locations. The most sensitive area you found was the meso-diencephalic junction, where the parafascicular nucleus is located. To my knowledge, there is no significant autonomic system localized to this area of the brain. What is located in this area which would explain the motor phenomena of jumping and "wet dog" shakes that were observed in your studies? There are no visceral systems located in this area; rather, they are situated more ventrally and rostrally in the hypothalamus. Himmelsbach pointed out long ago that most, if not all, of the signs of withdrawal are autonomic signs. Is the jumping response you observed in some way an autonomic event? Is the wet-dog shake an autonomic sign associated with thermal regulation?

Way: The injections we generally used were quite large and it is possible that the naloxone spread from the injection site. It is noteworthy, however, that we failed to obtain responses in a number of areas not too far removed from the effective sites. As we have mentioned, Shute and Lewis reported high acetylcholinesterase levels in this region and perhaps this area may influence extrapyramidal function.

Goldstein: You mentioned that you observed diarrhea following implantation of naloxone. Is this a consistent finding?

Way: We have not followed this response routinely since we find that wet shakes and jumping behavior are the most consistent signs of withdrawal in our animals.

Kerr: If we use a specific sign, are we studying the syndrome of morphine dependence? Can we extrapolate from a single sign to the general phenomenon of withdrawal in the morphine-dependent animal?

Way: I agree that we must be careful in extrapolating from evidence based on a single sign of morphine dependence to the general phenomenon itself. However, the systematic study using a single sign may provide us with the key to understanding the overall phenomenon.

Kerr: It is interesting that the most effective site of naloxone-precipitated abstinence coincides with the dorsal midline nociceptive input to the thalamus, rather than the ventro lateral visceral input into hypothalamus.

Lomax: Cutaneous sensory fibers also pass through this area.

De Wied: Just to make things a little more complicated, electrical stimulation of this area will increase active avoidance behavior and destruction of the parafascicular nucleus will destroy these responses.

Narcotics and the Hypothalamus, edited by
E. Zimmermann and R. George. Raven Press,
New York © 1974

The Role of the Lateral Hypothalamus in Opiate Dependence

Frederick W. L. Kerr

Department of Neurosurgery, Mayo Graduate School of Medicine, Rochester, Minnesota 55901

Dependence on narcotics is clearly due to involvement of the central nervous system, whether one considers the psychic aspect, i.e., craving for the drug, or the physical features which manifest themselves during the withdrawal syndrome.

In the approach to understanding the mechanisms responsible for dependence, two main avenues may be followed: (1) assume that the syndrome is due to widespread involvement of the brain from cerebral cortex to many or all of the subcortical nuclei or (2) regard the syndrome as an expression of involvement of restricted neuronal systems of the brain and consider the signs observed during withdrawal to be a reflection of disordered function of these specific systems. In essence, one can subscribe either to a holistic hypothesis or to one of localization. In this chapter I summarize my observations from studies on rats and monkeys in support of localization of the disorder to the hypothalamus.

The first question is, why the hypothalamus and not some other area such as the thalamus or perhaps the cerebral cortex?

There are several reasons for giving preferential consideration to the hypothalamus. One is the working hypothesis I have proposed, that the craving for morphine which the addict suffers from during withdrawal may be mediated by the same neuronal systems concerned with hunger that lie in the lateral hypothalamus (6).

Another clue is implicit in the work of Olds and associates (12, 13), who have shown that the lateral hypothalamus is a major locus for self-stimulation and is thus intimately related to mechanisms of reward. One may ask the question, is an opiate interpreted by these neurons as a chemical reward in the same way that an electrical stimulus to the area is satisfying to the subject? Finally, most of the signs of withdrawal are expressions of overactivity of the autonomic nervous system, as pointed out many years ago by Himmelsbach (5). Thus, one sees sweating, piloerection, excessive salivation, increased bowel motility, pallor of the skin, yawning, rhinorrhea, and lacrimation while somatic symptoms (such as muscle cramps) are negligible.

Although any or all of these could occur as a result of involvement of a number of segmental levels of the autonomic nervous system, the hypothalamus is a major autonomic center from which the gamut of vegetative responses may be elicited.

The irritability and jitteriness that occur in animals and man during withdrawal can, again, be elicited by appropriate lesions or stimulation of the hypothalamus in nonaddicted animals (3, 11). While the preceding phenomena can be made to correlate with the objective signs of withdrawal, such correlations are no more than speculation unless supported by experimental data. In this report I present some of the evidence assembled from studies in the rat and the macaque that is compatible with the concept of the hypothalamus being the major site at which morphine acts to produce the derangements of neural function manifested during withdrawal.

HYPOTHALAMIC NEURONAL RESPONSES TO MORPHINE AND ANTAGONISTS IN THE RAT

The experiments on rats were undertaken to obtain quantitative data on the activity of a number of single units recorded simultaneously in two separate nuclei of the hypothalamus, as well as from other structures such as the amygdala, ventral tegmental area, cerebral neocortex, and hippocampal cortex. Parts of this study have been reported elsewhere and in a detailed report (7).

Seventy-five adult Sprague-Dawley rats weighing 500 ± 50 g were used; of these, 45 were discarded from the analysis, 9 were naive, and 21 were made dependent on morphine and were tolerant to twice-daily intraperitoneal doses of 100 mg of morphine. The tolerant rats were studied at intervals ranging from 7 to 52 hr after the last dose of morphine had been administered and were in frank withdrawal. All dependent rats were also tested for their degree of dependence by challenging with intraperitoneal naloxone; only those graded as 3+ or better were used for the study.

The animals were anesthetized with urethane supplemented with 1% procaine in the ear canals and through the tympanic membrane, to assure that introduction of the ear bars of the stereotactic apparatus (Baltimore Inst. Co.) did not produce noxious sensation. Urethane at the dosage administered is entirely adequate for the other surgical procedures that were necessary, but we felt it was not completely satisfactory for the ear canals. An endotracheal tube was inserted and artificial respiration maintained with a Harvard respiratory pump regulated to cycle at the rate and volume maintained by the rat prior to administration of curare, which was the muscle blocking agent of choice in these experiments.

Stereotactically guided insulated steel microelectrodes with a tip exposure of approximately 7 μ were introduced bilaterally. One electrode entered the ventromedian nucleus and the other entered the contralateral lateral hypothalamic area; this was done for convenience in view of the proximity of the two nuclei. In one experiment both electrodes were introduced into the respective nuclei on one side and the results were, as anticipated, the same as with bilateral placement.

The potentials recorded by these electrodes were amplified in the conventional manner, viewed on a standard and on a slave storage oscilloscope, and stored on tape for subsequent processing. Each electrode recorded the activity of a number of units simultaneously, and by careful positioning it was possible always to obtain one large unit, usually one intermediate unit, and, commonly, several small voltage units. By using window discriminators, the activity of these units was separated into three channels of normalized pulses which were relayed to a C.D.C. 3500 computer. This was programmed to deliver firing-frequency histograms or post-stimulus time (PST) histograms which were displayed on the storage cathode ray oscilloscope and photographed on Polaroid film.

Morphine was injected intravenously in a dose of 10 mg for the naive rats and 75 mg for the dependent animals. Nalorphine and, later, naloxone were injected in doses calculated to neutralize the preceding dose of morphine; the dose of antagonist was 1.35 mg of nalorphine and 0.00135 mg of naloxone for each milligram of morphine that had been injected during the experiment. At the end of the experiments a lethal dose of pentobarbital was given and the recording continued after death to determine accurately the level of noise present, if any; in this manner unacceptable records were identified and removed from the study. All animals were perfused with 10% aqueous formalin at the end of the procedure; serial sections were made through the brain, stained with luxol fast blue, and examined histologically.

Results

All experiments began with a 2 to 5 min period of recording of resting activity. At the end of this time morphine was injected and the injection was completed within approximately 15 to 20 sec. The recordings were continuous from the beginning to the end of the experiment. Figure 1 illustrates the responses to morphine in the ventromedian and lateral hypothalamic nuclei of a naive rat weighing 550 g. It is important to note that after i.v. administration of 5 mg morphine the ordinate scale in the histogram recorded from the ventromedian nucleus has doubled automatically to accommodate the increase in number of spikes. This increase is evident and amounts to eight times the resting activity, or 365 spikes in 56 sec with a consequent drop in interspike interval to 153 msec. The lower histograms in Fig. 1 trace the simultaneous activity of a neuron in the lateral hypothalamic area which is seen to decrease its firing rate from 373/56 sec to 61/56 sec, a sixfold drop. These reciprocal effects of morphine were reversed by nalorphine.

UNIT RESPONSES IN HYPOTHALAMUS
TO MORPHINE 10 mg/kg BW

VENTROMEDIAN NUCLEUS

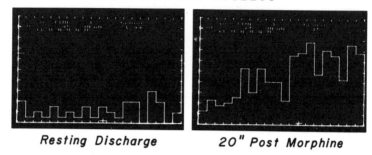

Resting Discharge   20" Post Morphine

LATERAL HYPOTHALAMIC AREA

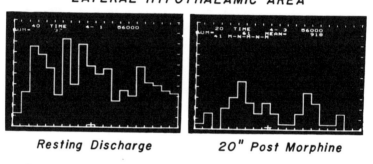

Resting Discharge   20" Post Morphine

FIG. 1. Firing frequency histograms of a single unit in the ventromedian nucleus and another unit in the lateral hypothalamic area recorded simultaneously. The resting activity of a neuron in the ventromedian nucleus is illustrated at top left. The ordinate scale indicates the number of spikes for each time bin in the abscissa; full scale on the ordinate corresponds to 20 spikes in this instance as indicated by the figure at the top left of the histogram and each time bin corresponds to 2.8 sec. The total number of spikes for the 56 sec represented is 45; the remaining 4 sec of each minute is utilized for computer time. The interspike interval is recorded at the top right of the histogram, below the duration, and is 1,244 msec. Five mg of morphine was administered intravenously beginning during the last 11 sec of the first histogram and ending during the first few seconds of the second histogram, at the top right of the figure. The resting discharge rate of the ventromedian unit was markedly accelerated while that of the lateral nucleus was profoundly inhibited (right) by i.v. administration of 5 mg of morphine.

Figure 2 illustrates the effect of morphine on the activity of neurons in the ventromedian and lateral hypothalamic area in a 460-g, dependent rat that received 100 mg of morphine twice daily until 52 hr prior to the recording. The sequence of events is similar to the previously described experiment. Again, morphine produced a marked increase in the firing rate of the ventromedian neuron and a precipitous drop in that of the lateral hypothalamic unit. The injection in this experiment was more prolonged than in the naive rats

UNIT RESPONSES IN HYPOTHALAMUS
Morphine Dependent Rat, 52 hours Withdrawal

VENTROMEDIAN NUCLEUS

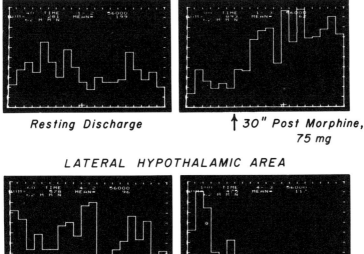

Resting Discharge   ↑ 30" Post Morphine,
                                              75 mg

LATERAL HYPOTHALAMIC AREA

Resting Discharge   ↑ 30" Post Morphine,
                                              75 mg

FIG. 2. Effect of 75 mg of morphine given i.v. on firing frequency of ventromedian and lateral hypothalamic units in a morphine-dependent rat in withdrawal. The arrows indicate the end of injection of morphine which had begun 30 sec earlier. Note the increase in ordinate scale for both sets of recordings. The reciprocal effects of morphine on the two nuclei are striking.

because of the larger volume of fluid needed for the 75-mg dose of morphine. The changes in firing rate were maintained until reversal by naloxone administered 5 min after the morphine.

Summary of Unit Recordings

The effects of morphine on the medial and lateral hypothalamus are diametrically opposite, the neurons in the ventromedian nucleus being strongly excited while those of the lateral hypothalamic area are powerfully inhibited. This response pattern is characteristic and virtually all neurons in each nucleus are affected in the same manner. Because of this reciprocal effect I have called this the push–pull phenomenon. The effects of antagonists on these nuclei are in the opposite direction in all respects, so that the lateral hypothalamus is excited while the ventromedian nucleus is inhibited.

The degree of specificity of these opposing responses is particularly emphasized by the fact that the firing aspects of the ventromedian nucleus and the lateral hypothalamic area are separated by a distance of 0.5 mm.

To study responses of other areas, recordings were obtained in the thalamus, other hypothalamic nuclei, the cerebral cortex, the amygdala, and the rostral midbrain (red nucleus and ventral tegmental area). Some nuclei followed the pattern of the ventromedian nucleus of excitation by morphine and inhibition by antagonists, others were affected similarly to the lateral hypothalamic area, and yet others, such as the nucleus gelatinosus of the thalamus, were excited by both morphine and naloxone. Other areas (for example, the cortex) were variably affected by morphine and antagonists. The complexity of central nervous system response to opiates cannot therefore be summarized in any comprehensive manner; rather, it is necessary to specify which nucleus is being considered and, in general, it appears that the pattern of response is then very consistent from animal to animal.

The latency of onset of the response in our experiments ranged between 20 and 30 sec from the beginning of injection.

It is also noteworthy that when the activity of neurons in the lateral hypothalamus of an animal in withdrawal was compared with that of neurons in the naive animal, the firing frequency of the former was significantly greater in most but not all instances, whereas there were no appreciable differences in the case of the ventromedian nucleus.

The preceding observations indicate that neurons have very specific and predictable responses to morphine, but do not clarify for us whether these nuclei are in fact primarily concerned with the phenomenon of dependence. It may well be that other nuclei which we have shown to be significantly excited or inhibited by morphine could in fact be the ones responsible for the syndrome of dependence–withdrawal. The experiments that follow were carried out on monkeys and give some clues regarding these questions.

EFFECT OF LESIONS OF THE LATERAL HYPOTHALAMUS ON SELF-ADMINISTRATION OF MORPHINE BY MONKEYS

Young adult female macaque monkeys kept in restraint chairs were trained to self-administer morphine by pressing a bar; some were also trained to self-administer 1-g food pellets by pressing another bar. The morphine was delivered in 10-mg doses in a volume of 1 ml of saline on a fixed schedule of 10:1. Once dependence was well established and the monkeys were self-administering the drug in a regular manner, a withdrawal test was carried out and the intensity of the response graded on a 0 to 4+ basis. Lesions were placed in the hypothalamus either by electrolytic destruction or by injection of 6-hydroxydopamine (6-OHDA).

In the first type of experiment, insulated steel electrodes were introduced stereotactically into the lateral hypothalamus and their positions checked by X-ray. Because of the great variations that exist in the stereotactic coordinates of the macaque's brain [Olszewski (14)], significant errors in electrode position, particularly in the anteroposterior and vertical planes, occurred in a number of animals (ventriculography is now used routinely to try to minimize this problem). An array of three electrodes, arranged in the saggital plane bilaterally, was used to lesion a large area. The electrode assembly was secured with screws and acrylic to the skull. Several days after the operative procedure, and only if a reliable baseline of morphine and pellet self-administration was being maintained, electrolytic lesions were made using a Grass lesion generator.

In the second type of experiment a 22-gauge spinal needle was introduced stereotactically into the lateral hypothalamus on each side and secured in the same manner as the electrodes. Chemical lesions were made with a fresh solution of 6-ODHA, prepared as follows. An 0.5% solution of ascorbic acid in saline was taken to a pH of 4.5 to 5.0 by adding NaOH. Nitrogen was bubbled through this solution for 5 min and the solution was kept chilled on ice. 6-OHDA was added just before injection into the hypothalamus. A total dose of 200 μg was injected into each lateral hypothalamic area.

Results

Electrolytic Lesions

Figure 3 illustrates the effect of bilateral electrolytic lesions in the lateral hypothalamic area in a morphine-dependent monkey. Prior to making the lesions, dependence was tested by challenge with nalorphine and by substituting saline for the morphine solution. As a result there was a great increase in bar pressing to a peak of 4,670 in 24 hr on the fourth day. Withdrawal without antagonist precipitation was repeated on the 47th day of dependence, resulting in a peak of 8,000 bar presses in 24 hr.

Bilateral lesions were made in the lateral hypothalamic area (Fig. 3) after morphine self-administration was resumed and an intake of between 130 and 260 mg per day requiring 130 to 260 bar presses on a fixed 10:1 ratio attained. Morphine was discontinued when the electrolytic lesions were made. As illustrated, there was a moderate increase in bar pressing to 670 in 24 hr on the third day. This was associated with a moderately intense withdrawal syndrome; bar pressing decreased to 290 on the fourth day. Morphine access ad libitum was then allowed on the fifth day. It was interesting that the intake of drug was reduced to between 30 and 50 mg per day for 5 days, followed by a further increase to approximately 80 mg per day for 3 days. Repeat withdrawal at this time showed a return toward previous high levels of bar pressing. The monkey's general condition deteriorated acutely on the 85th day and at postmortem acute pancreatic necrosis was found. Similar results have been obtained with other monkeys by lesioning the lateral hypothalamus. Lesions of the septal area have, however, had no influence on the course of dependence.

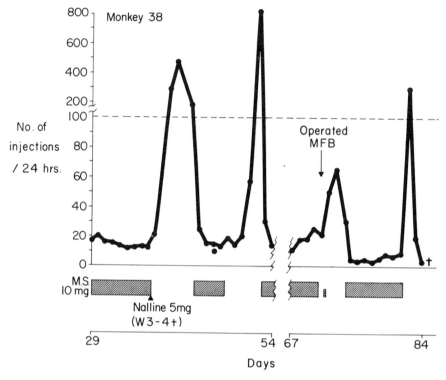

FIG. 3. Morphine self-administration by a dependent monkey, response to nalorphine (nalline) and to withdrawal, and effect of bilateral electrolytic lesions in the lateral hypothalamus (medial forebrain bundle). Note the 10-fold increase in the ordinate scale at interrupted line. Level of morphine intake was significantly depressed following the lesions. Ordinate = number of cycles (fixed ratio of 10:1) in 24 hr; each completed cycle resulted in the i.v. injection of 10 mg of morphine in 1 ml of saline or of 1 ml of saline alone during withdrawal.

It is important to note—and this comment applies to all the electrolytic and chemical lesions—that appetite is usually but not invariably affected in the same way as desire for morphine and that the animals showed no detectable disturbances of consciousness as a result of the lesions. They were normally alert and would actively push the examiner's hands away when they were handled. As shown in the graph, at the end of this period they resumed taking morphine and, in some instances, drug intake increased markedly over pre-lesional levels.

Serial sections of the brain showed that the lesions were located exactly in the lateral hypothalamus in the course of the median forebrain bundle.

Effects of 6-OHDA on the Lateral Hypothalamic Area in Morphine-dependent Monkeys

These effects will be divided into the immediate response to the injection and delayed effects.

6-OHDA in a dose of 200 μg dissolved in 0.10 ml of saline solution was injected over a 2-min period. Toward the latter part of the injection or within a minute or two of the end of administration of the drug, retching and vomiting occurred, at times of considerable intensity and lasting intermittently for approximately 10 min. Although these animals had had excellent appetites prior to the injection, immediately following it they refused any food offered them. In addition to the vomiting there was some vocalization of the same barking type seen during withdrawal in this species, associated at times with a mild degree of irritability.

The delayed effects are illustrated in Fig. 4, which shows the pattern of morphine self-administration and of food pellet intake by bar pressing prior to injection of 6-OHDA, and the sudden and profound drop in both which resulted from the injection. The decrease in morphine intake was approximately 10-fold for the first 48 hr and then rose to 100 to 130 mg per day which was approximately a third of the pre-injection requirement. This monkey was markedly anoretic during the first 3 days following administration of 6-OHDA and her appetite recovered as her morphine intake rose. However, on the sixth post-injection day she had a sudden violent seizure while eating

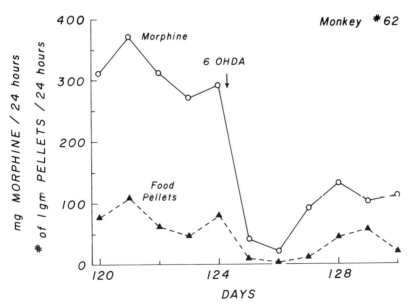

FIG. 4. Morphine and food pellet self-administration by a dependent monkey and effect of injection of 200 μg of 6-OHDA into the lateral hypothalamic area bilaterally. A precipitous drop of both morphine and food intake occurred immediately, but partial recovery of both is noted. The marked parallel between the appetite for morphine and for food is emphasized in these tracings.

and expired despite all efforts at resuscitation. Postmortem examination gave no explanation for this result.

Similar marked depression of morphine intake was obtained in two additional monkeys with administration of 6-OHDA, while in two monkeys in which the cannula position apparently was unsatisfactory, injection of 6-OHDA had neither immediate (retching or vomiting) nor delayed effects on morphine intake.

Summary of the Effect of Lesions in the Lateral Hypothalamus on Morphine Self-administration

Destruction of either neurons or tracts in the lateral hypothalamus produces a depression in the intake of morphine by these dependent monkeys which is usually but not invariably associated with a similar depression of appetite. This change lasts for several days to a little over a week, and although the number of experiments is as yet limited, a gradual return to previous levels of morphine intake has occurred. The two most likely possibilities that would account for this are that either the lesions have not been sufficiently extensive and therefore part of the nucleus or pathways has been spared, or there is another system which can substitute. Until histologic study is completed these suggestions can only be regarded as speculation.

DISCUSSION

In the foregoing account of efforts to determine the degree of localization and specificity of morphine effects on the central nervous system with particular reference to the phenomena of dependence, data have been acquired that provide support for the concept. This is exemplified by the specificity of single unit responses according to the nucleus and the conspicuous reciprocity of effects on lateral versus ventromedian hypothalamic nuclei, and by the significantly increased firing rate of lateral hypothalamic units in morphine-dependent rats during withdrawal.

These observations also indicate that morphine effects are specifically excitatory to some nuclei and inhibitory to others and that this is remarkably consistent from animal to animal. It is also clear that the effects of morphine are widespread and that most neurons are affected by this potent drug in either an excitatory or inhibitory manner. Thus, since the influence of morphine and its antagonists is particularly pronounced on the lateral and medial hypothalamus, and since the direction in which these effects is exerted is entirely compatible with the hypothesis that opiate dependence can be compared to appetitive drives and especially hunger, whose localization is to a major degree in the lateral hypothalamus (1, 2, 4), these observations are regarded as supportive but not conclusive evidence with reference to localization.

Conversely, the fact that many neurons in nuclei other than the hypothalamus are markedly influenced by morphine should not be considered conclusive evidence that the syndrome of morphine dependence has a widespread basis rooted in virtually the entire central nervous system.

The behavioral responses to electrolytic and chemical lesions of the lateral hypothalamus are suggestive of localization of the mechanism which underlies the drive or craving for opiates to this area. Furthermore, 6-OHDA, which has a relatively specific effect on dopamine-containing terminals, was injected into the lateral hypothalamus in an attempt to determine whether dopaminergic neurons are specifically concerned with the mechanism of craving for opiates. The results obtained do suggest that these pathways should receive major consideration as potentially underlying the mechanisms involved in craving for morphine. The parallel between depression of desire for morphine and for food by both electrolytic and chemical lesions also tends to favor the hypothesis that appetitive centers in the lateral hypothalamus are predominantly responsible for psychic dependence on opiates.

However, it is also necessary to maintain a cautious and critical attitude toward these findings. Thus, as noted earlier, the single unit studies, although demonstrating a striking specificity of effects of morphine on individual nuclei, do not restrict the influence of morphine to the hypothalamus; to the contrary, they indicate, as would be expected from behavioral observations on animals and man, that morphine affects the majority of central nervous system neurons in either an excitatory or inhibitory manner. But although such effects do occur, it seems more reasonable in view of what we know of localization of function in the central nervous system to assume as a working hypothesis that the signs and symptoms which occur during withdrawal are due to involvement of only some systems; the question is, how few or how restricted? That the effects of morphine on the hypothalamus are in fact limited to specific areas has been demonstrated clearly by Lomax and Kirkpatrick (8) and by Lotti, Lomax, and George (9, 10) in studies on the hypothermic effects of local administration of the drug.

Similarly, hypothalamic lesions, whether electrolytic or chemical, do indeed produce a striking decrease in voluntary drug intake. However, this effect has been limited to from 3 or 4 days up to 8 days so far, and its causes are difficult to determine even with so excellent an experimental animal as the monkey. We know that the decrease is not due to changes in levels of consciousness, since these changes are at most transient (being limited to 5 or 10 min of mild drowsiness in some cases immediately following injection of 6-OHDA). Drowsiness was not observed with the electrolytic lesions.

The observations of Wei, Loh, and Way (15) on the effect of injections of naloxone into the diencephalon of morphine-dependent rats are at variance with the hypothesis that the hypothalamus is a major locus of action of morphine insofar as the phenomena of dependence are concerned. Withdrawal signs did not occur when the antagonist was injected into the hypothalamus but did appear following injections into the medial thalamus. However, it is difficult to understand why the variety of autonomic signs these investigators described are elicited from an area of the brain such as the medial thalamus, which does not control visceral functions. The possibility that the antagonist entered the nearby ventricular system can be considered, in which case wide diffusion throughout the brain would occur.

ACKNOWLEDGMENTS

Supported in part by grant DA 00110 from the National Institute of Mental Health, U.S. Public Health Service. The single unit studies described above were done in collaboration with Drs. J. N. Triplett and G. W. Beeler (7).

REFERENCES

1. Anand, B. K., and Brobeck, J. Hypothalamic control of food intake in rats and cats. *Yale J. Biol. Med.,* 24:123–140, 1950.
2. Delgado, J. M. R., and Anand, B. K. Increased food intake induced by electrical stimulation of the lateral hypothalamus. *Am. J. Physiol.,* 172:162–168, 1953.
3. Hess, W. R. *Diencephalon, Autonomic and Extrapyramidal Function.* Grune and Stratton, New York, 1954.
4. Hetherington, A. W., and Ranson, S. W. Hypothalamic lesions and adiposity in the rat. *Anat. Rec.,* 78:149–172, 1940.
5. Himmelsbach, C. K. With reference to physical dependence. *Fed. Proc.,* 2:201–203, 1943.
6. Kerr, F. W. L., and Pozuelo, J., Suppression of physical dependence and induction of hypersensitivity to morphine by stereotaxic hypothalamic lesions in addicted rats. *Mayo Clin. Proc.,* 46:653–665, 1971.
7. Kerr, F. W. L., Triplett, J. N., and Beeler, G. W. Reciprocal (push–pull) effects of morphine on single units in the ventromedial and lateral hypothalamus and influences on other nuclei: With a comment on methadone effects during withdrawal from morphine. *Brain Res.,* 74:81–103, 1974.
8. Lomax, P., and Kirkpatrick, W. E. The effect of n-allyl-normorphine on the development of acute tolerance to the analgesic and hypothermic effects of morphine in the rat. *Med. Pharmacol. Exp.,* 16:165–170, 1967.
9. Lotti, V. J., Lomax, P., and George, R. Temperature response in the rat following intracerebral microinjection of morphine. *J. Pharmacol. Exp. Ther.,* 150:135–139, 1965.
10. Lotti, V. J., Lomax, P., and George, R. N-allyl-normorphine antagonism of the hypothermic effect of morphine in the rat following intracerebral and systemic administration. *J. Pharmacol. Exp. Ther.,* 150:420–425, 1965.
11. MacLean, P. D. The hypothalamus and emotional behavior. In: *The Hypothalamus,* edited by W. Haymaker, E. Anderson, and W. J. H. Nauta.
12. Olds, J. Hypothalamic substrates of reward. *Physiol. Rev.,* 42:554–604, 1962.
13. Olds, J. *The neurological basis of behavior.* Ciba Foundation Symposium, Churchill, London, 1958.
14. Olszewski, J. *The thalamus of the Macaca Mulatta.* S. Karger, Basel, 1952.
15. Wei, E., Loh, H. H., and Way, E. L. Neuroanatomical correlates of morphine dependence. *Science,* 177:616–617, 1972.

DISCUSSION

Wikler: Have you carried out studies using antagonists in morphine-dependent animals?

Kerr: Yes, we have and we find that naloxone administration causes an increase in firing rate of hypothalamic neurons.

Goldstein: Does naloxone alone have an excitatory action on these neurons?

Kerr: No. The increased firing rate seen following naloxone occurs only in animals pretreated with morphine. Naloxone alone does not produce this effect in the naive animal. I don't know, however, if the effect of naloxone is purely a reversal of the action of morphine or whether it represents an independent excitatory action of naloxone in the morphine-treated animal.

Deneau: We must remember that morphine has both excitatory and inhibitory effects and that naloxone antagonizes only the depressant actions of the drug.

Kerr: The data I have presented would suggest that some neurons are inhibited and others excited by morphine, and it does not appear that morphine has both excitatory and inhibitory effects on the same neuron. Further, naloxone appears to counteract both of these effects.

Mirsky: Were there any other behavioral manifestations of dopamine following the intraventricular administration of this agent in your animals?

Kerr: Yes. In several animals we have seen that within one to two minutes following the onset of the injection the animals start to eructate and vomit. They continue to do so for five to ten minutes and then stop.

Narcotics and the Hypothalamus, edited by
E. Zimmermann and R. George. Raven Press,
New York © 1974

Sites of Action of Narcotic Analgesics in the Hypothalamus

Peter Lomax and Marylouise Ary

Department of Pharmacology, School of Medicine and Brain Research Institute, University of
California, Los Angeles, California 90024

The narcotic analgesics possess one of the widest spectra of pharmacologic actions of all commonly used drugs, especially in relation to the central nervous system. Numerous studies have been undertaken to catalogue these effects, to assign specific sites of action, and to determine the mechanism by which the responses are mediated (see 1). Perhaps the least understood of all of these effects is the relief of pain, which constitutes the major clinical use of the drugs. To a large extent this stems from difficulty in measuring pain, either qualitatively or quantitatively, in experimental subjects, including man. Consequently there has been a tendency to study other aspects of the actions of the narcotic analgesics and to attempt to construct a general case from such data. Fortunately, for present purposes, the hypothalamus appears to participate in many of these actions and provides a fruitful field for investigation. The present discussion is restricted to only some of the effects involving hypothalamic mechanisms since other authors will be dealing with their own fields in greater detail.

In attempting to establish the specificity of a site of action in the central nervous system it is not enough that a given focal effect can be demonstrated; in addition the neurons involved ought to mirror the known pharmacologic responses to the drug in question. Such responses, in the case of the narcotic analgesics, include specific antagonism, the development of tolerance, and the phenomenon of dependence. The basic concept that all of these represent events at the neuronal level has been fundamental to our studies, even though the exact nature of the molecular changes cannot yet be defined.

EFFECTS ON BODY TEMPERATURE

In many species, including man, morphine and other narcotic analgesics cause a fall in body temperature. Some animals, including the felines, exhibit excitation after relatively low doses of morphine with an accompanying increase in core temperature. The responses in the rat vary with the dose administered; below 10 mg/kg i.v. moderate hyperthermia is seen, whereas larger doses cause a fall in temperature with the maximum effect being manifest at a dose level of 35 to 50 mg/kg i.v. (2, 3). Injection of morphine directly into the preoptic/anterior hypothalamic nuclei in doses ranging from 10 to 50 μg also lowers core temperature in rats (2, 4). Systemic injection of nalorphine (2 mg/kg i.v.) prevents the fall in temperature induced by systemic (50 mg/kg) or intracerebral (50 μg) injection of morphine (4). If nalorphine (3.3 μg) is injected into the preoptic region the hypothermic effect of morphine (25 mg/kg i.v.) is either terminated or prevented, depending on the sequence of drug administration (4). These last data indicate that the sole site of action of morphine in producing hypothermia in the rat is in the rostral hypothalamic thermoregulatory centers. The central site of action was further confirmed by the observation that the quaternary derivative, N-methyl morphine, was without effect on body temperature when injected systemically but caused marked hypothermia when injected into the rostral hypothalamus (5).

The hyperthermia induced by morphine in cats also appears to be mediated centrally. Intraventricular injection of morphine leads to shivering and a rise in temperature that can be prevented by prior intraventricular administration of nalorphine (6).

Taken together, these data indicate that the changes in core temperature induced by morphine are due to an action on the rostral hypothalamic thermoregulatory centers. As with other effects of morphine, there have been many studies to determine the role of brain amines in these thermoregulatory responses. Administration of depletors of brain serotonin (5-HT) abolishes the hypothermic effect of morphine in rats (7, 8). Lesions of the midbrain raphe, which reduce forebrain 5-HT concentrations, abolish the rise in temperature in rats after small doses of morphine (5 mg/kg i.p.) and the fall in temperature after larger doses (30 mg/kg i.p.) (9). Thus, it is possible that morphine is acting on the thermoregulatory centers indirectly through serotonergic inter-neurons. The observation that intraventricular injection of 5-HT lowers core temperature in the rat (10) would seem to support this concept. However, the contradicting data concerning the effect of 5-HT on body temperature in different species (11) render it unlikely that the mediation of serotonergic neurons represents a general case in relation to the central actions of morphine.

When the same dose of morphine is administered 3 to 4 hr after an initial intravenous dose, the fall in temperature is markedly attenuated or absent, indicating the development of acute tolerance (3). Similarly, acute tolerance after injection directly into the thermoregulatory centers can be demonstrated, and the dose must be increased to produce a comparable response (Fig. 1). These experiments would seem to indicate that the phenomenon of tolerance is the result of changes occurring directly at the neuronal level. The possibility that tolerance involves a generalized immune type of mechanism is not, however, ruled out, since even doses in the microgram range could induce such a reaction. If nalorphine (2 mg/kg i.v.) is administered immediately prior to morphine (25 mg/kg i.v.), the fall in body temperature is prevented and so is the development of tolerance, since a subsequent injection of morphine alone

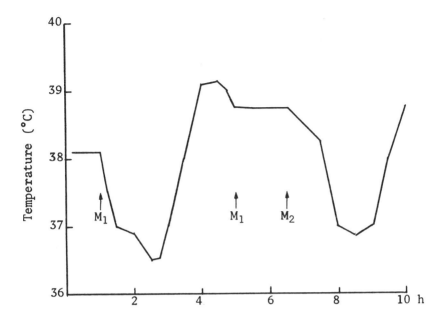

FIG. 1. Record of body temperature from a conscious rat. At M₁, morphine (15 μg) was injected unilaterally into the rostral hypothalamic thermoregulatory center (preoptic/anterior hypothalamic nuclei) via a chronically implanted guide. The second injection was ineffective in lowering the core temperature due to development of tolerance. When the dose was increased to 50 μg (M₂), a fall in temperature comparable to that following the first injection occurred.

causes hypothermia (12). Protection against the occurrence of acute tolerance to the hypothermic effect of morphine can also be afforded by injecting nalorphine (5 μg) directly into the rostral hypothalamus (12).

These results indicate that administration of morphine per se does not necessarily lead to the development of tolerance, and that nalorphine inhibits the mechanisms which cause tolerance to develop as well as some of the pharmacologic actions of morphine. In fact, it appears that morphine must first exert a particular effect before tolerance to that effect appears. In these experiments, because of the time course of the events, it was not feasible to measure temperature and analgesia concurrently, but observation of the animals in which the fall in temperature is prevented by intracerebral injection of nalorphine reveals all the signs of analgesia, exophthalmus, and catatonia normally associated with an initial systemic injection of morphine. Thus, if the phenomenon of tolerance is caused by some generalized antibody reaction, one would expect the animals to be tolerant to the hypothermic effect of a second dose of morphine in this experimental situation. It would appear, as far as the hypothermic effect of morphine is concerned, that tolerance is the result of changes at the neuronal receptor sites in the rostral hypothalamus.

It is of interest in this respect that, although injection of the quaternary analogue N-methyl morphine into the rostral hypothalamus of the rat leads to a fall in core temperature, tolerance does not occur with repeated injections (5). Possibly the charged quaternary species is restrained from an intracellular site to which the molecule must have access before tolerance occurs. Alternatively, tolerance to morphine may involve the formation of morphine conjugates and intracellular binding via the secondary amine group (13), which is unable to take place with the quaternary derivative.

Changes in thermoregulatory function are a marked feature of the withdrawal syndrome in many species. Abstinence from morphine in rats addicted to 80 mg/kg per day leads to a fall in body temperature and metabolic heat production (14); the fall in rectal temperature is more pronounced when withdrawal is precipitated by administration of nalorphine (15). Large falls in body temperature are seen in morphine-dependent rhesus monkeys when the drug is withdrawn or when nalorphine is administered, and are accompanied by other signs of withdrawal. The hypothermia was reversed by injection of morphine, meperidine, or levorphan (16, 17). In human addicts nalorphine causes shivering, a feeling of cold and gooseflesh, and an accompanying rise in rectal temperature. Sometimes sweating also occurs. These last effects suggest that there has been an upward setting of the hypothalamic thermostat.

Morphine withdrawal hypothermia in the rat can be prevented by a conditioned stimulus (e.g., ringing a bell) (18). Depletion of brain 5-HT levels reduces the hypothermic effect of morphine in naive rats but does not modify the fall following injection of naloxone in tolerant animals (8). From these observations it would appear that the mechanisms mediating the fall in temperature when morphine is administered to normal animals and when withdrawal occurs in addicted animals are fundamentally different, although in both instances they seem to be mediated by the central nervous system.

ANALGESIC EFFECTS

In spite of a large number of experimental studies, knowledge of the central sites and mechanisms of action of the antinociceptive effects of the narcotic analgesics is limited. The complex nature of pain perception renders it unlikely that any single brain structure constitutes a specific locus of action. From early studies involving serial transections of the brain at different levels only gross localization to structures, such as the spinal cord and thalamus, was possible. The later use of stereotactic techniques, whereby the drugs could be accurately injected into the cerebral ventricles and at specific points in the brain, has led to some conclusions concerning sites of analgesic action in several species.

Tsou and Jang (19) measured the threshold responses to radiant heating of the skin in rabbits after intraventricular or intracerebral injection of morphine. Analgesia was seen after intraventricular administration and when the drug was injected bilaterally into the periventricular gray matter within 1 to 2 mm of the third ventricle. No increase in threshold occurred when morphine was applied to the sensory cortex, midbrain reticular formation, thalamic nuclei, the septum, or the medial geniculate body. Nalorphine injected bilaterally into the periventricular region antagonized the analgesic effect of systemically administered morphine. Similar studies were carried out in rabbits, using electrical stimulation of the tooth pulp, by Herz and his co-workers (20). Morphine and fentanyl were injected into the ventricular system and the spread of the drugs was restricted to different areas. Both drugs inhibited the nociceptive response completely when the aqueduct and fourth ventricle were perfused; the analgesia was not so marked when the third ventricle was perfused and was absent when perfusion was restricted to the lateral ventricles. Injection directly into the diencephalic and mesencephalic periventricular structures caused analgesia, with the most pronounced effect occurring when the drugs were placed in the aqueductal region. Autoradiographic studies with ^{14}C-morphine showed the effective sites to be located in the ventricular walls at a depth of 1 to 2 mm from the cavity (21).

Using the response to pin prick in cats, Yanagida and Yamamura (22) found that fentanyl (compounded with droperidol under the trade name of Innovar®) caused deep sedation and analgesia when placed in the caudal hypothalamus, the centromedian thalamic nuclei, and ventromedial thalamic nuclei. No effect was seen when the injection sites lay in the mesencephalic and pontine reticular formations.

In the rat, injection of morphine (50 μg) at various sites in the medial hypothalamus caused analgesia (assessed by diminution of corneal reflexes and loss of tail withdrawal on pinching), but there did not appear to be specific localization of the effective areas (2). The data of Herz et al. (20) indicate, however, that diffusion of the drug to a common site could have occurred. Using the response to electric shock delivered through a grid in the bottom of the cage, Jacquet and Lajtha (23) studied the effect of intracerebral injection of morphine (10 μg) in rats. Injections into the caudal hypothalamus or third ventricle caused significant analgesia. When the drug was injected into the medial septum, the caudate nucleus, or the periaqueductal gray matter, "hyperalgesia" was noted. However, the "hyperalgesic" response is open to interpretation in this testing situation. Both fentanyl and sodium salicylate given subcutaneously protected against the nociceptive responses to electrical stimulation of the lateral hypothalamus in rats (24). As in the case of the hypothermic effect of morphine, lesions of the midbrain raphe which reduce the levels of 5-HT in the forebrain of rats also reduce the analgesic effect of the drug (25).

Kobayashi (26) failed to elicit analgesia in dogs by injecting morphine into the ventricles. The larger diffusion path, in view of the size of the brain, might account for these negative findings (20).

The sites of intracerebral injection of morphine causing analgesia to electrical stimulation of the foot pad have been mapped in the rhesus monkey (27). The periventricular and periaqueductal gray regions were the most effective of 300 sites tested.

These several studies suggest that the narcotic analgesics generate an essential part of the behavioral depression, including the decreased reaction to nociceptive stimuli, in structures close to the walls of the third and fourth ventricles and the connecting aqueduct. It is not yet clear whether these effects represent modification of afferent or efferent components of the measured responses.

PHYSICAL DEPENDENCE AND WITHDRAWAL

The concept has long been implied, if not explicitly stated, that the phenomena of dependence and withdrawal from the narcotic analgesics result from widespread involvement of cortical and subcortical structures of the central nervous system. More recently, a number of investigators have studied the alternative hypothesis that the addictive properties of these drugs are caused by effects on limited nuclear areas of the brain, including the hypothalamus.

On the basis that narcotic addiction represented a disorder of the hypothalamic nuclei regulating eating and drinking, Kerr and Pozuelo (28) studied the effect of electrolytic lesions of the hypothalamus on nalorphine- or naloxone-induced withdrawal in rats dependent on morphine (120 mg/kg i.p. b.d.). The severity of behavioral withdrawal signs was markedly reduced in animals in which the greater part of the ventromedial hypothalamic (VMH) nuclei had been destroyed. Lesions of similar size in other parts of the hypothalamus were ineffective in modifying withdrawal. Dependent rats exhibited marked sensitivity to small doses of morphine (30 mg/kg compared with preoperative doses of 120 mg/kg) after VMH lesions, and several animals had convulsions.

Rats undergoing withdrawal from morphine show characteristic repetitive shaking movements of the body. Similar signs are seen when the animals are immersed in ice water, and were described by Martin et al. (29) as "wet dog shakes." On the basis of studies involving the injection of crystalline naloxone (40 to 200 μg) directly into the brain or the transverse sectioning of the brain, Wei and his associates (30–33) concluded that certain aspects of morphine abstinence, including wet dog shakes, could be mediated by structures in the medial thalamus and in the diencephalic–mesencephalic junction.

The effect of injecting nalorphine into various parts of the ventricular system after 15 days of administration of morphine (to a final dose of 120 mg/kg per day i.m.) has been studied in the rabbit (34). As in the case of morphine analgesia (see above), the most effective site for eliciting withdrawal was the fourth ventricle. Withdrawal precipitated by intraventricular injection of nalorphine was often accompanied by tonic convulsions when the drug entered the fourth ventricle. Injection of nalorphine into the third ventricle produced only mild signs of withdrawal. It was concluded that structures located in the medullary and pontine regions of the brainstem are important sites of action of morphine for the development of physical dependence in the rabbit.

Physical dependence to repeated injections of morphine into the lateral ventricles was demonstrated after systemic or intraventricular administration of nalorphine in monkeys (35). The firing frequency of rostral hypothalamic neurons in morphine-dependent rats was studied by Eidelberg and Bond (36). Both morphine and naloxone increased the firing frequency of these cells although the pattern of firing was different, morphine causing a characteristic bursting type of discharge.

Hypothalamic neuronal activity in naive and morphine-addicted rats has been investigated by Triplett et al. (37). Intravenous morphine increased the activity of units in the VMH nuclei and inhibited those recorded in the lateral hypothalamic area (LHA) in both groups of animals. These effects were reversed by intravenous injection of nalorphine or naloxone. Morphine (10 mg/kg s.c.) suppressed self-stimulation of the medial forebrain bundle in rats after an initial injection. With repeated injections complete tolerance to this effect developed, and thereafter stimulation rates increased with the injections (38). Similar results were obtained by Glick et al. (39), who also showed that naloxone-precipitated withdrawal depressed the rate of self-stimulation. Self-stimulation during withdrawal had no effect on the accompanying weight loss, but when the animals were allowed to stimulate the medial forebrain bundle during the period of chronic morphine administration, withdrawal-induced weight loss was ameliorated. Lesions of the medial forebrain bundle, which decrease brain levels of norepinephrine and 5-HT, reduced withdrawal-induced weight loss in morphine-dependent rats. Measurements of hypothalamic levels of norepinephrine, 5-HT, and dopamine in rhesus monkeys failed to reveal any differences between normal animals, morphine-dependent animals, and animals undergoing withdrawal (40).

The suggestion, from these data, that at least part of the withdrawal syndrome may be mediated by hypothalamic structures is intriguing. The data of Wei and his associates do not strongly implicate the hypothalamus, but precise localization of central sites of action is difficult with relatively large (40 to 200 μg) amounts of drugs applied in crystalline form, since diffusion of fairly high concentrations from the injection site would be widespread. The medial thalamic area in the rat is less than 2 mm from the medial hypothalamic nuclei, and the studies of Herz and his co-workers (20) have demonstrated that lipid-soluble drugs freely penetrate brain tissue over such a distance. When the injections were made into the hypothalamus (see brain section diagrams in Wei et al., 31), these were placed somewhat lateral and dorsal to the VMH nuclei implicated by Kerr and Pozuelo (28).

In a series of experiments we have investigated the effect of injection of naloxone into the VMH nuclei in morphine-dependent rats. Bilateral guides for intracerebral cannulas were implanted into 21 rats; these guides were positioned so as to allow injection to be made into either the medial thalamus or the VMH nuclei since, according to the rat stereotactic atlas of König and Klippel (41), these structures lie in the same vertical plane. At least 10 days were allowed for postoperative recovery. Thereafter, either naloxone (1 μg in 1 μl 0.9% NaCl) or 0.9% NaCl (1 μl) was injected bilaterally into the VMH nuclei in some animals which were then observed over the following 15 min. The signs listed in Table 1 were recorded and graded as indicated.

TABLE 1. *Signs recorded for 15 min after bilateral intracerebral injection of naloxone or 0.9% NaCl.*

Sign	Severity grading
Piloerection	0 or 1
Wet dog shakes	1–4[a]
Chewing	1–3
Facial tremor	1–3
Grooming	1–3
Defecation	1–3
Licking floor of pan	0 or 1
Excitement	0–4
Loss of balance	0 or 1
Ejaculation	0 or 1

[a] Four was maximum number included.

The most consistent and pronounced effects were wet dog shakes, chewing (on anything presented to the animals), and grooming behavior (that appeared almost "compulsive").

The animals were then made dependent on morphine over the following 5 days by administering the drug twice daily intraperitoneally according to the schedule: 10 mg/kg b.d. first day, 20 mg/kg b.d. second day, 30 mg/kg b.d. third day, 50 mg/kg b.d. fourth and fifth day. On the sixth day morphine (50 mg/kg i.p.) was injected and, 2 hr later, naloxone (1 μg) or 0.9% NaCl (1 μl) was injected bilaterally into the VMH nuclei or (in four animals) into the medial thalamic nuclei. Again the signs were recorded over the ensuing 15 min. The severity of the withdrawal syndromes was assessed by determining the mean total score of the recorded signs in each group of animals. These data are shown in Fig. 2. Both saline (three animals) and naloxone (four animals) elicited some responses in nondependent animals and, although these were not pronounced, a definite wet dog shake was seen in one saline- and one naloxone-injected animal. However, in dependent animals the responses were much more dramatic and both saline and naloxone produced marked withdrawal signs, with mean scores of 6 (11 animals) and 10.5 (16 animals), respectively, following VMH nuclei injections (Fig. 2). Wet dog

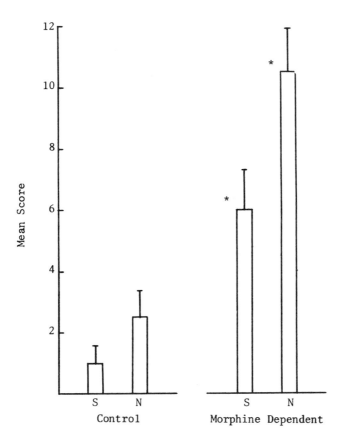

FIG. 2. Mean behavioral scores in groups of rats (for details of scoring system see Table 1 and text) with chronically implanted guides allowing bilateral injections into the ventromedial hypothalamic nuclei. S, 0.9% NaCl (1 μl); N, naloxone (1 μg in 1 μl 0.9% NaCl). Both 0.9% NaCl and naloxone produced signs of withdrawal significantly different (*$p < 0.05$) from those seen in corresponding animals prior to the development of dependence. Vertical bars represent SEM.

shakes were seen in almost all animals, and although 4 was the maximum number recorded, some animals exhibited continuous shaking during the 15-min period. The behavioral scores were significantly different ($p < 0.05$) from those in the corresponding animals prior to the injections of morphine. The mean scores in dependent animals injected with saline or naloxone were only marginally significantly different ($p < 0.10 > 0.05$, df 25). Injection of naloxone (1 μg) into the medial thalamic area in dependent animals had no significant effects (mean score 2.5 in four animals). The accuracy of placement of the injection sites was subsequently confirmed histologically.

These data support the concept that the VMH nuclei are involved in the genesis of some of the signs of the morphine withdrawal syndrome in the rat. The significant degree of withdrawal seen after injection of saline into the VMH nuclei of dependent animals, coupled with the results of Kerr and

Pozuelo (28) in which VMH nuclei lesions suppressed withdrawal, suggests that in some way the VMH are activated by the interaction with naloxone with consequent production of the associated withdrawal behavior. Repeated prior administration of morphine is necessary for the activation to occur, or for the activation to be effective at other sites in the brain, or possibly a combination of these conditions pertains. In some preliminary experiments this hypothesis has been tested by electrical stimulation of the VMH nuclei through bilateral electrodes in rats rendered dependent on morphine by subcutaneous pellet implantation (42). Stimulation on the third day after insertion of the pellets did not cause any signs of withdrawal, nor was the severity of withdrawal induced by systemic naloxone (0.5 to 1.0 mg/kg i.p.) dramatically modified by electrical stimulation. Some animals did exhibit behavioral changes when stimulated during withdrawal, but further experiments, using varied parameters of stimulation and different time courses, are required.

All of these investigations point to involvement of diencephalic structures in the withdrawal phenomena. As in the case of analgesia, hypothalamic structures may merely modify influences from other regions of the central nervous system, possibly by connections with the limbic system. Clearly, further studies are needed to settle these questions.

CONCLUSIONS

There are many studies to indicate that the effects of the narcotic analgesics on neuroendocrine function are mediated directly on hypothalamic structures regulating pituitary activity; these are discussed elsewhere in this volume. Undoubtedly, the thermoregulatory responses to these drugs are also caused by modification of hypothalamic thermoregulatory neurons. In the case of analgesia, dependence, and withdrawal, the role of the hypothalamus as the essential seat of these phenomena is far less certain, but undoubtedly these pharmacologic effects of the drugs are at least partly regulated by hypothalamic structures. It remains to be determined whether such effects result from direct drug–receptor interactions on the neurons and/or from indirect modification of neurotransmitter function.

SUMMARY

The evidence that the hypothalamus is involved in the hypothermic and analgesic effects of the narcotic analgesics is reviewed. In addition it is seen that the major pharmacologic characteristics of these drugs—specific antagonism, tolerance and dependence—can be demonstrated at the cellular level using the rostral hypothalamic thermoregulatory centers as a model neuronal system. Recent data concerning the role of hypothalamic nuclei in the phenomenon of withdrawal are discussed and experimental results obtained in our own laboratories are presented.

REFERENCES

1. Borison, H. L. The nervous system. In: *Narcotic Drugs, Biochemical Pharmacology,* edited by D. H. Clouet, pp. 342–365. Plenum Press, New York, 1971.
2. Lotti, V. J., Lomax, P., and George, R. Temperature responses in the rat following intracerebral microinjection of morphine. *J. Pharmacol.,* 150:135–139, 1965.
3. Lotti, V. J., Lomax, P., and George, R. Acute tolerance to morphine following systemic and intracerebral injection in the rat. *Int. J. Neuropharmacol.,* 5:35–42, 1966.
4. Lotti, V. J., Lomax, P. and George, R. N-allylnormorphine antagonism of the hypothermic effect of morphine in the rat following intracerebral and systemic administration. *J. Pharmacol.,* 150:420–425, 1965.
5. Foster, R. S., Jenden, D. J., and Lomax, P. A comparison of the pharmacologic effects of morphine and N-methyl morphine. *J. Pharmacol.,* 157:185–195, 1967.
6. Banerjee, U., Feldberg, W., and Lotti, V. J. Effect on body temperature of morphine and ergotamine injected into the cerebral ventricles of cats. *Br. J. Pharmac. Chemother.,* 32:523–538, 1968.
7. Haubrich, D. R., and Blake, D. E. Modification of the hypothermic action of morphine after depletion of brain serotonin and catecholamines. *Life Sci.,* 10:175–180, 1971.
8. Oka, T., Nozaki, M., and Hosaya, E. Effects of *p*-chlorophenylalanine and cholinergic antagonists on body temperature changes induced by the administration of morphine to nontolerant and morphine-tolerant rats. *J. Pharmacol.,* 180:136–143, 1972.
9. Somanin, R., Kon, S., and Garattini, S. Abolition of the morphine effect on body temperature in midbrain raphe lesioned rats. *J. Pharm. Pharmac.,* 24:374–377, 1972.
10. Feldberg, W., and Lotti, V. J. Temperature responses to monoamines and an inhibitor of MAO injected into the cerebral ventricles of rats. *Br. J. Pharmac. Chemother.,* 31:152–161, 1967.
11. Lomax, P. Drugs and body temperature. *Intern. Rev. Neurobiol.* 12:1–43, 1970.
12. Lomax, P., and Kirkpatrick, W. E. The effect of N-allylnormorphine on the development of acute tolerance to the analgesic and hypothermic effects of morphine in the rat. *Med. Pharmacol. Exp.,* 16:165–170, 1967.
13. Misra, A. L., Mitchell, C. L., and Woods, L. A. Persistence of morphine in central nervous system of rats after a single injection and its bearing on tolerance. *Nature,* 232:48–50, 1971.
14. Martin, W. R., Wikler, A., Eades, C. G., and Pescor, F. T. Tolerance and physical dependence on morphine in rats. *Psychopharmacologia,* 4:247–260, 1963.
15. Maynert, E. W., and Klinger, B. I. Tolerance to morphine. I. Effects on catecholamines in the brain and adrenal glands. *J. Pharmacol.,* 135:285–299, 1962.
16. Holtzman, S. G., and Villarreal, J. E. Morphine dependence and body temperature in rhesus monkeys. *J. Pharmacol.,* 166:125–133, 1969.
17. Holtzman, S. G., and Villarreal, J. E. Pharmacologic analysis of the hypothermic responses of the morphine-dependent rhesus monkey. *J. Pharmacol.,* 177:317–325, 1971.
18. Roffman, M., Reddy, C., and Lal, H. Control of morphine-withdrawal hypothermia by conditional stimuli. *Psychopharmacologia* 29:197–201, 1973.
19. Tsou, K., and Jang, C. S. Studies on the site of analgesic action of morphine by intracerebral micro-injection. *Scientia Sinica,* 13:1099–1109, 1964.
20. Herz, A., Albus, K., Metys, J., Schubert, P., and Teschemacher, Hj. On the central sites for the antinociceptive action of morphine and fentanyl. *Neuropharmacology,* 9:539–551, 1970.
21. Teschemacher, Hj., Schubert, P., and Herz, A. Autoradiographic studies concern-

ing the supraspinal site of the antinociceptive action of morphine when inhibiting the hindleg flexor reflex in rabbits. *Neuropharmacology,* 12:123–131, 1973.

22. Yanagida, H. and Yamamura, H. The site of action of Innovar in the brain. *Canad. Anaesth. Soc. J.,* 18:552–557, 1971.

23. Jacquet, Y. F., and Lajtha, A. Morphine action at central nervous system sites in rat: Analgesia or hyperalgesia depending on site and dose. *Science,* 183:490–492, 1973.

24. Dubas, T. C., and Parker, J. M. A central component in the analgesic action of sodium salicylate. *Arch. Int. Pharmacodyn. Therap.,* 194:117–122, 1971.

25. Samanin, R., and Bernasconi, S. Effects of intraventricularly injected 6-OH dopamine or midbrain raphe lesions on morphine analgesia in rats. *Psychopharmacologia,* 25:175–182, 1972.

26. Kobayashi, T. Drug administration to cerebral cortex of freely moving dogs. *Science,* 135:1126–1127, 1962.

27. Yaksh, T. L., and Pert, A. Localization in the primate brain of the antinociceptive action of morphine. *Abstracts Soc. Neurosci.,* 3rd Annual Meeting, p. 354, 1973.

28. Kerr, F. W. L., and Pozuelo, J. Suppression of physical dependence and induction of hypersensitivity to morphine by stereotaxic hypothalamic lesions in addicted rats. *Mayo Clin. Proc.,* 46:563–665, 1971.

29. Martin, W. R., Wikler, A., Eades, C. G., and Pescor, F. T. Tolerance to and physical dependence on morphine in rats. *Psychopharmacologia,* 4:247–260, 1963.

30. Wei, E., Loh, H. H., and Way, E. L. Neuroanatomical correlates of morphine dependence. *Science,* 177:616–617, 1972.

31. Wei, E., Loh, H. H., and Way, E. L. Brain sites of precipitated abstinence in morphine-dependent rats. *J. Pharmacol.,* 185:108–115, 1973.

32. Wei, E. Brain lesions attenuating "wet shake" behavior in morphine-abstinent rats. *Life Sci.,* 12:385–392, 1973.

33. Wei, E., Loh, H. H., and Way, E. L. Neuroanatomical correlates of wet shake behavior in the rat. *Life Sci.,* 12:489–496, 1973.

34. Herz, A., Teschemacher, Hj., Albus, K., and Zieglgänsberge, S. Morphine abstinence syndrome in rabbits precipitated by injection of morphine antagonists into the ventricular system and restricted parts of it. *Psychopharmacologia,* 26:219–235, 1972.

35. Eidelberg, E., and Barstow, C. A. Morphine tolerance and dependence induced by intraventricular injection. *Science,* 174:74–76, 1971.

36. Eidelberg, E., and Bond, M. L. Effects of morphine and antagonists on hypothalamic cell activity. *Arch. Int. Pharmacodyn. Therap.,* 196:16–24, 1972.

37. Triplett, J. N., Beeler, G. W., and Kerr, F. W. L. Effects of morphine and antagonists on hypothalamic neurone activity in naive and addicted rats. *Abstracts Soc. Neurosci.,* 3rd Annual Meeting, p. 353, 1973.

38. Adams, W. J., Lorens, S. A., and Mitchell, C. L. Morphine enhances lateral hypothalamic self-stimulation in the rat. *Proc. Soc. Exp. Biol. Med.,* 140:770–771, 1972.

39. Glick, S. D., Marsanico, R. G., Zimmerberg, B., and Charap, A. D. Morphine dependence and self-stimulation: Attenuation of withdrawal-induced weight loss. *Res. Comm. Chem. Pathol. Pharmacol.,* 5:725–732, 1973.

40. Segal, M., Deneau, G. A., and Seevers, M. H. Level and distribution of central nervous system amines in normal and morphine-dependent monkeys. *Neuropharmacology,* 11:211–222, 1972.

41. König, J. F. R., and Klippel, R. A. The rat brain. Williams and Wilkins, Baltimore, 1963.

42. Gibson, R. D., and Tingstad, J. E. Formulation of a morphine implantation pellet suitable for tolerance-physical dependence studies in mice. *J. Pharm. Sci.,* 59:426–427, 1970.

DISCUSSION

Way: The wet-shake response is triggered by many diverse stimuli and is not necessarily the result of implantation of an antagonist in a given brain area. Even blowing on the animal's ear will increase the incidence of the wet-shake response.

Lomax: I agree that there are many inputs which influence this particular withdrawal sign.

Taylor: The interaction of morphine and nalorphine with respect to temperature regulation is demonstrated nicely by your injections into anterior hypothalamus. Have you injected these agents into the thalamus or medial midbrain area and measured the interaction of these agents with respect to analgesia?

Lomax: No, we have not done that, but the studies of Dr. Herz and his co-workers have shown clearly that morphine, given systemically or intra-ventricularly, can act on structures adjacent to the ventricular system to produce analgesia, and this action of morphine is blocked by intraventricular administration of the antagonist. Our studies show that it is necessary to put the antagonist into the anterior hypothalamic preoptic area to get the fall in temperature. I think that the fall in temperature response to naloxone is a relatively simple interaction which is a quite well localized response of anterior hypothalamic thermoregulatory centers.

Kerr: With regard to localization of function in the hypothalamus, your studies on thermal regulation show further that there is compartmentalization of activity in the hypothalamus. However, we cannot be sure that the drug is acting there or on some secondary level of activity in the autonomic nervous system downstream.

Way: What is the serotonin input to the preoptic area, and where do you get the fall in temperature with naloxone? Is 5-HT involved in the mediation of this response?

Lomax: As you know, there is a considerable amount of 5-HT in this part of the hypothalamus, but thermal responses to implantation of 5-HT in this area are rather inconsistent in the rat. Although *p*CPA has been reported to block the hypothermic effect of 5-HT, it is difficult to interpret the results of such experiments since *p*CPA itself has profound effects upon the animal's thermoregulation.

de Wied: To what extent is this area in which you obtain the hypothermic response with naloxone related to the area in which one may elicit TSH secretion with morphine?

Lomax: They do not appear to be related responses since the area in which we obtained TSH release with implantation of morphine is located in the caudal hypothalamus.

Narcotics and the Hypothalamus, edited by
E. Zimmermann and R. George. Raven Press,
New York © 1974

Morphine Effects on Neurons of the Median Eminence and on Other Neurons

Donald H. Ford, Ralph K. Rhines, and Kytja Voeller*

Departments of Anatomy and *Neurology, Downstate Medical Center, 450 Clarkson Avenue,
Brooklyn, New York 11203

Recent concern over the abuse of literally hundreds of drugs has prompted a marked increase in investigations directed toward unraveling the underlying mechanisms which produce tolerance and dependence to a wide spectrum of narcotic and barbiturate drugs. Several aspects of the problems encountered in such investigations and the results obtained have been reviewed (1, 2).

While heroin, the 3,6-diacetyl derivative of morphine, today causes greater social addictive problems than morphine, investigators have generally used morphine in their studies because of the difficulty involved in governmental regulation of heroin. Although this might seem a disadvantage in determining the "how and why" of heroin addiction, it is probably not a real issue since the diacetylation apparently serves only to facilitate passage of morphine through the blood-brain barrier after which it is largely deacetylated, leaving morphine as the effective intraparenchymal agent. Accumulation of morphine within the central nervous system has been established (3–5), although there is no clear evidence that any particular site represents an important center in the tolerance—dependence diad. Pert and Snyder (6) suggest from their studies on the accumulation of ^{3}H-naloxone, a specific antagonist of morphine, that the caudate nucleus may be such a site because of the higher levels of naloxone in this area. This seems unlikely in view of the suggested role of the striatum in the cataleptic response to morphine (7). Thus, morphine-induced cataleptic posturing and the Straub tail response may be associated with such a regional localization.

Other investigators have linked the response to morphine to an alteration in protein synthesis (8–13). However, since cells other than neurons demonstrate similar responses (14), the effects on protein synthesis may be nonspecific and only indirectly related to the tolerance and dependence in that the alterations in protein synthesis may alter other functions of the neurons. This could be associated with the synthesis or degradation of the various catechol- and indoleamine neurotransmitter substances, which also appear to be influenced by morphine treatment (15–20) and which appear to play a role in analgesia and tolerance. However, not all investigators agree that this may be so. Lesion studies (21) suggest that various regions of the diencephalon may have particular relevance in the morphine-addictive pattern. Other observations suggest that the hypothalamus as well as various components of the limbic system would be appropriate sites to look for changes in neurons which could be involved in the development of addiction. Numerous reports on changes in circulating hormones after morphine treatment (review, 22) suggest the possibility of specific effects on hypothalamic neurons, possibly those associated with releasing factors.

These and other considerations led us to undertake an electron microscopic investigation of the central nervous system in morphine-treated animals. Further, since it is generally considered that morphine influences protein metabolism and probably exerts its action on neurons rather than on glia, an attempt was made to determine quantitatively the effect of morphine on amino acid incorporation into neuronal protein compared with what occurs in blocks of neural tissue (cerebral cortex, cerebellar cortex, tuber cinereum, spinal cord gray, and whole dorsal root ganglia).

ELECTRON MICROSCOPIC INVESTIGATION

Five control and seven morphine-treated male Wistar rats were used for this study. All animals were injected with saline or morphine in saline intraperitoneally (23). Thirty min before killing by perfusion with the buffered aldehyde fixative, the animals were injected i.p. with 0.5 ml of heparin to prevent blood clotting. Each animal was then lightly anesthetized with ether and the heart and jugular veins exposed. Perfusion was performed through the heart with a buffered aldehyde (pH 7.4) fixative (24, 25). The jugulars were cut just prior to perfusion to permit blood and perfusate to escape. The rate of perfusion was 30 ml per min for 15 min. The brain was removed after fixation, and small blocks of the median eminence-arcuate region, preoptic area, hippocampus, sensorimotor cortex, and medial reticular nucleus of the medulla were postfixed in 2% osmium tetroxide. Blocks were embedded in an Epon mixture and thin sections were cut and stained with saturated uranyl acetate or lead citrate and examined under a Siemens Elmiskopf 1A electron microscope. Photographic plates were generally taken at a magnification of 20,000, which was enlarged to 60,000 × during printing.

Two of the morphine-treated animals were examined after a 5-day sequence of increasing morphine dosages (30, 50, 70, 90, and 120 mg/kg twice daily except for the last dose which was only given once, 2 hr before killing the animal). Three animals were killed 2 hr after a single 60 mg/kg dose of morphine and two were killed 24 hr after a single 60 mg/kg dose of the drug. [With the Wistar rats obtained from Carworth Farms, a single intravenous 40 mg/kg dose produces anesthesia to the hot plate test (13) in 100% of the animals for over 2 hr plus catatonic posturing, the Straub tail response, and hyperacusia.]

All the morphine-treated animals showed the presence of whorls consisting

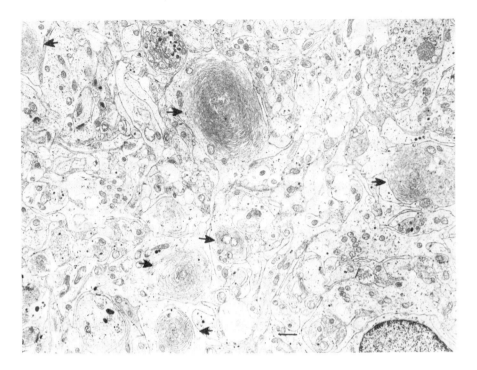

FIG. 1. Low-power (4,300 ✕) micrograph of a field from the median eminence-arcuate region of a rat chronically treated with morphine. The arrows indicate the locations of the numerous whorl structures that appeared in the field. In the micrographs (Figs. 1–4), the line in each figure represents a length of 1 micron, and the following abbreviations have been employed: er = endoplasmic reticulum, m = mitochondria, r = ribosome, S = synapse, V = synaptic vesicle, and WH = whorl. Permission to use Figs. 1–4 has been granted by the editors of *J. Neurobiol.* (see ref. 23).

of membranes (Figs. 1–3) which appeared to be derived from the endoplasmic reticulum (ER), comparable to the whorls described by Brawer in castrate males (26) and by King et al. (27) in females during diestrus. We observed them in the soma and in the processes of neurons. In some instances more than one whorl was present in the neuronal soma. In one of the 5-day treated rats, there were seven such whorls seen in single field at a magnification of 9,000 ✕ (Fig. 1). Of the various regions examined, only the median eminence-arcuate area routinely demonstrated the whorl configuration of smooth ER. A survey of several thousand microscopic fields in the cortex, hippocampus, and medulla revealed no comparable membranous structure. However, one of the 5-day treated rats did show similar configurations in the preoptic area. In all five controls, only one animal had ER whorls and these were much reduced in number.

Changes in other cytoplasmic organelles were sought among the Golgi apparatus and mitochondria and in dense bodies, vessels, and glia, etc., but were not found. This differs from the observations cited by Roizen et al. (28)

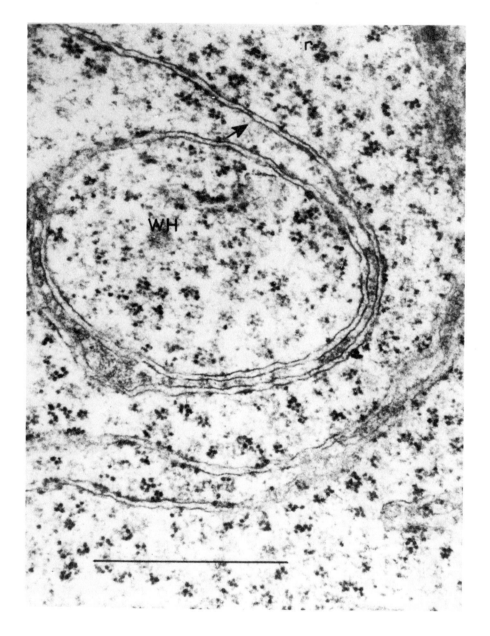

FIG. 2. Micrograph at 38,400 × demonstrating what appears to be a whorl just as it begins to form from the endoplasmic reticulum.

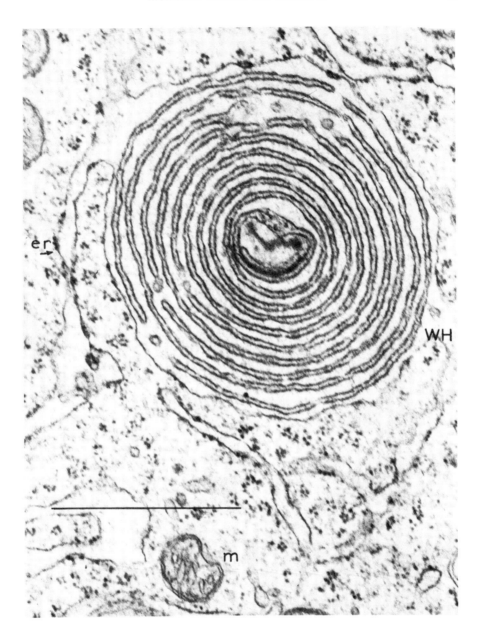

FIG. 3. Micrograph demonstrating a well-formed whorl formed of smooth endoplasmic reticulum which appears to have become invaginated in a cisternal space. 38,400 ×.

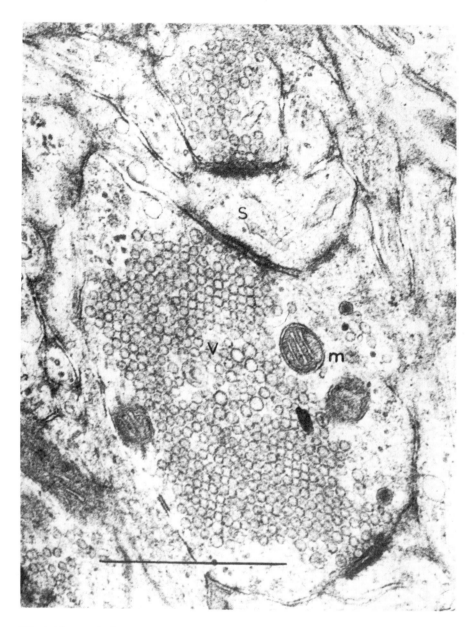

FIG. 4. Micrograph illustrating a synapse containing very densely packed synaptic vesicles which have become compressed into what appears as a crystalline array. 38,400 ×.

in human addicts and in animals subjected to very long exposure to the drug.

In examining the synapses, three general states of organization were noted: a general clustering of vesicles; synaptic endings with an increased number of vesicles, often packed to present an effect of crystalline organization; and increased pleomorphism of the vesicles within a single synapse (Fig. 4). These patterns were observed in both control and experimental animals. It was noted, however, that there was an increase in synapses with pleomorphic vesicles (from 12.62 to 19.18%) and vesicles packed in crystalline arrays (from 4.43 to 11.02%) in the morphine-treated rats. Synapses with vesicles mostly of the same size with regular packing occurred in only 25.67% of the synapses counted in drug-treated rats, compared with 36.86% in controls. The number of dense core vesicles were examined in the two groups and did not differ.

The finding of a particular structural change only in the median eminence-arcuate region suggests a specific site-related relationship, which could be associated with tolerance and/or dependence. However, the response may equally relate to the effect of morphine on pituitary function, and the observed changes in these neurons may reflect only on an action on neurons associated with the production of hypothalamic hormones (releasing or inhibiting factors). Further, it is not yet clear if this is a specific response to morphine or one that may occur with any addictive drug.

EFFECT OF MORPHINE ON ACCUMULATION OF ^{3}H-L-LYSINE INTO NEURONS

In this investigation both the labeled lysine (Schwarz/Mann, Orangeburg, N.Y., specific activity 41.6 C/mM injected in a dose of 3.5 μg/kg, 1.0 mC/kg) and the morphine sulfate (40 mg/kg) were injected via previously implanted indwelling intravenous cannulas (29) in unanesthetized animals. Animals were killed by injecting 0.5 ml of a 50% solution of phenobarbital 2 or 24 hr after morphine and at various time intervals after lysine (15, 30, 45, and 60 min). There were 14 control rats, 12 morphine-treated rats killed 2 hr after the drug, and 14 animals killed 24 hr after the drug was administered. All were males. Blood samples taken when the animals were killed were analyzed to determine the levels of ^{3}H-L-lysine in the whole plasma as well as in the free and bound fractions. Similar determinations were made for the cerebral gray matter in the animals killed 2 hr after morphine. The remainder of the brain and spinal cord was fixed in 10% neutral formalin for the animals killed 2 hr after morphine. For the 24-hr group, only the spinal cord and dorsal root ganglion neurons were examined for amino acid accumulation. Ventral horn motoneurons and dorsal root ganglion, supraoptic, hippocampal, and Purkinje neurons were dissected from the fixed brain (Fig. 5) (30–32) and processed by liquid scintillation counting techniques as previously described (13). Only supraoptic neurons were dissected from the hypothalamus because the others are too small.

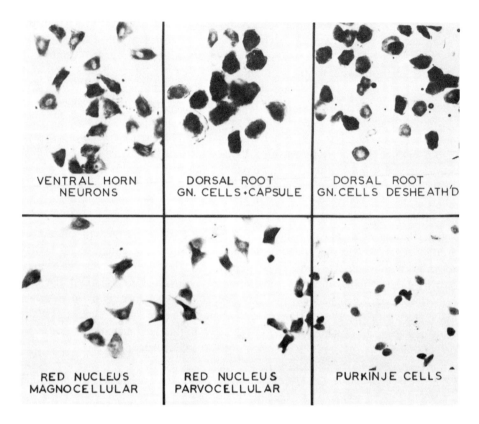

FIG. 5. Neurons of young adult male rats, dissected from formalin-fixed neural tissue after staining with methylene blue (magnification about 250 ×). Hippocampal pyramidal neurons and supraoptic neurons are about the same size as the perikarya of Purkinje cells. The cells from the red nucleus represent other neurons which may be dissected from brain. Cerebral cortical and all motor neurons can also be dissected from formalin-fixed material if desired. Permission to use this figure has been granted by the editor of *J. Neurol. Sci.* (see 9:483–490, 1973).

In animals killed 2 hr after morphine, the distribution of ^{3}H-L-lysine in plasma was significantly elevated in the free amino acid fraction and depressed in the plasma proteins (Fig. 6). A comparable elevation of labeled lysine was noted in the free pool in cerebral cortex (Fig. 7), with an accompanying decrease in the protein fraction (obtained from neurons, glia, and vessels as well as from nerve fibers).

An analysis of the size of the total free lysine pool (Levi and Ford, *unpublished*) showed that it was elevated in the plasma of morphine-treated rats but essentially unchanged in the brain at both the 2- and 24-hr intervals after morphine. Thus, the results on the distribution of labeled lysine in plasma and brain, and on the size of the lysine pool, indicate a real dislocation in the metabolism and distribution of lysine which may apply to other amino acids as well. The decreased accumulation into the plasma proteins

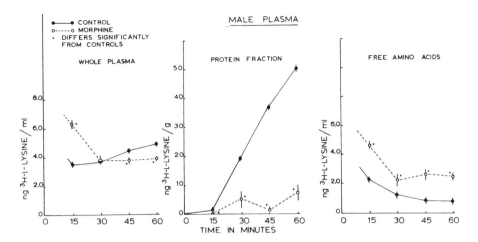

FIG. 6. The levels of plasma ^{3}H-L-lysine in male rats treated with morphine sulfate 2 hr before death. The vertical lines indicate the standard error and the + symbols indicate time intervals where there was a significant difference between the morphine-treated and the control groups in Figs. 6–11. In all figures the time elapsed after injection of the ^{3}H-L-lysine is indicated in the abscissa. The levels of ^{3}H-L-lysine accumulated are indicated by the ordinate. Permission to use Figs. 6 and 7 has been granted by the editors of Acta Neurol. Scand. (see ref. 13).

suggests an interference in liver synthesis of plasma protein that may have an important effect on the availability of plasma protein binding sites for many biologically active compounds. Finally, the changes noted in brain, where the size of the free lysine pool is unchanged while the specific activity is elevated in conjunction with a decreased labeling of brain protein, imply that the synthesis of at least some brain protein is altered. With this information at hand on the incorporation of lysine into some cellular element of brain, an analysis of how the drug specifically influences neuronal accumulation of lysine seemed relevant.

The data obtained from lysine incorporation into neurons (Figs. 8–11) indicate that there is a significant change in amino acid incorporation into neurons (persumably into protein; see 33–36) which varies somewhat between different neuronal types. All neurons accumulated label [in a previous experiment identified as lysine (31)] rapidly during the first 15 min after injection of ^{3}H-L-lysine, attaining concentrations per gram of neuron that are considerably higher than for brain gray matter. This reflects the relatively low levels of radioactive amino acids detectable in neuropil as compared with neuronal perikarya after pulse-injecting a labeled amino acid. In ventral horn motoneurons (Fig. 7), there was a depressed accumulation of lysine at either 2 or 24 hr after morphine treatment. Moreover, the curves for these 2- and 24-hr morphine-treated groups also differ from each other. It would appear, therefore, that turnover of ^{3}H-L-lysine in the neurons from the 24-hr morphine group proceeds at a different rate from that observed in animals

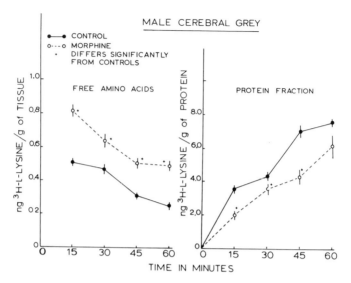

FIG. 7. The levels of ³H-L-lysine in the free and bound amino acid (protein fraction) pools of the cerebral gray matter of male rats treated with morphine sulfate 2 hr before death.

killed 2 hr after morphine or in controls. The depressed lysine accumulation 24 hr after morphine varies from reports by Clouet and co-workers (1, 8–12), who note an increased labeling of protein in *brain* (mixed cell types) 24 hr after morphine. Since the neuropil surrounding the neurons makes up about 90% of the volume of tissue in gray matter (37), the changes described here in neurons, which may reflect increased protein turnover, could well have been obscured by examining whole brain (gray mixed with white).

Cells obtained from the supraoptic nucleus and hippocampus also demonstrated a decreased accumulation of lysine compared with controls (Fig. 9). However, it is also apparent from the appearance of the graphs that controls attain maximal concentration earlier than do the experimental animals, and that this point is followed by a loss (presumably through degradation) which is not occurring in the morphine-treated group during the time intervals covered by the study. This then suggests that turnover is being depressed as well as accumulation. Note that blocks of tissue from the tuber cinereum showed no effect of treatment and that at 45 min after lysine injection, accumulation of lysine in cerebral cortex was actually elevated in the drug-treated group. In both instances the difference in response between neurons and whole tissue is believed to result from the great heterogeneity of tissue elements in gray matter in conjunction with the relatively small volume occupied by neuronal soma.

Purkinje cells (Fig. 10) obtained from cerebellar cortex demonstrate a significant depression in ³H-L-lysine accumulation in morphine-treated animals at all time intervals. Whole blocks of cerebellar cortex showed a mor-

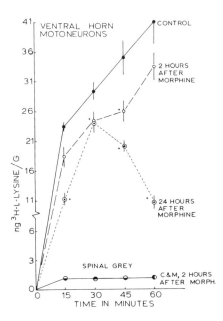

FIG. 8. The levels of ³H-L-lysine accumulated in control (C) and morphine-treated (M) male rats in ventral horn motoneurons and spinal cord gray matter 2 or 24 hr after drug treatment.

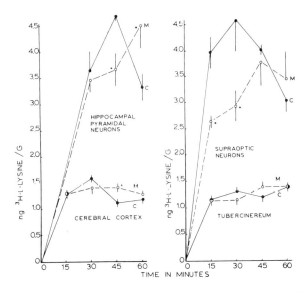

FIG. 9. The levels of ³H-L-lysine accumulated in control (C) and morphine-treated (M) male rats in hippocampal pyramidal and supraoptic neurons cerebral cortex, and tuber cinereum 2 hr after drug treatment.

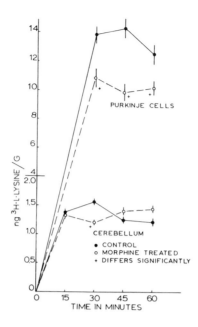

FIG. 10. The levels of ^{3}H-L-lysine accumulated in control (C) and morphine-treated (M) male rats in Purkinje neurons and cerebellar cortex 2 hr after drug treatment.

phine effect at only one time interval. It should be noted that cerebellar cortex is the only region wherein a block of gray matter showed a depressed uptake of lysine after morphine treatment. Cerebral cortex showed a significant elevation at one point. [For additional details on morphine effects in regional lysine uptake see Ford et al. (13).]

Cells obtained from dorsal root ganglia 2 or 24 hr after morphine injection appear much less influenced by drug treatment than central nervous system neurons (Fig. 11), there being only one significant point for each group as compared to controls. Further, the patterns of the accumulation curves imply no marked difference in turnover rates of lysine in the proteins of these neurons. However, since whole ganglia do demonstrate a significant depression of uptake in animals killed 2 hr after morphine and a significant elevation in animals killed 24 hr after morphine, it is apparent that the tissue surrounding the neurons (presumably the satellite cells which encapsulate the neurons) responds differently to morphine than do the neurons.

Thus, the data obtained from neurons dissected from the central and peripheral nervous systems reveal different responses to morphine in relation to whether or not amino acid accumulation is depressed or elevated. Further, the time course of accumulation or loss appears different between experimental and control neurons as well as between different neuronal types. The marked differences in accumulation between different types of neurons and the gener-

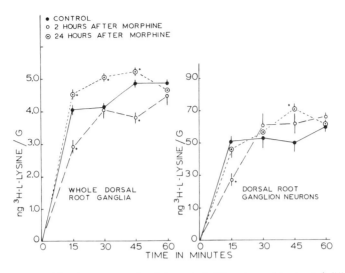

FIG. 11. The levels of ³H-L-lysine accumulated in control (C) and morphine-treated (M) male rats in whole dorsal root ganglia and in the dorsal root ganglion neurons 2 and 24 hr after drug treatment.

ally higher levels of accumulation compared with brain gray matter should also be noted. These data make it apparent that various types of neurons synthesize protein at different rates, and it is conceivable that the proteins are probably not completely comparable between different neuronal types. Furthermore, it seems likely that these changes in lysine accumulation into cortical or neuronal protein are nonspecific in relation to the tolerance–dependence diad, since morphine is known to interfere with protein synthesis in other cell types which subsequently become tolerant to any given dose of morphine (14). However, the morphine effect on neuronal protein synthesis may have indirect effects. These could be related to the roles played by enzymes concerned with transmitter synthesis and degradation and to the maintenance of neuronal membranes. The changes observed in the ultrastructure of arcuate neurons also suggest a change in protein synthesis that could be related to the releasing factors produced by neurons in this area. However, these changes might also reflect some more specific response restricted to cells in this area which could relate to the behavioral effects of morphine.

SUMMARY

This investigation, combining a morphologic with a biochemical approach, provides evidence for morphine having different effects on different types of neurons. The effect on lysine accumulation into neurons of the central nervous system, which are essentially depressive, is probably nonspecific and relates to an overall general interference in metabolic activity. This could, in an indirect way, have some role in the production of tolerance or dependence through its effect on the synthesis of those enzymes involved in synthesis of neurotransmitters, which could then influence the physiologic role of specific neurons. The failure of peripheral neurons to demonstrate a comparable response only serves to indicate further that different neurons have biochemical mechanisms which, although similar, may not be identical.

The electron microscopic study, which focuses on the median eminence-arcuate area, also indicates that different neurons respond differently to any particular alteration in their environment. Thus, only the neurons of the median eminence routinely demonstrated changes in the ER with the production of smooth ER whorls. Only a small percentage of the cells in this area responded (probably less than 5%). Do these then represent neurons associated with the development of dependence, or are they neurons related to production of releasing factors. Further, both lines of investigation indicate that if one wishes to determine the effect of any agent on neurons, one can determine the response only by devising an experimental model that permits observation of what happens in neurons, as distinct from models wherein organelles of one cell type are admixed with another or where a number of cell types are considered together.

ACKNOWLEDGMENTS

The work reported in this study was supported by U.S. Public Health Service grant 5 RO1 DA 0014–03. The authors also wish to express their appreciation to Miss Bruna Callegari for her excellent electron microscopic preparations.

REFERENCES

1. Clouet, D. H., editor. *Narcotic Drugs, Biochemical Pharmacology.* Plenum Press, New York, 1971.
2. Mulé, S. J., and Brill, H., editors. *Chemical and Biological Aspects of Drug Dependence.* C.R.C. Press, Cleveland, Ohio, 1972.
3. Mulé, S. J., and Woods, L. A. Distribution of N-C^{14}-methyl labeled morphine: I. In central nervous system of nontolerant and tolerant dogs. *J. Pharmacol. Exp. Ther.,* 136:232–241, 1962.
4. Miller, J. W., and Elliott, H. W. Rat tissue levels of carbon-14 labeled analgesics as related to pharmacological activity. *J. Pharmacol. Exp. Ther.,* 113:283–291, 1955.
5. Muraki, T. Uptake of morphine-3-glucuronide by choroid plexus *in vitro. Eur. J. Pharmacol.,* 15:393–395, 1971.
6. Pert, C. B., and Snyder, S. H. Opiate receptor: Demonstration in nervous tissue. *Science,* 179:1011–1014, 1973.
7. Kuschinsky, K., and Hornykiewicz, O. Morphine catalepsy in the rat with relation to striatal dopamine metabolism. *Eur. J. Pharmacol.,* 19:119–122, 1972.
8. Clouet, D. H. Effect of morphine on protein and ribonucleic acid metabolism in brain. In: *Drug Abuse: Social and Psychopharmacological Aspects,* edited by J. O.

Cole and K. Wittenborn, pp. 153–163. Charles C Thomas, Springfield, Illinois, 1969.

9. Clouet, D. H. The effect of drugs on protein synthesis in the nervous system. In: *Protein Metabolism of the Nervous System*, edited by A. Lajtha, pp. 699–713. Plenum Press, New York.

10. Clouet, D. Protein and nucleic acid metabolism. In: *Narcotic Drugs, Biochemical Pharmacology*, edited by D. H. Clouet, pp. 216–228. Plenum Press, New York, 1971.

11. Clouet, D. H., and Neidle, A. The effect of morphine on the transport and metabolism of intracisternally injected leucine in the rat. *J. Neurochem.*, 17:1069–1074, 1970.

12. Clouet, D., and Ratner, H. The effect of morphine on the incorporation of ^{14}C-leucine into protein in cell free systems from rat brain and liver. *J. Neurochem.*, 15:17–23, 1968.

13. Ford, D. H., Weisfuse, D., Levi, M., and Rhines, R. K. Accumulation of ^{3}H-L-lysine by brain and plasma in male and female rats treated acutely with morphine sulfate. *Acta Neurol. Scand.*, 50:57–75, 1974.

14. Simon, E. J. Single Cells. In: *Narcotic Drugs, Biochemical Pharmacology*, edited by D. H. Clouet, pp. 310–341. Plenum Press, New York, 1971.

15. Akil, H., and Mayer, D. J. Antagonism of stimulation-produced analgesia by p-CPA, a serotonin synthesis inhibitor. *Brain Res.*, 44:692–697, 1972.

16. Ho, I. K., Lu, S. E., Tolman, S., Loh, H. H., and Way, E. L. Influence of p-chlorophenylalanine on morphine tolerance and physical dependence and regional brain serotonin turnover studies in morphine tolerant-dependent mice. *J. Pharmacol. Exp. Ther.*, 182:155–165, 1972.

17. Knapp, S., and Mandell, A. J. Narcotic drugs: Effect on the serotonin biosynthetic systems of the brain. *Science*, 177:1209–1211, 1972.

18. Shen, F. H., Loh, H., and Way, E. L. Brain serotonin turnover in morphine tolerant-dependent mice. *J. Pharmacol. Exp. Ther.*, 140:149–154, 1970.

19. Large, W. A., and Milton, A. S. The effect of acute and chronic morphine administration on brain acetylcholine levels in the rat. *Br. J. Pharmacol.*, 38:451, 1970.

20. Pozuelo, J., and Kerr, F. W. L. Suppression of craving and other signs of dependence in morphine-addicted monkeys by administration of alpha-methyl-para-tyrosine. *Mayo Clin. Proc.*, 47:621–628, 1972.

21. Kerr, F. W. L., and Pozuelo, J. Suppression of physical dependence and induction of hypersensitivity to morphine by stereotaxic lesions in addicted rats. *Mayo Clin. Proc.*, 46:653–665, 1971.

22. George, R., and Lomax, P. Hormones. In: *Chemical and Biological Aspects of Drug Dependence*, edited by S. J. Mulé and H. Brill, p. 524. C.R.C. Press, Cleveland, Ohio, 1972.

23. Ford, D. H., Voeller, K., Callegari, B., and Gresik, E. Changes in neurons of the median eminence-arcuate region of rats induced by morphine treatment: An electron microscopic study. *J. Neurobiol.*, 4:1–11, 1974.

24. Sotelo, C., and Palay, S. C. The fine structure of the lateral vestibular nucleus in the rat. I. Neurons and neuroglial cells. *J. Cell Biol.*, 36:151–179, 1968.

25. Cohen, E. B., and Pappas, G. D. Dark profiles in the apparently normal central nervous system: A problem in the electron microscopic identification of early antegrade axonal degeneration. *J. Comp. Neurol.*, 136:375–387, 1969.

26. Brawer, J. O. R. The role of the arcuate nucleus in the brain-pituitary gonad axis. *J. Comp. Neurol.*, 143:411–446, 1971.

27. King, J. C., Williams, T. H., and Gekall, A. A. Ultrastructural transformation in rat arcuate neurons during the estrous cycle. *Anat. Rec.*, 175:358, 1973.

28. Roizin, L., Halpern, M., Baden, M. M., Kaufman, M., Hashimoto, S., Liu, J. C., and Eisenberg, B. Neuropathology of drugs of dependence. In: *Chemical and Biochemical Aspects of Drug Dependence*, edited by S. J. Mulé and H. Brill, pp. 390–411. C.R.C. Press, Cleveland, Ohio, 1972.

29. Bleecker, M., Ford, D. H., and Rhines, R. K. A comparison of ^{131}I-triiodothyronine accumulation in ethanol-treated and control rats. *Life Sci.*, 8:267–275, 1969.

30. Ford, D. H., Pascoe, E., and Rhines, R. K. The effect of high pressure oxygen on

the uptake of DL-lysine-H³ by brain and other tissues of rat. *Acta Neurol. Scand.,* 43:129–148, 1967.

31. Ford, D. H., and Rhines, R. K. Accumulation of (^{3}H) lysine in various types of neurons in male rats. *J. Neurol. Sci.,* 10:179–183, 1970.

32. Ford, D. H., and Rhines, R. K. The effect of multiple exposure to high pressure oxygen on the accumulation of (^{3}H) lysine into spinal cord grey matter, retina and various types of neurons. *J. Neurol. Sci.,* 19:483–490, 1973.

33. Benditt, E. P., Martin, G. M., and Platter, H. Application of freeze-drying and formaldehyde-vapor fixation to radiographic localization of soluble amino acids. In: *The Use of Radioautography in Investigating Protein Synthesis,* edited by C. P. Leblond, pp. 65–75. Academic Press, New York, 1965.

34. Bergman, M., and Droz, B. Analyse critique des conditions de fixation et de preparation des tissues pour la detection radioautographique des proteines neo-formes en microscopic electronique. *J. Micros.,* 7:51–62, 1968.

35. Droz, B., and Warshawsky, H. Reliability of the radioautographic technique for the detection of newly synthesized proteins. *J. Histochem. Cytochem.,* 11:426–435, 1963.

36. Peters, T., and Ashley, C. An artefact on radioautography due to binding of free amino acids to tissue by fixation. *J. Cell Biol.,* 33:53–60, 1967.

37. Ford, D. H. Selected changes in the developing rat brain. In: *Development and Aging in the Nervous System,* edited by M. Rockstein and M. S. Sussman, pp. 63–88. Academic Press, New York, 1973.

DISCUSSION

Way: Have you compared the cells of the substantia nigra and the caudate nucleus?

Ford: The cells of the substantia nigra are large enough for us to dissect. However, those of the caudate nucleus are quite small. We are working with a new technique involving ultrasonic breakdown of tissue block, hoping to get these very small caudate cells out so we can study them. We have succeeded in dissecting cells of the red nucleus, the deep nuclei of the cerebellum, and the lateral vestibular nucleus. Almost any motor nucleus can be dissected because the cells in it are quite large, the only problem being that the number of cells available in any given nucleus may be quite small.

Mirsky: Have you tried to use enzymatic dispersion of brain cells?

Ford: Yes. We have tried a variety of techniques described by others and, in general, find that most of them work well for isolating glial cells, but the nerve cell preparations have not been particularly successful.

Goldstein: Isn't it possible that in studies such as yours, lysine could be taken up into the brain cells without necessarily being incorporated into brain protein?

Ford: Yes, this is possible. However, our measurements reflect only the accumulation uptake of labeled amino acid which remains in tissue after prolonged fixation has leached out most of the free amino acids present.

Narcotics and the Hypothalamus, edited by
E. Zimmermann and R. George. Raven Press,
New York © 1974

Theoretical Problems in Localizing Drug Actions and Origins of Withdrawal Syndromes in the Central Nervous System: The Glass-Eye Booby Trap

Abraham Wikler

Departments of Psychiatry and Pharmacology, University of Kentucky Medical Center, Lexington, Kentucky 40506

Long ago, as a resident in psychiatry at the U.S. Public Health Service Hospital in Lexington, Kentucky, I was responsible for the management of drug withdrawal in patients physically dependent upon opioids (usually morphine or heroin). On arriving on the ward one morning, I found a newly admitted patient who complained of "kicking a bad habit". Examination disclosed typical signs of the primary opioid abstinence syndrome including mydriasis which, however, was confined to one eye; the diameter of the other eye was much smaller. Extraocular movements of both eyes were quite normal but the smaller pupil did not react to light or in accommodation, and application of the ophthalmoscope soon confirmed my suspicion that that eye was a prosthesis.

This observation is rather trivial but it does raise an important question. How do we know that if a sign (or group of signs) of opioid action or opioid withdrawal disappears following placement of a lesion in the *central* nervous system, that the site of the lesion *is* the site of drug action or origin of the drug withdrawal signs in question? The lesion, per se, may have impaired the physiologic function at a locus "distal" to that on which opioids or opioid withdrawal exert their effects. Or, to take another case, suppose that the lesion, per se, altered the physiologic function in the same direction as that produced by morphine or morphine withdrawal in the nonlesioned subject. How can we conclude that the locus of the lesion *is not* a site of drug action or origin of a drug withdrawal sign?

To illustrate one method for beginning to answer these questions, allow me to cite some data from our study, "Limbic System and Opioid Addiction in the Rat" (1). In this study, we were concerned with the effects of lesions placed bilaterally in the cingulum bundle, dorsomedial thalamic nucleus, anterior temporal lobe, or the septum, upon selected, quantifiable morphine withdrawal signs and "relapse tendencies" in the rat. The lesions were placed stereotactically 17 to 19 days before drug treatments were started, and the measurements of the "primary" (24 hr) morphine abstinence syndrome were made 70 to 84 days after initiation of drug treatments. The data, therefore, deal with the effects of "chronic" rather than "acute" lesions; this issue will be discussed later.

Our measurements of the primary morphine abstinence syndrome included the following: (a) No-choice drinking of etonitazene, 5 μg/ml, without prior water deprivation (etonitazene is a benzimidazole derivative with morphine-like properties, but is about 1,000 times as potent as morphine for analgesia in the rat); rats in primary morphine abstinence drink significantly *greater* volumes of etonitazene, 5 μg/ml, than normal rats. (b) No-choice drinking of water without prior water deprivation; rats in primary morphine abstinence drink significantly *less* water than normal rats. (c) The difference between the consumption of etonitazene, 5 μg/ml, and water. (d) "Wet-dog" shake frequency A (the number of wet-dog shakes during the first 15 min after transfer of the rat from home cage to large glass observation jars) and wet-dog shake frequency B (the number of wet-dog shakes 50 min after transfer); rats in primary morphine abstinence show significantly *higher* wet-dog A shake frequencies and higher (sometimes not significant) wet-dog B shake frequencies than control rats. (e) Colonic temperature (telethermometer inserted 4 cm into the colon and retained there for at least 2 min); rats in primary morphine abstinence shows significantly *lower* colonic temperatures than control rats. The drinking tests were conducted from 8:00 P.M. (12 hr after the last injection of morphine or saline) to 8:00 A.M. (24-hr morphine abstinence), whereas the measurements of wet-dog shake frequencies and of colonic temperature were made at 24-hr morphine abstinence.

The experimental design was based on concomitant observation of four groups of rats: lesioned, morphine-abstinent · (LM); lesioned, saline-"abstinent" (LS); nonlesioned morphine-abstinent (NLM); and nonlesioned saline-"abstinent" (NLS). Because the same concurrent control groups (LS and NLS) were used for two of the studies (on the effects of lesions in the cingulum and dorsomedial thalamic nucleus), a standard analysis of variance could not be applied to the data. Instead, we applied an unweighted means analysis, computing for each study on the effects of a given limbic lesion the "grand effect," the "lesion effect," the "morphine withdrawal effect," and "interaction" from the four cell-block means obtained for each measure. The relationships between the cell-block means and these effects are given by the following equations:

$$\overline{LM} = \text{grand} + \text{lesion} + \text{morphine withdrawal} + \text{interaction}$$
$$\overline{NLM} = \text{grand} - \text{lesion} + \text{morphine withdrawal} - \text{interaction}$$
$$\overline{LS} = \text{grand} + \text{lesion} - \text{morphine withdrawal} - \text{interaction}$$
$$\overline{NLS} = \text{grand} - \text{lesion} - \text{morphine withdrawal} + \text{interaction}$$

For example, let us take no-choice drinking of etonitazene, 5 μg/ml, in the case of the cingulum bundle lesions. The four group means (in ml) are given in the square:

	L	NL
M	70.9	59.8
S	31.2	37.5

Adding all four means and dividing by four yields the grand effect, 49.9. Subtracting NL from L for M and for S, adding these differences and dividing by four yields the "lesion effect," 1.2. Subtracting S from M for L and NL, adding these differences and dividing by four yields the morphine withdrawal effect, 15.5. Computing interactions by the equations given above for LM, NLM, LS, and NLS separately and averaging them yields an interaction of 4.35 for the cingulum bundle lesion data. Because the N's of the four groups were unequal, the standard error estimate was computed by adding the squares of the separate standard errors of each of the four groups, taking the square root of the sum, and dividing this by four. This computation yielded a standard error value of 2.72 for the cingulum bundle lesion study. The number of degrees of freedom utilized for estimating levels of significance from Student's t distribution was computed by use of a modified form of the Satterthwaite approximation (2), viz:

$$\text{E.D.F.} = \frac{\left(\sum_{i=1}^{4} a_i\right)^2}{\sum_{i=1}^{4} a_i^2 \Big/ \left(n_i - 1\right)}$$

where a_i = squared standard error of the average of group i; and n_i = the number of subjects in group i. For the cingulum bundle lesion study, this equation yielded 14 degrees of freedom. From Student's t distribution, the lesion effect is nonsignificant, whereas the morphine withdrawal effect is significant ($t = 15.5/2.72 = 5.698$) at a level of $p < 0.001$. From this we may conclude that cingulum bundle lesions did not alter this particular morphine withdrawal sign, namely, increased drinking of etonitazene, 5 μg/ml.

Inspection of Table 1 reveals that none of the limbic system lesions unequivocally altered any of the morphine abstinence signs measured except the anterior temporal lobe lesion, which abolished the increase in wet-dog shake frequency B (both morphine withdrawal and lesion effects are nonsignificant). However, the lesions in the dorsomedial nucleus produced significantly positive morphine withdrawal *and* lesion effects on wet-dog shake frequency B, and this lesion, as well as the anterior temporal lobe lesion, produced significantly negative morphine withdrawal *and* lesion effects on no-choice

TABLE 1. Primary (24 hr) morphine abstinence syndrome

Measures (signs)	Lesion site[1] (bilateral)	Effects of conditions				Standard error	Degrees of freedom (est.)
		grand	lesion	morphine withdrawal	inter-action		
No-choice intake of	C	49.9	1.20	15.5[f]	4.35	2.72	14
etonitazene,	DTN	45.5	−3.20	8.15[e]	−3.00	2.29	22
5 µg/ml[2] (increase)	ATL	34.9	−3.13	5.72[a]	1.68	2.59	27
	S	46.5	0.15	9.25[b]	−4.80	3.38	28
No-choice intake of	C	22.6	−0.28	−9.22[f]	−2.17	1.36	18
water (decrease)	DTN	20.1	−2.78[a]	−7.52[f]	−0.47	1.31	17
	ATL	18.5	−3.00[d]	−7.55[f]	−0.70	0.91	35
	S	26.2	−0.03	−17.8[f]	−2.58	1.72	30
Difference, etonita-	C	27.3[f]	1.47	24.7[f]	6.52[a]	2.99	18
zene-water	DTN	20.1[f]	−0.43	15.7[f]	−2.53	2.57	26
(increase)	ATL	18.5[f]	−0.13	13.3[f]	2.37	2.59	27
	S	26.2[f]	0.27	27.0[f]	−2.22	3.52	35
Wet-dog shake	C	3.55	−0.30	3.05[e]	−0.20	0.69	10
frequency A[3]	DTN	5.07	1.22	4.42[d]	1.17	1.00	8
(increase)	ATL	4.25	0.40	2.85[f]	0.30	0.52	28
	S	2.22	−0.23	1.82[f]	−0.42	0.34	34
Wet-dog shake	C	0.67	−0.13	0.67[d]	−0.13	0.19	17
frequency B[4]	DTN	1.55	0.75[a]	1.55[f]	0.75[a]	0.29	10
(increase)	ATL	1.30	−0.30	0.70	0.30	0.17	19
Colonic temperature[5]	C	37.8	−0.03	−0.38[f]	−0.03	0.06	25
(decrease)	DTN	37.8	−0.08	−0.47[f]	−0.13	0.07	27
	ATL	37.8	−0.02	−0.27[f]	−0.02	0.04	39
	S	37.8	−0.07	−0.53[f]	−0.03	0.06	33

[1] C, cingulum; DTN, dorsomedial thalamic nucleus; ATL, anterior temporal lobe; S, septum.

[2] 12-hr period, 12–24 hr morphine-abstinent.

[3] 0–15 min after transfer to observation jar, 24-hr morphine-abstinent.

[4] 50–65 min after transfer to observation jar, 24-hr morphine-abstinent.

[5] Immediately after completion of measurement of wet-dog shake frequency B.

Significance levels (2-tailed): [a] = 0.05; [b] = 0.02; [c] = 0.01; [d] = 0.005; [e] = 0.002; [f] = 0.001. For "grand" effects, significance levels are of interest only with reference to the measure "Difference, etonitazene-water"; hence, significance levels for grand effects are not displayed elsewhere in Tables 1 and 2.

Reprinted with permission from Wikler, A., Norrell, H., and Miller, D., Exp. Neurol., 34:543–557, 1972.

intake of water; hence, we cannot be sure that these lesions did not attenuate these particular morphine abstinence signs.

"Relapse" tests were made by conducting "choice" 12-hr (8:00 P.M.– 8:00 A.M.) drinking tests (etonitazene, 5 µg/ml, versus water) on the ninth postwithdrawal day and at intervals of 2 to 5 weeks thereafter. Interpretation of these data is more difficult because of the arbitrariness of the definition of relapse and because of the complications introduced by the "secondary" (or "protracted") abstinence syndrome, one feature of which is increased consumption of water. We have used a rather rigorous definition of relapse, namely, significantly greater intakes of etonitazene by post-addict rats compared with previously saline-injected rats, provided that the intake of water by the two groups is not significantly different. Accordingly, a determinate result is said to have been obtained on any given choice drinking test if the "previous-dependence effect" is both positive in sign and significant with respect to intake of etonitazene, $5\mu g/ml$, but not both positive and significant with respect to water intake. Given a determinate effect, inspection of the lesion effects reveals whether it was the LM or NLM group or both that relapsed. LM is said to have relapsed to a degree equal to NLM if the lesion effects on both etonitazene and water intake are nonsignificant, and to a degree greater than NLM if the lesion effect is significantly positive with respect to water intake. On the other hand, LM is said not to have relapsed, or to have relapsed to a lesser degree than NLM if the lesion effect is significantly negative with respect to etonitazene intake but not significantly negative with respect to water intake.

Inspection of Table 2 reveals only one significant lesion effect, namely, decreased water intake on the first relapse test (9 days postwithdrawal) in the dorsomedial thalamic nucleus study. However, this finding is irrelevant, inasmuch as the previous-dependence effect was indeterminate (both etonitazene and water intake are significantly positive). Such an indeterminate result is also seen for the first relapse test in the cingulum bundle lesion study, in both cases probably due to the increased water intake associated with the secondary morphine abstinence syndrome. Similarly, the criteria for a determinate result are not met in the second relapse test for the cingulum bundle group because the previous-dependence effect on etonitazene intake, although larger than that on water intake, is not statistically significant. The results obtained on the third relapse test in the cingulum bundle group, the second and third on the dorsomedial thalamic nucleus group, and all three relapse tests in anterior temporal lobe and septum lesion groups were determinate, and the absence of significant lesion effects indicates that LM and NLM relapsed to comparable degrees.

It has already been noted that these studies were conducted on animals with *chronic* lesions in the limbic system (roughly 100 days after making the lesions), and Tables 1 and 2 show that few significant lesion effects were observed, at least insofar as the functions measured are concerned. This raises the question of whether or not "restitution" of these functions had occurred after an initial disruption of them, and whether or not the practically unchanged morphine withdrawal effects might have been altered if the lesions had been "acute" ones. It seems to me that in the case of *either* the acute *or* chronic lesion, one may conclude that the lesioned area was necessary for the morphine withdrawal to occur if, and only if, the following criteria are met: (a) the lesion produces no change in physiologic "base line" and the pertinent morphine withdrawal sign fails to occur, or (b) the lesion does produce a change in base line, the pertinent morphine withdrawal sign fails

TABLE 2. *Relapse tests (choice intake of etonitazene or water) after permanent withdrawal of morphine*

Lesion site[1] (bilateral)	Test no.	Days with-drawal	Fluid[2]	Grand	Lesion	Previous depend-ence	Inter-action	Standard error	Degrees of freedom (est.)
C	I	9	E	21.5	3.88	7.32[b]	−0.82	2.46	13
			W	38.5	−2.85	8.90[c]	−0.10	2.97	28
	II	37	E	15.8	4.45	7.80	4.35	3.57	9
			W	27.0	−1.05	2.80	−0.35	3.90	13
	III	72	E	13.4	1.30	4.75[a]	2.60	2.23	23
			W	31.7	0.20	2.75	−2.30	2.79	27
DTN	I	9	E	18.3	0.67	8.72[f]	0.57	1.81	26
			W	35.4	−5.95[a]	6.45[a]	−2.55	2.88	22
	II	37	E	12.8	1.47	5.77[d]	2.32	1.74	18
			W	28.2	0.15	−0.45	−3.60	3.41	18
	III	72	E	14.7	2.67	5.42[g]	3.27	2.59	18
			W	27.2	−4.30	1.05	−4.00	2.52	28
ATL	I	9	E	17.6	−0.30	9.35[f]	−1.65	2.00	29
			W	27.3	−5.18	1.53	0.97	2.63	28
	II	30	E	16.8	−2.35	7.10[d]	−4.00	2.12	30
			W	29.6	0.67	1.58	1.42	2.18	33
	III	44	E	15.0	0.90	6.90[d]	−1.10	2.05	28
			W	30.7	−2.17	1.17	−0.27	2.18	26
S	I	9	E	21.7	3.05	6.00[a]	−4.40	2.84	38
			W	30.0	−0.20	4.50	1.10	3.05	37
	II	23	E	19.2	0.50	6.30[b]	−1.30	2.53	45
			W	31.9	−3.23	0.08	−0.83	2.72	44
	III	51	E	17.2	1.95	7.20[d]	−1.20	2.35	32
			W	32.4	−2.77	−4.98	−1.42	2.89	34

[1] C, cingulum; DTN, dorsomedial thalamic nucleus; ATL, anterior temporal lobe; S, septum.
[2] Choice intake of etonitazene (E), 5 μg/ml, or water (W).
Significance levels (2-tailed): [a] $= 0.05$; [b] $= 0.02$; [c] $= 0.01$; [d] $= 0.005$; [e] $= 0.002$; [f] $= 0.001$.
Reprinted with permission from Wikler, A., Norrell, H., and Miller, D., *Exp. Neurol.,* 34:543–557, 1972.

to occur, *and* the morphine withdrawal sign does occur in an intact animal whose physiologic base line had been altered in the same direction as in the lesioned animal, by means other than making the lesion. In the case of an animal in which a lesion produces a temporary change in base line and in which the morphine withdrawal sign fails to occur, but, after the passage of time, the physiologic base line returns to normal (i.e., it is restituted) and then the morphine withdrawal sign does occur, either of the following conclusions may be drawn: (a) the initial effect (absence of a morphine withdrawal sign) was due to artifact (edema or hemorrhage, diaschisis or sudden removal of tonic neurochemical influences on other areas involved in the manifestation of the function), or (b) the area lesioned *may* have been necessary for the morphine withdrawal sign to occur, but other areas, normally not critically involved in the expression of that function, "took over" that function after a lapse of time and were sites of origin of the morphine withdrawal sign in question. At present, I see no operational way of distinguishing between these two possibilities and I can therefore conclude that acute or chronic lesions are useful in localizing drug actions or drug withdrawal signs only if the previously mentioned criteria are met.

In our experiments, bilateral *chronic* lesions in the cingulum bundle, the dorsomedial thalamic nucleus, the anterior temporal lobe, or the septum failed, by and large, to alter the specific morphine abstinence phenomena measured or to attenuate relapse tendencies. If the lesions had been acute, and if they had *not* altered the physiologic base lines against which the morphine withdrawal effects are measured, then it could be assumed that no restitution would have occurred with further lapse of time and that the morphine withdrawal phenomena and relapse tendencies observed in the animals with chronic lesions would have occurred also after acute lesions. On the other hand, if the lesions had been acute ones which *altered* the physiologic base lines, and if the morphine withdrawal phenomena and relapse tendencies had failed to occur in such animals, then the results would have been ambiguous—knowing that after further lapse of time the physiologic base line returned to normal and both the morphine withdrawal phenomena and relapse tendencies then did occur, we would not be able to decide whether the absence of the latter in the animal with acute lesions was due to artifact or was indicative of a "locus of origin" of the withdrawal phenomena and relapse tendencies.

From these considerations, it appears that our data do not prove that the lesioned areas are not sites of action of morphine or sites of origin of morphine withdrawal phenomena; to prove this, it would have been necessary to show that acute lesions did not alter the physiologic base lines against which the morphine withdrawal phenomena are measured, and that such acute lesions did not alter the withdrawal signs measured. Our purpose in studying the effects of chronic lesions was a practical one, namely, to determine if such lesions would *permanently* attenuate the specific signs of opioid withdrawal and relapse tendencies. Obviously, our conclusions were in the negative.

This discussion has some bearing on our concepts of how the nervous system is organized, to the extent that such concepts are based on the effects of lesions. It appears that we have two such concepts, one based on acute effects, and another on chronic effects of lesions. In general, those based on acute effects are at best ambiguous, whereas those based on chronic effects are subject to the reservations already made. There is no "pure" neurophysiology, and the "impurities" in it are due mainly to the vagaries of the concepts of diaschisis and restitution.

Many of the difficulties in interpreting the effects of lesions on opioid actions can be avoided by the technique of introducing narcotic antagonists into restricted portions of the central nervous system in animals previously treated with opioids. Herz (3) and his collaborators injected nalorphine or levallorphan into restricted portions of the ventricular system (e.g., third and lateral ventricles, fourth ventricle, or cisterna cerebellomedullaris) in rabbits previously treated with one or more doses of morphine parenterally. They found that injection of the narcotic antagonist into the fourth ventricle, but not more rostrally or caudally, antagonized an analgetic effect of parenterally-administered morphine (a licking reaction elicited by electrical stimulation of the tooth pulp) and evoked morphine withdrawal phenomena, namely, a characteristic motor excitation and, with higher doses, convulsive symptoms (4) said to be similar to those evoked by narcotic antagonists given systemically in morphine-dependent rabbits. They conclude that structures located very probably in the medullary and pontine parts of the brain are important sites of action of morphine and for the origin of morphine withdrawal phenomena (3, 4).

However, Wei et al. (5) found that features of the naloxone-precipitated abstinence syndrome, notably leaping from the observation jar and wet-dog shakes but also, though less prominently, teeth chattering, swallowing movements, ptosis, ear blanching, and diarrhea, could be elicited by microinjection of 0.04 to 0.2 mg of naloxone into the medial regions of the thalamus (region surrounding the nucleus parafascicularis) and the rostral portions of the midbrain, but not into the neocortex, dorsal hippocampus, and medial mesencephalic and hypothalamic regions in rats 70 to 76 hr after morphine pellet implantations.

The findings of Herz and his collaborators and of Wei et al. indicate that the medial thalamus, the rostral part of the mesencephalon, and the floor of the fourth ventricle are *among* the sites of action of morphine, antagonism of which releases *certain* of the morphine withdrawal phenomena, namely, those measured. The loci of origin of the morphine withdrawal phenomena observed are not established by these techniques. Furthermore, a distinction must be made between acute and chronic physical dependence on morphine. As Martin and Eades (6) and Martin (7) have demonstrated, chronic spinal dogs made "acutely" morphine-dependent by a 7-hr infusion of morphine, 3 mg/kg/hr, show withdrawal phenomena after nalorphine, 20 mg/kg s.c., both above the level of spinal cord transection (lacrimation, rhinorrhea, salivation, tremors, mydriasis, increased heart rate, elevated body temperature) and below this level (mild hyperactivity of the flexor and crossed exterior reflexes, depression of the exterior thrust, and occasional running movements). In chronic spinal dogs made "chronically" morphine-dependent (subcutaneous doses of morphine increasing to 10 mg/kg twice daily over periods of 43 to 120 days), nalorphine, 20 mg/kg s.c., precipitated all of the withdrawal phenomena mentioned, but those below the level of spinal cord transection are very much enhanced, running movements occur almost always, and the entire abstinence syndrome is more prolonged than in the acutely morphine-dependent chronic spinal dog (Table 3). It may be re-

TABLE 3. *A summary and comparison of the actions and interactions of morphine and nalorphine in the nondependent, acutely dependent, and chronically dependent chronic spinal dog*

Effects of treatment	Morphine	Nalorphine	Nalorphine followed by morphine	Morphine infusion followed by nalorphine	Nalorphine in the chronically dependent dog
Lacrimation	+[1]		+	+	+
Rhinorrhea	+		+	+	+
Salivation	+		+	+	+
Urination				+	+
Tremors				+	+
Emesis	+		+	Occ	Occ
Restlessness	+ → −	−	+	+	+
Pupillary diameter	↓	↓		↑	↑
Heart rate	↓		↑	↑	↑
Body temperature	↓		↓	↑	↑
Respiratory rate	↑ → ↓		↑		↑
Flexor reflex	↓	↓		↑	↑ ↑
Crossed extensor reflex	↓	↓		↑	↑ ↑
Ipsilateral extensor thrust	↑	↓		↓	↓
Running movements	Occ		Occ early	Occ	almost always
No. signs similar to precipitated abstinence in chronically dependent dog	7	1	8	14	15

[1] +, the sign is commonly produced by the treatment; −, the sign is decreased by the treatment condition; ↑, the level of function is increased by the treatment condition; ↓, the level of function is decreased by the treatment condition; Occ, occasionally.

Reprinted with permission from W. R. Martin Chapt. XVI (p. 216) in: *The Addictive States*, edited by A. Wikler, *Res. Publ. Assn. Nerv. Ment. Dis.*, Vol. 46, Williams and Wilkins, Baltimore, 1968.

marked that the findings of Martin and Eades (6) on the nalorphine-precipitated abstinence syndrome in the chronically morphine-dependent chronic spinal dog are very similar to the morphine withdrawal syndrome both in the chronically morphine-dependent chronic spinal dog (8) and in a chronically morphine-dependent chronic spinal man (9) except for time course, i.e., the morphine withdrawal syndromes are more drawn out.

The demonstration of morphine effects and of morphine withdrawal phenomena in the hindlimbs of chronic spinal dog and man demonstrates that the spinal cord, at least after restitution, is a site of morphine action and a locus of origin of morphine abstinence signs. Whether or not this would be true in the absence of restitution is impossible to determine because transection of the spinal cord in dogs and higher mammals produces a profound degree of "spinal shock," recovery from which takes days or weeks. Nor does this demonstration prove that the central nervous system above the level of transection plays no role in the modification of the actions of morphine or of morphine withdrawal on spinal reflexes. Indeed, Houde and Wikler (10) have shown that the effects of morphine on the skin twitch in the dog are due to depression of this reflex at the spinal segmental level, coupled with augmentation of supraspinal inhibition. However, the differences in acutely and chronically morphine-dependent chronic spinal dogs with regard to the nalorphine-precipitated abstinence syndrome shown by Martin and Eades (6) illustrate limitations on conclusions that may be drawn regarding sites of origin of morphine withdrawal phenomena from studies, such as those of Wei et al. (5), on "acutely" morphine-dependent animals.

According to Martin and Eades (6), withdrawal phenomena precipitated by nalorphine in acutely morphine-dependent subjects represent the responses of resensitized and *normalized* homeostatic systems to an abnormal internal environment that developed as a consequence of the depressant effects of morphine. In contrast, the withdrawal phenomena precipitated by nalorphine in chronically morphine-dependent subjects represent the activities of *hyperexcitable* homeostatic systems in a less abnormal internal environment, when the depressant effects of morphine have been antagonized. Furthermore, Martin (11) has proposed that the hyperexcitability of such homeostatic systems can be ascribed to hypertrophy of circuits that are pharmacologically "redundant" under normal conditions, but which "take over" the functions that are depressed or inhibited by morphine when this drug is administered chronically. Hence, while intracerebral microinjection of narcotic antagonists may assist in localizing the sites of action of morphine, it cannot establish the loci of origin of morphine withdrawal phenomena, which differ in the acutely and chronically morphine-dependent organism. These must still be investigated by other means, including the lesion technique, subject to all the provisos discussed.

SUMMARY

Signs of drug action or drug withdrawal may be altered or abolished by lesions which impair the function measured at a site "distal" to the actual site of drug action or locus of origin of a drug withdrawal sign. To prove that the lesion is at the site of drug action or locus of the withdrawal sign, it is necessary to demonstrate (a) that the lesion did not alter the function measured, while the drug phenomenon was altered, or (b), that the lesion altered the function measured, the drug phenomenon was altered, and the drug phenomenon remains unchanged in normal animals in which the function measured is altered by means other than a lesion in the same direction as that observed in animals with the lesion. If an "acute" lesion alters the function measured and "restitution" occurs after a lapse of time, then demonstration of the unaltered drug phenomenon in the restituted animal does not, per se, prove that the lesioned area was not a site of drug action or locus of origin of the drug withdrawal sign; however, in such cases, interpretation of the effects of "acute" lesions is ambiguous because of local edema, hemorrhage, or diaschisis. In part, these problems may be resolved by comparing four subject groups: lesioned, drug-treated; lesioned, non–drug-treated; nonlesioned, drug-treated; nonlesioned, non–drug-treated. Illustrations are presented from a previous study of the limbic system and opioid addiction in the rat. Introduction of narcotic antagonists into restricted areas of the brain in animals pretreated with narcotic agonists may assist in localizing sites of morphine action, but they cannot determine loci of origin of morphine withdrawal signs. Furthermore, such loci of origin may differ in acutely and chronically morphine-dependent subjects, as illustrated by consideration of the results of studies on chronic spinal dogs in the literature.

REFERENCES

1. Wikler, A., Norrell, H., and Miller, D. Limbic system and opioid addiction in the rat. *Exp. Neurol.,* 34:543–557, 1972.
2. Anderson, R. L., and Bancroft, T. A. *Statistical Theory in Research.* New York, McGraw-Hill, 1952, p. 83.
3. Herz, A. Central nervous sites of action of morphine in dependent and nondependent rabbits. In: *Fifth International Congress on Pharmacology, San Francisco, 23–28 July 1972,* Abstracts of Invited Presentations, pp. 148–149.
4. Herz, A., Teschemacher, Hj., Albus, K., and Zieglgänsberger, S. Caudal brain stem structures mediating the precipitated morphine abstinence syndrome. In: *Twenty-fifth Congress of Physiology, Munich, 1971,* Abstract No. 725.
5. Wei, E., Loh, H. H., and Way, E. L. Neuroanatomical correlates of morphine dependence. *Science,* 177:616–617, 1972.
6. Martin, W. R., and Eades, C. G. A comparison between acute and chronic physical dependence in the chronic spinal dog. *J. Pharmacol. Exp. Ther.,* 146:385–394, 1964.
7. Martin, W. R. A homeostatic and redundancy theory of tolerance to and dependence on narcotic analgesics. In: *The Addictive States,* edited by A. Wikler, Vol. 46, pp. 206–225. Williams and Wilkins, Baltimore, 1968.
8. Wikler, A., Frank, K. Hindlimb reflexes of chronic spinal dogs during addiction to morphine and methadone. *J. Pharmacol. Exp. Ther.,* 94:382–400, 1948.
9. Wikler, A., and Rayport, M. Lower limb reflexes of a chronic "spinal" man in cycles of morphine and methadone addiction. *Arch. Neurol. Psychiat.,* 71:160–170, 1954.
10. Houde, R. W., and Wikler, A. Delineation of the skin-twitch response in dogs and the effects thereon of morphine, thiopental and mephenesin. *J. Pharmacol. Exp. Ther.,* 103:236–242, 1951.
11. Martin, W. R. Pharmacological redundancy as an adaptive mechanism in the central nervous system. *Fed. Proc.,* 29:13–18, 1970.

DISCUSSION

Way: I don't think there is any question that morphine acts throughout the central nervous system and that manifestations of withdrawal can be traced to diverse areas. However, there are sites which are more sensitive than others to certain effects of the drug, and localized injection technique can help identify these more sensitive areas.

Kerr: The points that Dr. Wikler brings up are enormously challenging and extremely frustrating when trying to localize sites of action in the central nervous system. There is no question that morphine affects both the central nervous system and the peripheral nervous system. It is extremely difficult to respond to such a well-thought out paper. The effects of morphine, however, are different when you have long-term administration in contrast to short-term injection of the drug. And the withdrawal syndrome is different in each case. There are constellations of withdrawal signs which are quite likely integrated at various levels within the nervous system. If we can agree that these signs reflect the function of integrated central circuitry and that it is possible to interrupt this circuitry with localized lesions, then we can learn something about the central organization of these withdrawal responses with appropriately placed lesions and in that way study the localization of the specific signs in question. It is another question to wonder how and at what level these signs are generated. I think we can learn a great deal about the central organization without having to identify the prime mover in each case.

Wikler: It is true, however, that if a lesion destroys an effector system then one can draw no conclusions regarding the central organization of the particular sign in question.

Goldstein: I think that when we talk about the site of morphine action on the one hand, and the origin of a withdrawal sign on the other, we may be talking about two different things. The theories for morphine tolerance and dependence that have been advanced in the past may be grouped into two categories. The first is in the tradition of Himmelsbach and of Seevers and Tatum, which holds that the signs of withdrawal of opiates are attributable to systems which are different from those involved in the primary action of the drug. These systems serve to counterbalance or counteract the disturbance created in those systems which respond to the primary action of the drug. On the other hand, the theories advanced by Schuster and by Goldstein and by Collier maintain that systems responding to the primary action of the drug are the same systems which are responsible for tolerance and physical dependence. It should be possible with proper experiments to distinguish between these two types or categories of explanations or theories of tolerance and physical dependence. The second class of theories would necessarily maintain that naloxone implantation, as proposed by Dr. Way, would precipitate withdrawal when implanted into the location at which the site of dependence on the drug is located.

Narcotics and the Hypothalamus, edited by
E. Zimmermann and R. George. Raven Press,
New York © 1974

Effects of Drugs of Abuse on Motivated Behavior and Magnocellular Neuroendocrine Cells

James N. Hayward

Departments of Neurology and Anatomy, Reed Neurological Research Center and Brain Research Institute, UCLA School of Medicine, Los Angeles, California 90024

INTRODUCTION

Drugs of abuse exert profound effects on motivated behavior and on the neuroendocrine system. In some species morphine induces sedation and sleep while in others excitement ensues. The antidiuretic response to morphine is thought to be due, at least in part, to a release of vasopressin from the neurohypophysis. Whether this morphine-induced activation of supraoptic neurons is due to a direct stimulatory action on these magnocellular neuro-endocrine cells, or is mediated indirectly by an alteration in the "behavioral" state, by a change in "osmometric" or "volumetric" thresholds, or by some other mechanism, is not known at the present time. In this essay I shall comment on the pertinent factors relating morphine to motivated behavior and to vasopressin release.

MAGNOCELLULAR NEUROENDOCRINE CELLS

The magnocellular neuroendocrine cells of the hypothalamic supraoptic and paraventricular nuclei in mammals are often presented as a uniform population of simplified neurons with abbreviated dendrites, a cytoplasmic biochemical apparatus for synthesizing and packaging neurohypophysial hormones and carrier proteins into 1,500 Å neurosecretory granules. Each neuron is said to furnish a single, unmyelinated axon along which these neuro-secretory packets are transported for storage and/or release of both hormones and carrier proteins by some unknown release mechanism involving the depolarization of the nerve endings in conjunction with an action of calcium and the process of "exocytosis" (1, 2). Recent evidence suggests that synaptic input on dendritic, somatic, and axonal membranes of these neurosecretory neurons may involve not only cholinergic and noradrenergic (3) but also histaminergic transmitters (4). Furthermore, the presence of mast cells in the posterior pituitary gland at the junction between the magnocellular neuro-endocrine nerve terminals and the capillaries (5), and the presence of high levels of histamine in the posterior pituitary gland (4) suggest a possible "glandular" role for histamine in vasopressin release. The histaminergic link between morphine and vasopressin release is determined by the fact that morphine is known to be a selective releaser of histamine from isolated rat mast cells (6) and by the fact that in morphine-treated man (7) and monkeys the intense itching seen can be attributed to histamine release. In favor of a central site of action of morphine on histaminergic vasopressin release are the ability of morphine to pass slowly across the blood-brain barrier (8) and its ability to release vasopressin when injected directly into the supraoptic nuclei. Direct injections of histamine into the third ventricles (9) or into the supraoptic nuclei (10) produce the vasopressin type of antidiuretic responses. In favor of a peripheral (posterior pituitary) histaminergic release of vasopressin by morphine is the evidence of Blackmore and Cherry (11) who, infusing small doses (2.5 μg/kg/min) of histamine, did not produce renal hemodynamic changes but did obtain vasopressin type of antidiuretic responses.

To determine the possible histaminergic or other mechanisms of morphine-induced stimulation of vasopressin release it is important to know if there are specialized types of magnocellular neuroendocrine cells. Recent evidence suggests that the magnocellular neuroendocrine cells are not a uniform and homogeneous population of neurons, but rather are a heterogeneous group of cells with quite different morphologic, functional, and chemical characteristics (1, 12–17). I find three morphologic types of Procion yellow-filled magnocellular neuroendocrine cells in the preoptic nucleus of the goldfish. *Cell Type I* is a large (37 μm), multipolar neuron, 48 μm from the ependyma, with fine "dendrites" projecting into the lateral hypothalamus and within the preoptic nucleus, with multiple branched "axons" (12). *Cell Type II* is a large (31 μm), multipolar neuron, 24 μm from the ependyma, with a coarse "dendrite" to the ependyma and fine dendrites within the preoptic nucleus, and with limited "axonal" branching. *Cell Type III* is a small (18 μm), multipolar neuron, 46 μm from the ependyma, with fine dendritic processes distributed within the preoptic nucleus and with limited axonal branching. In the unanesthetized monkey we find three functional magnocellular neuroendocrine types in the supraoptic nucleus and the internuclear zone: silent, continuously active, and burster neurons (13). These three cell types are randomly distributed in the supraoptic nucleus and the internuclear zone, with each type receiving specific input connections. All three functional cell types are osmosensitive to intracarotid hypertonic sodium chloride (14) and hypertonic D-glucose (16) and can be driven by nociceptive stimuli, the firing patterns modified by the state of motivated behavior (15, 18).

CENTRAL SITES AND MECHANISMS OF ACTION OF MORPHINE

Limbic-Midbrain Areas

Morphine crosses the blood-brain barrier slowly (8) and is probably selectively bound by a proteolipid or other type of receptor (19, 20), at least one of which has its highest concentration in the anterior amygdala, followed by periaqueductal area of midbrain, medial thalamus, hypothalamus, and head of caudate. In our own studies of vasopressin release by electrical stimulation of the brain we found the amygdala, periaqueductal area of midbrain, hypothalamus, and other limbic-midbrain sites effective releasers of vasopressin (21, 22). Deneau and Takori (see Domino, 23) demonstrated in the monkey that morphine (3 to 9 mg/kg s.c.) elevated the electrical threshold for amygdala-induced chewing and licking, but not the threshold for hippocampal afterdischarge or electroencephalographic and behavioral arousal to reticular formation stimulation.

Hypothalamus

Morphine injected systemically and directly into the hypothalamus produces antidiuretic hormone release and hypothermia, the latter probably by action on the thermoregulatory centers located within the anterior hypothalamus and as a result of a reduction in metabolic heat production (24). Eidelberg and Bond (25) found that morphine depressed the firing patterns of units in the anterior hypothalamus of naive, urethane-anesthetized rats. In morphine-dependent rats, morphine produced an accelerated bursting pattern in these hypothalamic neurons. We found that preoptic cooling in the unanesthetized monkey inhibited vasopressin release, produced behavioral arousal, and elevated the arterial blood pressure (26).

Brainstem

Morphine, by its action on the brainstem, depresses the response of the respiratory center to carbon dioxide, produces a reduction of arterial blood pressure, and depresses baroreceptor reflexes in the regulation of blood volume (27). Vasopressin release may occur in response both to a reduction in blood volume and to hypoxic stress (28, 29). Morphine specifically stimulates the chemoreceptor trigger zone in the area postrema of the medulla oblongata to initiate a specific behavioral effect, namely vomiting (27). Emesis induced by apomorphine, copper sulfate (30), or laboratory-induced motion sickness (31) was consistently accompanied by an inhibition of water diuresis of the vasopressin type.

Nociceptive Pathways

Microinjections of morphine into the posterior hypothalamus (10 μg) resulted in significant analgesia, whereas the same dose injected into the medial septum, the caudate, or the periaqueductal gray matter yielded hyperalgesia (32). Nociceptive and emotional stimuli can release vasopressin (15, 33). Mills and Wang (34) found that morphine blocked the release of antidiuretic hormone by electrical stimulation in the medulla or of the ulnar nerve, whereas the release brought about by central vagal stimulation was unaffected. They concluded, therefore, that morphine inhibits vasopressin secretion in two ways: (a) by inhibiting responses to nociceptive stimulation, and (b) by an action at a site rostral to the midbrain.

MORPHINE, MOTIVATED BEHAVIOR, AND VASOPRESSIN RELEASE

Fujimoto (35) carefully reviewed most of the available literature on the antidiuretic effect of morphine in animals and man. Many of these studies are contradictory, depending on the species and dosage employed, route of administration, presence or absence of anesthetic agents, and the development of tolerance. Studies showing convincing vasopressin release by morphine were performed in the dog (36, 37, 38) and rat (39), but studies in man

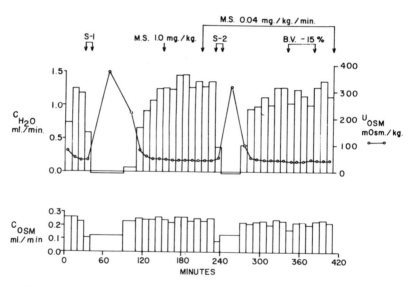

FIG. 1. Effects of electrical stimulation of the amygdala, of infusion of morphine sulfate, and of reduction of blood volume on motivated behavior and antidiuretic hormone release in the monkey. During a sustained water diuresis (left to right), electrical stimulation of the amygdala (S-1, 400 μA, 30 Hz, 1 mA, 30 sec on-off, 10 min) produces arousal, looking upward, turning of the head, and apnea followed by 100 min of antidiuretic response with a rise of urine osmolality to 375 mosmol/kg. Next, a rapid infusion of a second dose (initial dose 1 mg/kg 5 hr earlier) of morphine sulfate (1 mg/kg) causes mild sedation (increase of slow-wave sleep from 5 to 20% during subsequent 10 min) without change in renal parameters. During a constant infusion of morphine sulfate (0.04 mg/kg/min, 200 min, total dose 8 mg/kg) there are no changes in renal parameters but there is a progressive sedation (increase of slow-wave sleep from 15 to 50% at end). Amygdala stimulation S-2 (same parameters as S-1) during morphine infusion produces a 50-min period of antidiuresis with urine concentration to 325 mosmol/kg with essentially the same behavioral effects. Removal of 15% blood volume for 40 min and replacement did not change renal or behavioral parameters. *Abbreviations:* C_{H_2O}, free water clearance; C_{osm}, osmolal clearance; U_{osm}, urine osmolality; S, electrical stimulation of the amygdala; M.S., morphine sulfate; B.V., blood volume.

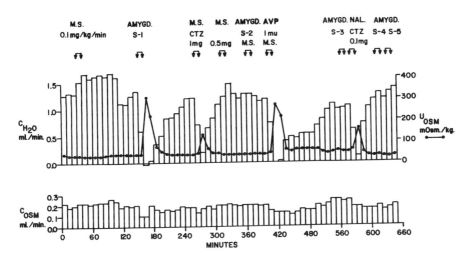

FIG. 2. Excitatory and inhibitory effects of morphine and nalorphine on motivated behavior, limbic system thresholds, and vasopressin release in the monkey. During a sustained water diuresis (left to right), an initial infusion of morphine sulfate (0.1 mg/kg/min, 10 min, total dose 1 mg/kg) produces mild tranquility, hypothermia, and a water diuresis followed by a rebound return to control levels of water excretion, shivering, restlessness, and intense scratching of the hairy skin. Amydala stimulation S-1 (300 μA, 30 Hz, 1 mA, 30 sec on-off, 10 min) produces arousal, looking upward, turning the head, and apnea as well as a 50-min period of antidiuresis with rise in urine osmolality to 300 mosmol/kg. A high rate of morphine infusion (1 mg/kg/min, 10 min, total dose 10 mg/kg) produces retching, salivation, vomiting (chemoreceptor trigger zone) with sustained arousal during and immediately after infusion, and antidiuretic response with over 50% reduction in free water clearance and urinary concentration to 132 mosmol/kg. Shivering alternating with slow-wave sleep ensues in the subsequent periods. Infusion of morphine at intermediate rates (0.5 mg/kg/min, 10 min, total dose 5 mg/kg) produces increased slow-wave sleep (control 30 to 60% during infusion), a transient water diuresis, and supression of shivering with hypothermia. Amygdala stimulation S-2 (same parameters as S-1) during intermediate morphine infusion (0.5 mg/kg/min) produces arousal, looking upward, and apnea but no antidiuretic response. The renal tubules are still responsive to vasopressin infusion (1 mU/kg/min) during intermediate morphine treatment (0.5 mg/kg/min). After a total dose of 26 mg/kg of morphine, slow-wave sleep increases from 40 to 80%, shivering is supressed, and hypothermia increases. Amygdala stimulation S-3 (same parameters as S-1) produces arousal and apnea but no change in water excretion. Infusion of nalorphine HCl (0.1 mg/kg/min, 10 min, 1 mg/kg) produces transient arousal, retching, salivation, vomiting (chemoreceptor trigger zone), and an antidiuretic response with rise in urine osmolality to 158 mosmol/kg. Amygdala stimulations S-4 (same parameters as S-1) and S-5 (400 μA, 30 Hz, 1 mA, 30 sec on-off, 10 min) produce brief arousal and apnea but no change in water excretion. Abbreviations: AVP, arginine vasopressin; NAL, nalorphine, CTZ, chemoreceptor trigger zone; otherwise the same as in Fig. 1.

show either a primary change in renal hemodynamics (40, 41) or a diuretic effect (35).

I have examined some of the possible mechanisms involved in the excitatory and inhibitory effects (Figs. 1 and 2) of morphine and nalorphine on motivated behavior, limbic system and "volumetric" thresholds, and vasopressin release in the chronically prepared adult female rhesus monkey. Animal preparation consisted of implanted bipolar, concentric stainless steel stimulating and recording electrodes in the amygdala, hypothalamus, and mid-brain reticular formation; biparietal and bifrontal silver-silver chloride cortical electroencephalographic electrodes; stainless steel periorbital wires for re-cording extraocular movements; and two silicon-rubber cannulas implanted into the right atrium for remote drug and fluid infusion and blood withdrawal according to previously published methods (21, 22, 26). During study the animal was isolated in an environmental chamber with one-way glass and TV monitor, in a primate restraining chair, with a Foley catheter in the blad-der for 10-min urine collections and with continuous recordings of electro-encephalogram, electromyogram, body movements, and electrical activity of multiple deep brain sites (21, 22, 26). Water diuresis was induced by a con-tinuous infusion of intraatrial-infused, sterile pyrogen-free solution of 5% D-glucose and water by means of a Harvard constant infusion pump. Total solute concentration (osmols/kg plasma or urine) was determined cryoscop-ically with a Fiske osmometer, thus allowing calculation of osmolal (C_{osm}) and free water clearance (C_{H_2O}) (21, 22, 26).

Inhibitory Effects of Morphine

In the chronically prepared, unanesthetized, naive monkey undergoing a water diuresis, intravenous administration of low doses (1 mg/kg) of mor-phine sulfate either as single injections or as infusions over a 10-minute period (0.1 mg/kg/min) produces a mild tranquilizing effect, an associated enhanced water diuresis (see Fig. 2), and hypothermia. These "inhibitory" effects may last between 30 and 90 min and are gradually replaced by rest-lessness, shivering, intense scratching of all areas of the hairy skin, and a return of water diuresis to control levels. It is presumed that these sedative effects and hypothermia may be due to hypothalamic (24, 32) or possibly amygdaloid effects (20). The enhanced water diuresis is reminiscent of a similar enhanced urine flow produced by low doses of morphine sulfate in the dog (38) and man (35).

In a non-naive monkey previously treated (1 to 5 hr) with a low dose (1 mg/kg) of morphine, a subsequent infusion (0.04 to 0.5 mg/kg/min) may have very little effect on water diuresis despite producing a recurrence of the behavioral sequence of tranquility, sedation, enhanced slow-wave sleep, and hypothermia, followed by shivering, restlessness, and intense scratching. Progressively larger doses of morphine sulfate tend to lessen the behavioral effects of amygdala stimulation such as arousal, looking upward, turning, facial movements, licking, vocalization, and apnea. In the doses studied, mor-phine never completely abolishes the behavioral concomitants of amygdala stimulation. Low doses of morphine (3 to 5 mg/kg) produce minimal change in the amygdala-induced antidiuretic response (see Fig. 1); high doses of morphine (greater than 10 mg/kg) completely block the antidiuretic effects of amygdala stimulation despite the persistence of some of the behavioral effects including arousal, looking upward, and apnea (see Fig. 2). Since one of the postulated mechanisms of amygdala-induced vasopressin release was based on hypoxia secondary to apnea (42), the persistence of apnea but without vasopressin release perhaps indicates that the effects of morphine on the respiratory center are somehow involved (7, 27). Lack of antidiuresis from amygdala stimulation is not due to any change in renal responsiveness to arginine vasopressin, because infusion of this pituitary hormone yields a dramatic antidiuretic response (see Fig. 2). The marked reduction in osmolal clearance during arginine vasopressin-induced antidiuresis suggests a sensitization of sodium retention or renal vasculature by morphine.

The behavioral effects of increasing doses of morphine in the monkey are increasing periods of sedation as represented by a type of slow-wave sleep with high-voltage, slow waves from which the monkey can be aroused. At accumulated morphine doses of 5 to 10 mg/kg the sleep time runs between 20 and 50%; at accumulated doses of 10 to 30 mg/kg it runs between 50 and 100% (see legends for Figs. 1 and 2).

Under low doses of morphine—3 to 5 mg/kg—a 15% reduction in blood volume that would produce a 15 to 25% reduction in water diuresis in the unanesthetized monkey fails to make any significant change in free water clearance. Up to the present time the effects of morphine on osmometric thresholds of vasopressin release have not been studied.

Excitatory Effects of Morphine and Nalorphine

Following intravenously administered low doses of morphine (1 mg/kg), the inhibitory effects (mild sedation, hypothermia, diuresis) yield in 30 to 90 min to an excitatory phase (restlessness, shivering, intense scratching of the hairy skin, and return to control level of water excretion) (Fig. 2). One might speculate whether the restlessness, shivering, and intense itching are due to excitation of posterior hypothalamus, periaqueductal gray or midline thalamus (20, 24, 32), or to the peripheral release of histamine (6, 7).

Rapid infusion of morphine and nalorphine in high cumulative doses may trigger an antidiuretic response which is associated with arousal, salivation, retching, and vomiting. The mechanism of vasopressin release is undoubtedly connected to the opiate stimulation of the area postrema chemoreceptor trigger zone and the initiation of emesis (27). What medullary-hypothalamic pathways and neurotransmitters convey this emetic drive from the medulla to the magnocellular neuroendocrine cells is not well understood.

SUMMARY

Drugs of abuse exert profound effects on motivated behavior and on the regulation of the release of vasopressin from the magnocellular neuroendocrine cells. These neurosecretory neurons are of three morphologic and functional types and are under the control of osmometric, volumetric, and motivated behavioral neural mechanisms. The amygdala may be an important site not only for regulation of vasopressin release but also for mediation of the excitatory and inhibitory actions of morphine on motivated behavior and vasopressin release. In the monkey the inhibitory effects of morphine include sedation, hypothermia, mild water diuresis, elevation of electrical threshold for amygdala-induced release of vasopressin, and elevation of volumetric threshold for vasopressin release. The excitatory effects of morphine include rebound restlessness, shivering, intense scratching, emesis, and an antidiuretic response. Nalorphine induces emesis and an antidiuretic response.

ACKNOWLEDGMENTS

The work was supported in part by grants from N.I.N.D.S. (NS-05638 and NS-10129) and the Ford Foundation. I thank Mrs. Rubye Lawrence and Mr. Michael Sofronieu for valuable technical assistance. Preparation of this article was supported in part by Research Grant DA 00044 from the National Institute of Drug Abuse with funds from the Special Action Office for Drug Abuse Prevention.

REFERENCES

1. Hayward, J. N. Neurohumoral regulation of neuroendocrine cells in the hypothalamus. In: *Recent Studies of Hypothalamic Function,* edited by K. Lederis and K. E. Cooper. S. Karger, Basel, 1974 (*in press*).
2. Dreifuss, J. J. Mécanismes de sécrétion des hormones neurohypophysiaires. Aspects cellularies et sub-cellularies. *J. Physiol. (Paris),* 67:5A–52A, 1973.
3. Shute, C. C. D., and Lewis, P. R. Cholinergic and monaminergic pathways in the hypothalamus. *Brit. Med. Bull.,* 22:221–226, 1966.
4. Snyder, S. H., and Taylor, K. M. Histamine in the brain: A neurotransmitter? In: *Perspectives in Neuropharmacology,* edited by S. H. Snyder, pp. 43–73. Oxford University Press, New York, 1972.
5. Bodian, D. Cytological aspects of neurosecretion in opossum neurohypophysis. *Bull. Johns Hopkins Hosp.* 113:57–93, 1963.
6. Ellis, H. V., Johnson, A. R., and Moran, N. C. Selective release of histamine from rat mast cells by several drugs. *J. Pharm. Exp. Therap.,* 175:627–631, 1970.
7. Jaffe, J. H. Narcotic analgesics. In: *The Pharmacological Basis of Therapeutics,* edited by L. S. Goodman and A. Gilman, pp. 237–275. MacMillan, New York, 1970.
8. Oldendorf, W. H., Hyman, S., Braun, L., and Oldendorf, S. Z. Blood-brain barrier: Penetration of morphine, codeine, heroin and methadone after carotid injection. *Science,* 178:984–986, 1972.
9. Bhargava, K. P., Kulshrestha, V. K., Santhakumri, G., and Srivastava, Y. P. Mechanism of histamine induced antidiuretic response. *Brit. J. Pharmacol.,* 47:700–706, 1973.
10. Bennett, C. T., Pert, A., Gall, K., and Blair, J. Histaminergic release of vasopressin. *Fed. Proc.,* 32:221, 1973.
11. Blackmore, W. P., and Cherry, G. R. Antidiuretic action of histamine in the dog. *Amer. J. Physiol.,* 180:596–598, 1955.
12. Hayward, J. N. Physiological and morphological identification of hypothalamic magnocellular neuroendocrine cells in goldfish preoptic nucleus. *J. Physiol. (Lond.),* 239:103–134, 1974.
13. Hayward, J. N., and Jennings, D. P. Activity of magnocellular neuroendocrine cells in the hypothalamus of unanesthetized monkeys. I. Functional cell types and their

anatomical distribution in the supraoptic nucleus and the internuclear zone. *J. Physiol. (Lond.)*, 232:515–543, 1973.

14. Hayward, J. N., and Jennings, D. P. Activity of magnocellular neuroendocrine cells in the hypothalamus of unanesthetized monkeys. II. Osmosensitivity of functional cell types in the supraoptic nucleus and the internuclear zone. *J. Physiol. (Lond.)*, 232:545–572, 1973.
15. Hayward, J. N., and Jennings, D. P. Influence of sleep-waking and nociceptor-induced behavior on the activity of supraoptic neurons in the hypothalamus of the monkey. *Brain Research* 57:461–466, 1973.
16. Hayward, J. N., and Jennings, D. P. Osmosensitivity of hypothalamic magnocellular neuroendocrine cells to intracarotid hypertonic D-glucose in the waking monkey. *Brain Res.*, 57:467–472, 1973.
17. Zimmerman, E. A., Hzu, K. C., Robinson, A. G., Carmel, P. W., Frantz, A. G., and Tannenbaum, M. Studies of neurophysin secreting neurons with immunoperoxidase techniques employing antibody to bovine neurophysin I. Light microscopic findings in monkey and bovine tissues. *Endocrinology*, 92:931–940, 1973.
18. Hayward, J. N., and Murgas, K. Sensory input and firing patterns of antidromically identified supraoptic neurons in unanesthetized monkey. *Program and Abstracts of 3rd Meeting of Society for Neuroscience*, 3:120, 1973.
19. Lowney, L. I., Schulz, K., Lowery, P. J., and Goldstein, A. Partial purification of an opiate receptor from mouse brain. *Science*, 183:749–752, 1974.
20. Kuhar, M. J., Pert, C. B., and Snyder, S. H. Regional distribution of opiate receptor binding in monkey and human brain. *Nature*, 245:447–450, 1973.
21. Hayward, J. N., and Smith, W. K. Influence of limbic system on neurohypophysis. *Arch. Neurol.*, 9:171-177, 1963.
22. Hayward, J. N., and Smith, W. K. Antidiuretic response to electrical stimulation in brain stem of the monkey. *Amer. J. Physiol.*, 206:15–20, 1964.
23. Domino, E. F. Sites of action of some central nervous system depressants. *Ann. Rev. Pharmacol.*, 2:215–250, 1962.
24. Lotti, V. J. Body temperature responses to morphine. In: *Pharmacology of Thermoregulation*, edited by E. Schonbaum and P. Lomax, pp. 382–394. S. Karger, Basel, 1973.
25. Eidelberg, E., and Bond, M. L. Effects of morphine and antagonists on hypothalamic cell activity. *Arch. Internat. Pharmacodynam. Therap.*, 196:16–24, 1972.
26. Hayward, J. N., and Baker, M. A. Diuretic and thermoregulatory responses during preoptic cooling in the monkey. *Amer. J. Physiol.*, 214:843–850, 1968.
27. Borison, H. L. The nervous system. In: *Narcotic Drugs: Biochemical Pharmacology*, edited by D. H. Clouet, pp. 366–393. Plenum Press, New York, 1971.
28. Cross, B. A., and Silver, I. A. Electrophysiological studies on the hypothalamus. *Brit. Med. Bull.*, 22:254–260, 1966.
29. Share, L. Extracellular fluid volume and vasopressin secretion. In: *Frontiers in Neuroendocrinology*, edited by W. F. Ganong and L. Martini, pp. 183–210. Oxford University Press, New York, 1969.
30. Andersson, B., and Larson, S. Inhibitory effects of emesis on water diuresis in the dog. *Acta Physiol. Scand.*, 32:19–27, 1954.
31. Taylor, N. B. G., Hunter, J., and Johnson, W. H. Antidiuresis as a measurement of laboratory induced motion sickness. *Canad. J. Biochem.*, 35:1017–1027, 1957.
32. Jacquet, Y. F., and Lajtha, A. Morphine action at central nervous system sites in rat: Analgesia or hyperalgesia depending on site and dose. *Science*, 182:490–492, 1973.
33. Verney, E. B. The antidiuretic hormone and the factors which determine its release. *Proc. Roy. Soc. B*, 135:25–106, 1947.
34. Mills, E., and Wang, S. C. Liberation of antidiuretic hormone: Pharmacologic blockade of ascending pathways. *Amer. J. Physiol.*, 207:1405–1410, 1964.
35. Fujimoto, J. M. The kidney. In: *Narcotic Drugs: Biochemical Pharmacology*, edited by D. H. Clouet, pp. 366–393. Plenum Press, New York, 1971.
36. DeBodo, R. C. The antidiuretic action of morphine and its mechanism. *J. Pharmacol. Exp. Therap.*, 82:74–85, 1944.
37. Duke, H. N., Pickford, M., and Watt, J. A. The antidiuretic action of morphine:

Its site and mode of action in the hypothalamus of the dog. *Quart. J. Exp. Physiol.,* 36:149–158, 1951.

38. Handley, C. A., and Keller, A. D. Changes in renal function produced by morphine in normal dogs and dogs with diabetes insipidus. *J. Pharmacol. Exp. Therap.,* 99: 33–37, 1950.
39. George, R., and Way, E. L. The role of the hypothalamus in pituitary-adrenal activation and antidiuresis by morphine. *J. Pharmacol. Exp. Therap.,* 125:111–115, 1959.
40. Papper, S., and Papper, E. M. The effects of preanesthetic, anesthetic and post-operative drugs on renal function. *Clin. Pharmacol. Ther.,* 5:205–215, 1964.
41. Habif, D. V., Papper, E. M., Fitzpatrick, H. F., Lowrance, P., Smythe, C. McC., and Bradley, S. E. The renal and hepatic blood flow, glomerular filtration rate and urinary output of electrolytes during cyclopropane, ether, and thiopental anesthesia, operation, and the immediate postoperative period. *Surgery,* 30:241–255, 1951.
42. Hayward, J. N. The amygdaloid nuclear complex and mechanisms of release of vasopressin from the neurohypophysis. In: *Neurobiology of the Amygdala,* edited by B. E. Eleftheriou, pp. 685–749. Plenum Press, New York, 1972.

DISCUSSION

Kerr: Do you have any information on the effects of morphine on the renal tubule?

Hayward: Based on changes in osmolal clearance studies following administration of vasopressin in morphinized animals, it would appear that morphine may sensitize the renal tubule to either a vasoconstrictor or a sodium-retaining effect of vasopressin. This makes interpretation of our results very difficult since we may get the same results with inulin clearance studies. To resolve this matter, we need radioimmunoassay data on vasopressin levels in morphine-treated animals.

Kerr: I asked this question because we have seen in two of our monkeys a marked polydipsia and high urine output. When these animals received morphine, both drinking behavior and urine output dropped considerably. This suggests that morphine has a depressant action on fluid intake. The level at which this effect is exerted, be it cortical, hypothalamic, or renal, is not known and we have not tried to work this out.

Weiner: Do monkeys kept in an experimental chair show increased water intake simply as a nervous habit?

Mirsky: Normal monkeys adapted to the chair show no disturbances in fluid intake or output. In contrast, monkeys kept in isolation during infancy show a stupendous water intake and urine output and they sometimes even go into frank water intoxication. It's not clear what role vasopressin plays in this phenomenon.

Ganong: Were you able to identify any recurrent collaterals?

Hayward: No, I was not able to identify recurrent collaterals in our studies. One problem is that it is very difficult in this preparation to distinguish between axons and dendrites. As you know, the only clear demonstration of recurrent collaterals is in the motoneuron of the spinal cord.

Narcotics and the Hypothalamus, edited by
E. Zimmermann and R. George. Raven Press,
New York © 1974

A New Technique for Studying Neuroendocrine Systems

Bernard H. Marks, Kakuichi K. Sakai, Jack M. George,* and
Adalbert Koestner**

Department of Pharmacology, Wayne State University, Detroit, Michigan 48201 Departments of
* Medicine and ** Veterinary Pathobiology, The Ohio State University, Columbus, Ohio 43210

Several years ago we surveyed various rat brain regions for estrogen binding activity by measuring the estradiol binding by soluble cytosol protein. In doing so, we included the pineal body, and were impressed by the magnitude of the estradiol binding in this structure—about the same order of magnitude as the adenohypophysis (1). In an effort to learn more about the effect of estrogens upon the pineal, we were led to develop a method which may be useful in examining other neuroendocrine transducers, which typically consist of very small cellular masses.

The method consists in isolating neuroendocrine tissues, either acutely, as in the case of the pineal, or by long-term organ culture, which we have done in the case of the supraoptic nucleus. The isolated tissue is transferred to a small chamber and superfused with Krebs-Henseleit buffer at 37°C, or with the same buffer containing known concentrations of drugs whose effects one desires to evaluate (2). After a period of equilibration, the tissue is penetrated with microelectrodes to record cell membrane potentials and, in the supraoptic nucleus organ cultures, action potentials and action potential frequency (Fig. 1).

Using this method, one can ask questions about the relationship of membrane events to the unique functions of that particular neuroendocrine system. In the case of the pineal, for example, we find that the same concentrations of norepinephrine that are effective in inducing N-acetyl transferase activity (3) can influence the membrane potential of the pineal parenchymal cell (2). In a continuous microelectrode impalement, it is possible to determine the concentration–response relationship in a single cell by superfusing with a series of norepinephrine solutions (Fig. 2). The cell is not damaged during such an experiment, since its norepinephrine responsiveness at the end of a series of drug exposures is the same as it was at the beginning. The response to norepinephrine is hyperpolarization, from the initial resting potential of approximately -25 mV. The response is specific for beta-adrenergic agonists (Fig. 3), phenylephrine producing no membrane response. There is competitive inhibition by the beta-adrenergic antagonist propranolol, but no effect of an alpha-adrenergic antagonist. The effect of propranolol is rapidly reversed upon washing out the drug.

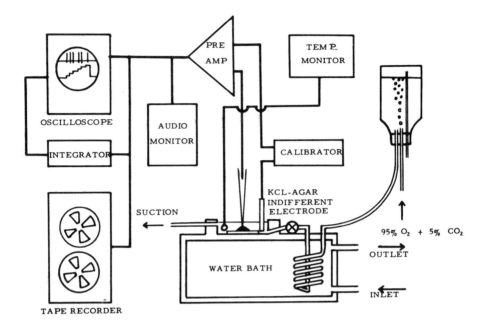

FIG. 1. Block diagram of microelectrode recording system for tissues *in vitro*. Reprinted with permission of *J. Pharmacol. Exp. Ther.*

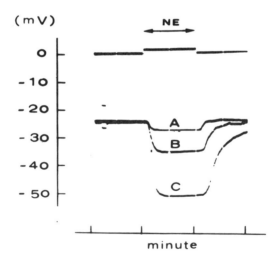

FIG. 2. Superimposed oscilloscope tracings showing the effect of 10^{-7}, 10^{-6}, and 10^{-5} M norepinephrine (NE) (curves A, B, and C, respectively) on pineal parenchymal cell membrane potential. Superfusion medium is Krebs-Henseleit buffer, 37°C. Reprinted with permission of *Life Sci.*

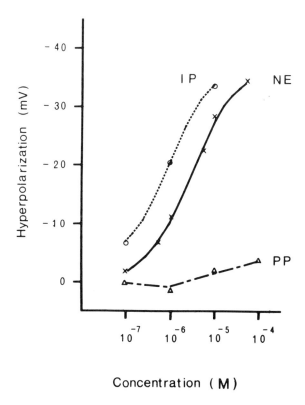

FIG. 3. Concentration–response relationships of isoproterenol (IP), norepinephrine (NE), and phenylephrine (PP) on membrane potential of pineal cells; means ± SE. Reprinted with permission of *Life Sci.*

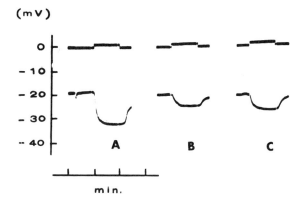

FIG. 4. Effects of estradiol (10^{-6} M) on the pineal cell membrane response to norepinephrine (NE) (10^{-6} M). A, NE alone; B, NE in the presence of estradiol; C, NE several minutes after washing out the estradiol. Reprinted with permission of *Life Sci.*

It is interesting that estradiol also attenuates the hyperpolarizing effect of norepinephrine (Fig. 4). Unlike propranolol, however, the effect of estradiol is not rapidly removed by washing (2). Thus, the membrane effect of estradiol resembles the effect of estradiol in inhibiting the adenyl cyclase activation produced by norepinephrine in the pineal (4). One might assume, therefore, that drugs which prevent hyperpolarization would prevent the accumulation of cyclic 3′,5′-adenosine monophosphate (cyclic AMP) in the pineal, and

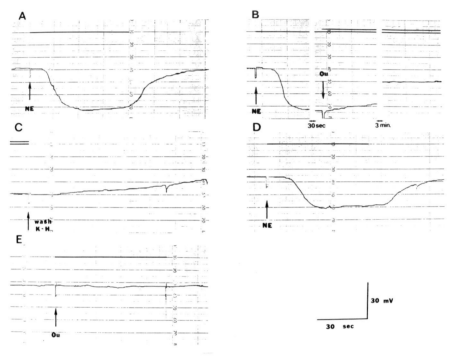

FIG. 5. Effect of 10^{-6} M ouabain (Ou) on the pineal cell membrane potential response to norepinephrine (NE) (10^{-6} M) superfusion.

the consequent induction of serotonin N-acetyltransferase (5). Recently, however, in collaboration with Dr. David Klein, we have found that several agents appear to dissociate or uncouple cyclic AMP production from N-acetyltransferase induction. For example, 10^{-6}M ouabain, which had no effect on pineal membrane potential, considerably reduced the hyper- polarizing effect of norepinephrine (Fig. 5). This same concentration of ouabain had no effect on the cyclic AMP accumulation in the pineal in re- sponse to norepinephrine, but very markedly inhibited the N-acetyltransferase induction response to norepinephrine (6). This same effect was observed with high potassium treatment. It appears, therefore, that there may be a relation- ship between the mechanisms involved in membrane hyperpolarization and the enzyme induction responses to norepinephrine. This relationship may center upon the presence of a factor which interferes with the activity of cyclic AMP both upon the membrane and upon protein synthesis, thereby uncoupling the synthesis of cyclic AMP from the biological effects of cyclic AMP. Thus, cyclic AMP in the perfusion medium itself will cause membrane hyperpolarization, and ouabain will attenuate this response, much as it attenuates the response to norepinephrine (Fig. 6).

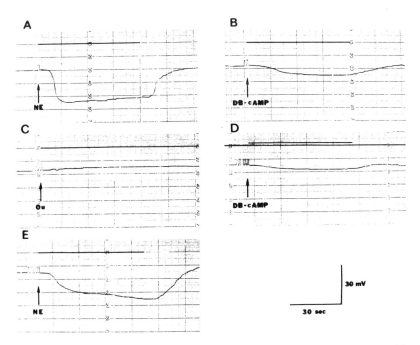

FIG. 6. Effect of 10^{-6} M ouabain (Ou) on the pineal cell membrane potential response to dibutyryl cAMP (DB-cAMP) (10^{-4} M) superfusion.

The biochemical meaning of these observations is still obscure, but the observations are presented to illustrate that microelectrode methods provide an additional dimension for the study of secretory systems.

Another application of this same approach has been made to the study of the supraoptic nucleus, when it was found that explants of puppy supraoptic nucleus could be maintained in organ culture for periods of several weeks (7). This allows time for degeneration and removal of afferents to supraoptic nucleus neurons, and permits direct study of these cells with minimal interference from modulating neuronal circuitry. The neurosecretory neurons themselves sprout new axons and show typical fine structural features of active synthesis and transport of neurosecretory material. The vasopressin content of the explants, measured by immunoassay (8), is approximately 39 pg per explant; spontaneous leakage of vasopressin into the culture medium is usually not measurable after the first week of organ culture, being at or below the limits of sensitivity of the assay (9).

For study with microelectrodes, the ideal period is apparently after 2 to 3 weeks of organ culture, since the measured resting membrane potentials appear to fall slowly after this time. Cover slips containing the explants are transferred to a 0.5-ml superfusion chamber containing oxygenated Krebs-Henseleit buffer, and the same buffer is allowed to flow through the chamber at 2 ml/min. The nerve cell bodies in the explant are penetrated with glass microelectrodes to record the resting membrane potential, action potentials, and action potential frequency. Cell penetrations are accepted as representing neurosecretory neurons if the cell responds typically to exposure to 10^{-6} M glutamate and 10^{-6} M nicotine in the superfusion medium. Drug exposures of approximately 1 min duration are usual. The cells are known not to have been damaged, since their response to glutamate at the end of a series of drug exposures is the same as it was at the start.

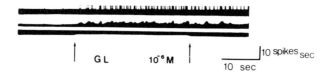

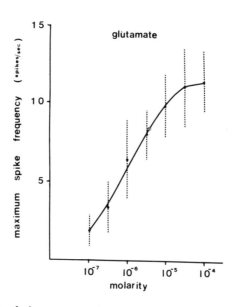

FIG. 7. Effects of glutamate on spiking activity of organ-cultured canine supraoptic nucleus cells. Above, marked increase in spike frequency during 10^{-6} M glutamate (GL) superfusion (top line, spikes; second line, spikes/sec). Below, concentration–response relationship for glutamate; means ± SE. Reprinted with permission of J. Pharmacol. Exp. Ther.

The resting membrane potential of these organ-cultured supraoptic neurons averaged −36 mV. These cells are quiescent, with spontaneous action potentials occurring with a frequency of less than 1 spike/sec. When exposed to glutamate, they respond immediately with a sustained increase of spike frequency (Fig. 7) whose magnitude is dependent on the glutamate concentration (9).

Acetylcholine superfusion also initiated concentration-dependent spiking activity, but the concentration–response relationship was bell-shaped (Fig. 8), suggesting more than one mechanism of response. The presence of a

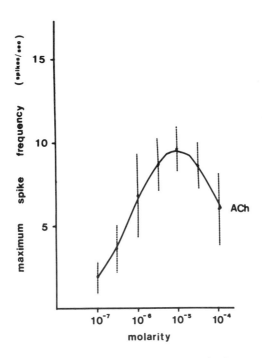

FIG. 8. Acetylcholine concentration–response relationship for spike frequency induced in organ-cultured supraoptic nucleus neurons by acetylcholine superfusion; means ± SE. Reprinted with permission of J. Pharmacol. Exp. Ther.

nicotinic receptor blocking drug, dihydro-beta-erythroidine, blocked acetylcholine-induced spiking activity, and a muscarinic receptor blocking drug, atropine, increased acetylcholine-induced spiking activity (Fig. 9). In contrast to acetylcholine, however, nicotine superfusion showed conventional sigmoid concentration–response relationships. These results support the conclusion that there is a stimulatory nicotinic receptor and an inhibitory muscarinic receptor mechanism in the same supraoptic nucleus cells. When the cholinergic agonist carbachol is superfused along with glutamate, the inhibitory cholinergic response is clearly observed (Fig. 10).

A

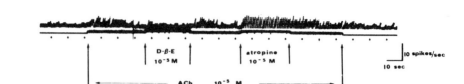

B

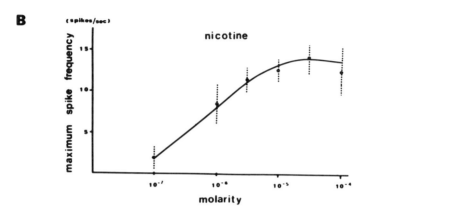

FIG. 9. A, Effect of a nicotinic receptor blocking drug, dihydro-beta-erythroidine (D-β-E), and a muscarinic receptor blocking drug, atropine, on the spiking frequency induced in an organ-cultured supraoptic nucleus neuron by acetylcholine (ACh 10^{-5} M) superfusion. B, Concentration–response relationship for spike frequency induced in organ-cultured supraoptic nucleus neurons by nicotine superfusion; means $\pm$ SE. Reprinted with permission of *J. Pharmacol. Exp. Ther.*

Neither gamma-aminobutyric acid nor norepinephrine initiates nerve cell firing. Both of these agents, superfused along with glutamate or nicotine, inhibit spiking activity. In the case of norepinephrine, the inhibition is also produced by other agents with beta-adrenergic agonist activity, and is blocked only by adrenergic beta-blocking agents (Fig. 11).

Of some interest in relation to ideas about regulation of vasopressin secretion is the observation that at least one polypeptide, not normally considered a neurotransmitter, is very active in initiating spiking activity in these organ-cultured supraoptic neurons. This is angiotensin II, which has been known to have important effects within the central nervous system (10). This peptide initiates concentration-dependent spiking, with an ED_{50} of approximately 3×10^{-7} M (Figs. 12 and 13). Peptide analogues of angiotensin II which are known to block the vascular effects of angiotensin II also block these neuronal effects (Fig. 14), but block the effects of neither glutamate nor nicotine (11). Thus, we feel that there is a unique, specific angiotensin receptor mechanism in these supraoptic nucleus neurosecretory neurons, which may play a part in the integrated response to osmotic stresses.

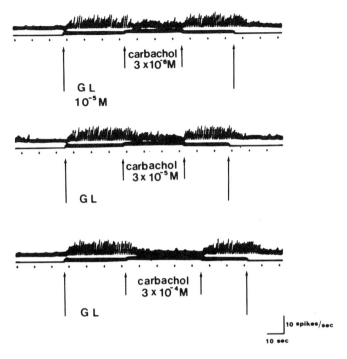

FIG. 10. Effect of three concentrations of carbachol when added to glutamate (GL) (10^{-5} M) superfusion of an organ-cultured supraoptic nucleus neuron. Reprinted with permission of *J. Pharmacol. Exp. Ther.*

Finally, we have made some efforts to identify membrane effects of morphine in the organ-cultured supraoptic nucleus, since it is well known that morphine initiates vasopressin secretion (12). However, in preliminary experiments in neurons that respond normally to glutamate, we have not observed any direct membrane activity of morphine in supraoptic nucleus organ cultures. Thus, if there are synaptic effects of morphine in this system, they may be indirect or presynaptic rather than direct postsynaptic effects.

To summarize, the use of intracellular microelectrode methods with isolated neuroendocrine tissues *in vitro* provides a technique for obtaining quantitative cellular responses which appear to be meaningful in relation to the neuroendocrine transducer function. Thus, in the case of the pineal, membrane responses appear to be more closely related to the control of N-acetyltransferase induction by norepinephrine than is the tissue cyclic AMP content. In the case of the supraoptic nucleus, we have found that the organ culture technique combined with microelectrode methods allows us to obtain quantitative data about neural activity which appears to be closely related to what is known of the response of these cells *in vivo* (13). Therefore, we are encouraged to continue to use this system to study the control of the neurosecretory functions themselves.

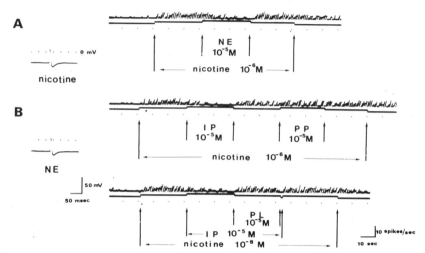

FIG. 11. Adrenergic effects on an organ-cultured supraoptic nucleus neuron. A, Spike configuration during nicotine superfusion. B, Spike configuration with norepinephrine (NE) added to a nicotine superfusion. C, Top tracing: NE reduces spike frequency induced by nicotine. Middle tracing: isoproterenol (IP) reduces spike frequency induced by nicotine, while phenylephrine (PP) is inactive. Bottom tracing: the effect of isoproterenol on spiking frequency is reversed by propranolol (PL). Reprinted with permission of J. Pharmacol. Exp. Ther.

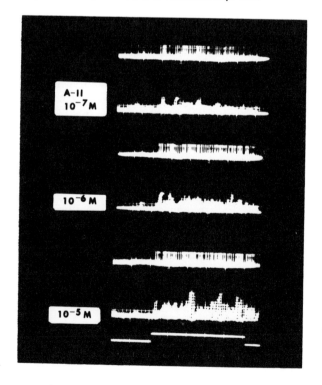

FIG. 12. Effect of three concentrations of angiotensin II (A–II) on spiking activity of an organ-cultured supraoptic nucleus cell. Reprinted with permission of Life Sci.

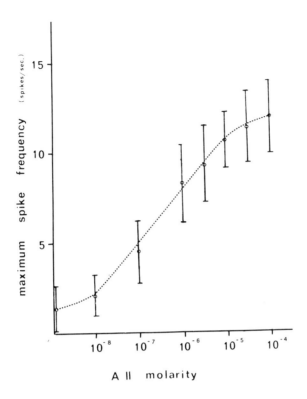

FIG. 13. Concentration–response relationship for angiotensin II (A–II) effect on spiking frequency of organ-cultured supraoptic nucleus neurons; means $\pm$ SE. Reprinted with permission of *Life Sci.*

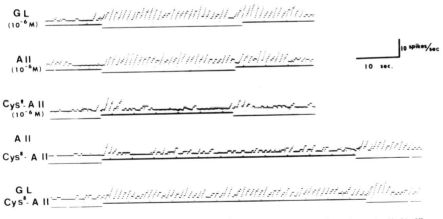

FIG. 14. Reversal by cysteine-8-angiotensin II (Cys[8]-A-II) of the effect of angiotensin II (A–II) on spiking activity of an organ-cultured supraoptic neuron, and failure of cysteine-8-angiotensin II to reverse the effect of glutamate (GL) on this same neuron. Reprinted with permission of *Life Sci.*

SUMMARY

Initial results are presented using intracellular microelectrode measurements from isolated rat pineal glands and isolated organ-cultured explants of canine supraoptic nucleus. Receptor mechanisms in neuroendocrine systems can be described using such a technique.

REFERENCES

1. Marks, B. H., Wu, T. K., and Goldman, H. Soluble estrogen binding protein in the rat pineal gland. *Res. Comm. Chem. Path. Pharmacol.,* 3:595–600, 1972.
2. Sakai, K. K., and Marks, B. H. Adrenergic effects on pineal cell membrane potential. *Life Sci.,* 11:285–291, 1972.
3. Klein, D. C., Berg, G. R., and Weller, J. Melatonin synthesis: Adenosine 3'5' monophosphate and norepinephrine stimulate N-acetyltransferase. *Science,* 168:979–980, 1970.
4. Weiss, B., and Crayton, J. Gonadal hormones as regulators of pineal adenylcyclase activity. *Endocrinology,* 87:527–533, 1970.
5. Klein, D. C., and Weller, J. Adrenergic-adenosine 3',5'-monophosphate regulation of serotonin N-acetyltransferase activity and the temporal relationship of serotonin N-acetyltransferase activity to synthesis of N-acetyl-serotonin and melatonin in the rat pineal gland. *J. Pharmacol. Exp. Ther.,* 186:516–527, 1973.
6. Parfitt, A., Weller, J., Sakai, K. K., Marks, B. H., and Klein, D. C. Depolarizing agents block the post-synaptic adrenergic-cAMP (3'–5') induction of pineal acetyl coA: Serotonin N-acetyltransferase activity. *Mol. Pharmacol.,* 1974 (*submitted*).
7. Koestner, A., George, J. M., and Lang, J. F. Neurosecretory activity of the canine supra-optic nucleus in vivo and in vitro. *J. Neuropath. Exp. Neurol.,* 31:194, 1972.
8. George, J. M., Capen, C. C., and Phillips, A. S. Biosynthesis of vasopressin in vitro and ultrastructure of a bronchogenic carcinoma. *J. Clin. Invest.,* 51:141–148, 1972.
9. Sakai, K. K., Marks, B. H., George, J. M., and Koestner, A. The isolated organ-cultured supra-optic nucleus as a neuro-pharmacological test system. *J. Pharmacol. Exp. Therap.,* 1974 (*in press*).
10. Severs, W. B., and Daniels-Severs, A. E. Effects of angiotensin on the central nervous system. *Pharmacol. Rev.,* 25:415–449, 1973.
11. Sakai, K. K., Marks, B. H., George, J., and Koestner, A. Specific angiotensin II receptors in organ-cultured canine supra-optic nucleus cells. *Life Sci.,* 14:1337–1344, 1974.
12. Giarman, N. J., and Condouris, G. A. The antidiuretic action of morphine and some of its analogs. *Arch. Int. Pharmacodyn.,* 97:28–33, 1954.
13. Barker, J. L., Crayton, J. W., and Nicoll, R. A. Noradrenaline and acetylcholine responses of supra-optic neurosecretory cells. *J. Physiol.,* 218:19–32, 1971.

DISCUSSION

Marks: In our limited experience using opiates in this *in vitro* supraoptic nucleus preparation, we have not been able to demonstrate either agonistic or antagonistic effects using reasonable concentrations of the opiates. Thus, if morphine stimulates vasopressin secretion, our data would suggest that it exerts this effect via one or another of the indirect inputs to the supraoptic nucleus described by Dr. Hayward earlier in this meeting, rather than by a direct action on the cells of this nucleus.

Hayward: Is there a possibility that histamine might play a role in the stimulation of your supraoptic cells *in vitro?*

Marks: We have done a number of electron micrographs of these cultured supraoptic cells and have not seen anything that resembles a mast cell. However, there is reported to be non-mast cell histamine in the hypothalamus so we can't be sure about this. We find histamine to be a very weak agonist in this system; it is nowhere near as effective in stimulating supraoptic cells as are the other biogenic amines we have studied. Serotonin and dopamine are also very weak agonists in our experience.

McCann: I am interested in the specificity of the estrogen effects on pinealocytes. Have you tried other steroids?

Marks: Testosterone and corticosteroids in similar concentrations do not exert the effects observed here with estrogen. We have not tried progesterone.

Mirsky: Have you tried cyclic GMP in this system?

Marks: Yes, we have tried this and, although we feel that cyclic GMP may be a modulator of some of the responses we have observed, we did not see any effect when exogenous cyclic GMP was added to explanted pineal gland preparations.

Narcotics and the Hypothalamus, edited by
E. Zimmermann and R. George. Raven Press,
New York © 1974

Trans-Hypothalamic Effects of Drugs of Abuse on the Secretion of Pituitary Hormones

P. Brazeau, W. Vale, and R. Guillemin

The Salk Institute, La Jolla, California 92037

Several recent reports have demonstrated that anesthetic doses of sodium pentobarbital cause acute secretion of radioimmunoassayable rat growth hormone (GH) (1–3). The GH response to this drug is rapid, with significant increases occurring within a few minutes following the injection (5 to 10 min, depending on the mode of injection being used). More recently, morphine sulfate was also seen to trigger an acute secretion of GH in the rat (3). These observations are important in that they suggest the existence of mechanisms for an acute release of GH in species in which most stimuli have been described to cause inhibition of secretion of this hormone (2, 4–7).

In addition to morphine, other narcotic drugs have also been described as potent inducers of GH release; methadone and codeine, to name only two, have recently been shown to initiate GH secretion in the rat (8). Heroin (diacetylmorphine) was also seen to trigger a constant elevation of radioimmunoassayable plasma GH in humans, and addicts have shown a uniformly elevated insulin response to a glucose tolerance test (9).

The effects of narcotic analgesics on the acute secretion of other pituitary hormones have also been studied. Morphine sulfate, methadone, and codeine have been reported to stimulate corticotropin (ACTH) secretion measured indirectly by corticosterone evaluation (8). It should be noted, however, that this secretion happens only at doses two to four times higher than that required to trigger GH secretion. These drugs are known to have both depressing and stimulating effects in rodents. The stimulating action of morphine sulfate on ACTH secretion is probably mediated by a direct effect on the hypothalamus and/or by a nonspecific stress effect, whereas the elevated GH secretion could be due to a dual action on the releasing and release-inhibiting factors of GH, the presence of which has been demonstrated in hypothalamic tissues. Pentobarbital was also claimed to inhibit ACTH, prolactin, and luteinizing hormone (LH) secretion, but follicle-stimulating hormone (FSH) secretion was unaffected (10). Chronic methadone administration had no effect on the hypothalamic-pituitary-thyroid axis (11).

We first became interested in the properties of pentobarbital and morphine stimulation of GH secretion while attempting to isolate somatotropin release-inhibiting factor (SRIF) in 1971–72. Pentobarbital provided us with a good means of inducing GH secretion against which we were able to assay the inhibiting potencies of different preparations of SRIF and its analogues.

In this chapter we present our results on the use of pentobarbital and morphine and describe a mode of action of these drugs of abuse proposed by some very recent studies.

Because we decided to use rats pretreated with pentobarbital as a means of triggering GH secretion, we first investigated a full scale of procedures and modes of injection in order to obtain maximum sensitivity, optimal responsivity, and best conditions for repetition. It first became obvious to us that intravenous rather than intraperitoneal injection of the drug was far more convenient based on these criteria; in our hands, intraperitoneal injection gives erratic response in terms of time and intensity. Moreover, injection into the jugular vein provides an acute and sharp response within 10 min, which is ideal for assaying (intravenously or subcutaneously) SRIF and its analogues.

Figure 1 shows the effect of intravenous pentobarbital (2 mg/100 g body weight) on circulating levels of GH in male Sprague-Dawley rats (100 to 120 g body weight) studied at 3:00 P.M. in a quiet, well-ventilated room. The barbiturate was injected into the jugular vein within 30 sec following ether anesthesia, and blood was withdrawn from the exposed vein at 0, 5, 10, 20,

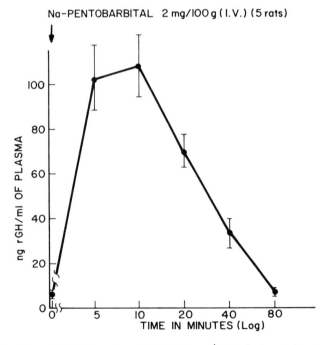

FIG. 1. Effect of i.v. administration of pentobarbital (2 mg/100 g body weight) on plasma levels of GH in ether-anesthetized male rats. In this and in subsequent figures the mean ± SEM are plotted.

40, and 80 min after injection. Similar results have been obtained when trunk blood was collected following decapitation at various times after pentobarbital injection.

The ether-anesthetized, pentobarbital-treated rat preparation described above was used to assay *in vivo* the biological potency of different SRIF preparations. Blood for GH determination was obtained 15 min following injection of the barbiturate. The results obtained when various doses of SRIF were injected subcutaneously within 1 min after intravenous administration of pentobarbital show that SRIF causes dose-dependent inhibition of the pentobarbital-stimulated rise in plasma GH (Fig. 2).

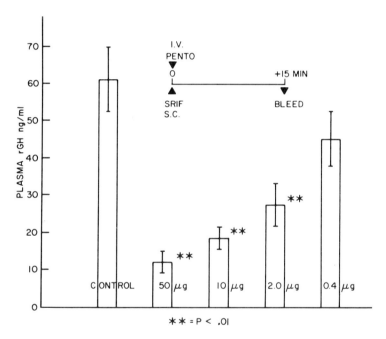

FIG. 2. Effects of various doses of s.c. SRIF on the 15-min GH response to i.v. pentobarbital in ether-anesthetized male rats.

To study effects of intravenous administration of SRIF on the pentobarbital-induced rise in plasma GH, we treated male rats with ether and pentobarbital as described above. After 10 min, SRIF (2 or 5 μg) was injected intravenously, and 5 min later the animals were decapitated and trunk blood was collected. The results (Fig. 3) show dose-dependent suppression by SRIF of the pentobarbital-induced rise in plasma GH levels.

Since ether is known to be a stressful stimulus which can inhibit GH secretion (2), it was of interest to study effects of SRIF on GH levels in unanesthetized rats. To minimize the stressful effects of handling and injection,

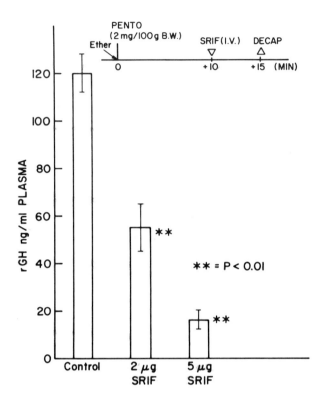

FIG. 3. Effects of i.v. administration of SRIF (2 or 5 μg) on pentobarbital-induced GH levels in ether-anesthetized male rats.

rats (70 to 80 g body weight) were gentled by handling for 2 min and by being injected subcutaneously with 0.5 ml saline twice daily for 7 to 10 days. On the day of the assay various doses of SRIF were injected subcutaneously. Fifteen min later each rat was taken to an adjacent room and quickly decapitated, and trunk blood was collected for subsequent determination of plasma GH levels. The results (Fig. 4) indicate that SRIF produced dose-related suppression of plasma GH levels in unanesthetized, gentled rats. These results are consistent with evidence that SRIF acts at the pituitary level to inhibit GH secretion (12, 13).

Morphine sulfate has recently been reported to be a potent stimulus for GH secretion in the rat (3). Using a protocol similar to that described above for pentobarbital, we have been able to confirm this finding. Male Sprague-Dawley rats were anesthetized with ether, an external jugular vein was exposed, and morphine sulfate (1 mg/100 g body weight) was injected intravenously. At 0, 5, 10, 20, 40, and 80 min following injection, a 0.4-ml blood sample was withdrawn from the vein and subsequently assayed for GH concentrations. The results (Fig. 5) show that after a 5-min latent period, mor-

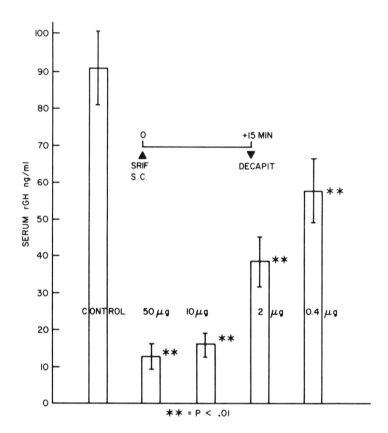

FIG. 4. Effects of various doses of s.c. SRIF on plasma GH levels in gentled, unanesthetized male rats.

phine produced a marked rise in plasma GH levels to peak values at 20 to 40 min following injection. By 80 min, GH levels had returned to preinjection concentrations.

To study effects of SRIF on the morphine-induced rise in plasma GH levels, we treated rats as described in the preceding paragraph except that 25 μg of synthetic linear (reduced) SRIF was injected both intravenously and subcutaneously immediately following the intravenous administration of morphine. Blood was obtained 20 and 40 min later for determination of GH levels. As shown in Fig. 6, SRIF completely blocked the GH response to morphine. Results similar to these have been obtained recently with SRIF in male rats bearing an indwelling intravenous cannula (J. B. Martin, *personal communication,* January 1974).

Until quite recently, little was known about the site(s) or mechanisms by which pentobarbital stimulates GH secretion in the rat. Martin (14–16) has

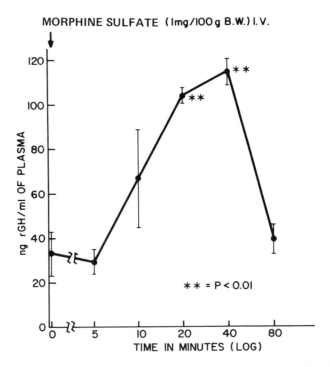

FIG. 5. Effect of i.v. morphine sulfate on plasma GH levels in ether-anesthetized male rats.

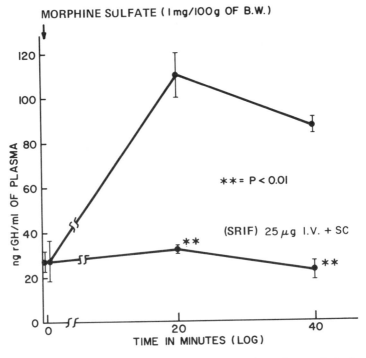

FIG. 6. Effect of SRIF on morphine-induced rise in plasma GH levels in ether-anesthetized male rats.

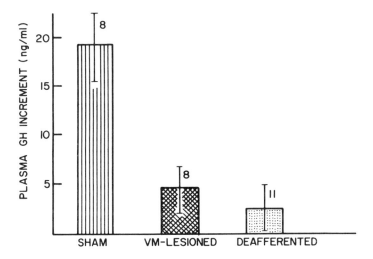

FIG. 7. Effect of ventromedial lesions or hypothalamic deafferentation on GH levels in pentobarbital-treated male rats. From Martin (15).

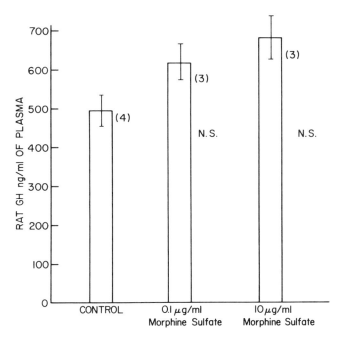

FIG. 8. Effect of morphine on GH secretion of cultured rat anterior pituitary cells. Numbers in parentheses denote the number of dishes.

presented evidence that pentobarbital triggers GH secretion via the central nervous system. He found that either electrolytic lesions in the ventromedial nucleus or deafferentation of the hypothalamus blocked the rise in plasma GH levels 10 min after intraperitoneal administration of pentobarbital (5 mg/100 g body weight) (Fig. 7). On the other hand, stimulation of the ventromedial and arcuate nuclei or of the hippocampus and basolateral nucleus of the amygdala triggered GH release. In contrast to Martin's findings, Halasz and his associates (17) and Mitchell and his co-workers (18) found that surgical deafferentation of the hypothalamus did not suppress growth or plasma or pituitary levels of GH. Nevertheless, we feel there is adequate evidence to suggest that extrahypothalamic areas, including limbic structures or their connections with the hypothalamus, are involved in triggering the GH response to pentobarbital.

There has been some suggestion that, unlike pentobarbital, morphine stimulates GH secretion by a direct action on the pituitary (Martin, *personal communication*). Working with our monolayered cultured pituitary cell assay (12, 13), we have been unable to confirm this possibility. As shown in Fig. 8, morphine added to cultured rat anterior pituitary cells failed to increase significantly the concentration of GH in the medium. On the other hand, lesions of the ventromedial nuclei or deafferentation of the hypothalamus had only a very marginal effect on the GH response to morphine.

In conclusion it can be said that pentobarbital initiates GH secretion through the nervous system via extrahypothalamic pathways. The recent findings of Martin (14–16 and *personal communication*) lead us to believe that at least the dorsal portion of the hippocampus region is involved in the triggering of GH secretion through the fornix pathways. This could trigger the arcuate nuclei in the hypothalamic region, which is known to have an effect on GH secretion when stimulated directly. The basal lateral amygdaloid region might also be involved. As far as morphine is concerned, it seems to act directly on the hypothalamo-pituitary axis to cause GH release. The fact that destruction of ventromedial nucleus or the total deafferentation of the medial basal hypothalamus had only a marginal effect would suggest that only a direct effect at the pituitary level and/or the arcuate nuclei could explain the increase in GH secretion in response to morphine. Nevertheless, no effect of morphine was seen *in vitro* on monolayered cultured pituitary cells. It is clear that further studies are needed to clarify the role of the medial basal hypothalamus in the GH response to morphine.

ACKNOWLEDGMENTS

The authors wish to thank Dr. Jean Rivier for the synthesis of the SRIF, Misses Kathy Setbacken and Carolyn Otto for their excellent technical assistance, and Mrs. Janice Bowman for her secretarial assistance.

REFERENCES

1. Howard, H., and Martin, J. M. A stimulatory test of growth hormone release in the rat. *Endocrinology*, 88:497, 1971.
2. Takahashi, K., Daughaday, W. H., and Kipnis, D. M. Regulation of immunoreactive growth hormone secretion in male rats. *Endocrinology*, 88:909, 1971.
3. Kokka, N., Garcia, J. F., George, R., and Elliott, H. W. Growth hormone and ACTH secretion: Evidence for an inverse relationship in rats. *Endocrinology*, 90: 735, 1972.
4. Schalch, D. S., and Reichlin, S. Plasma growth hormone concentration in the rat determined by radioimmunoassay: Influence of sex, pregnancy, lactation, anesthesia, hypophysectomy and extrasellar pituitary transplants. *Endocrinology*, 79:275, 1966.
5. Schalch, D. S., and Reichlin, S. Stress and growth hormone release. In: *Growth Hormone*, edited by A. Pecile and E. E. Muller, p. 211. Excerpta Medica, Amsterdam, 1968.
6. Garcia, J. F., and Geschwind, I. I. Investigation of growth hormone secretion in selected mammalian species. In: *Growth Hormone*, edited by A. Pecile and E. E. Muller, p. 267. Excerpta Medica, Amsterdam, 1968.
7. Muller, E. E. Analogous pattern of bioassayable and radioimmunoassayable growth hormone in some experimental conditions of rat and mouse. In: *Growth and Growth Hormone*, edited by A. Pecile and E. E. Muller, p. 283. Excerpta Medica, Amsterdam, 1972.
8. Kokka, N., Garcia, J. F., and Elliott, H. W. Effects of acute and chronic administration of narcotic analgesics on growth hormone and corticotrophin (ACTH) secretion in rats. In: *Progress in Brain Research*, Vol. 39, edited by E. Zimmermann, W. H. Gispen, B. Marks, and D. de Wied, p. 347. Elsevier, Amsterdam, 1973.
9. Reed, J. L., and Ghodse, A. H. Oral glucose tolerance and hormonal response in heroin-dependent males. *Brit. Med. J.*, 2:582, 1973.
10. Ajika, K., Kalra, S. P., Fawcett, C. P., Krulich, L., and McCann, S. M. The effect of stress and Nembutal on plasma levels of gonadotropins and prolactin in ovariectomized rats. *Endocrinology*, 90:707, 1972.
11. Shenkman, L., Massie, B., Mitsuma, T., and Hollander, C. S. Effects of chronic methadone administration on the hypothalamic-pituitary-thyroid axis. *J. Clin. Endocrinol. Metab.*, 35:169, 1972.
12. Vale, W. Premieres observations sur le mode d'action de la somatostatin, un facteur hypothalamique qui inhibe la sécrétion de l'hormone de croissance. *C.R. Acad. Sci. (Paris)*, 275:2913, 1972.
13. Brazeau, P., Vale, W., Burgus, R., Ling, N., Butcher, M., Rivier, J., and Guillemin, R. Hypothalamic polypeptide that inhibits the secretion of immunoreactive pituitary growth hormone. *Science*, 179:77, 1973.
14. Martin, J. B., Kontor, J., and Mead, P. Plasma GH responses to hypothalamic hippocampal and amygdaloid electrical stimulation: Effects of variation in stimulus parameters and treatment with alpha-methyl-*p*-tyrosine (alpha-MT). *Endocrinology*, 92:1354, 1973.
15. Martin, J. B. The role of hypothalamic and extrahypothalamic structures in the control of growth hormone secretion. In: *Advances in Human Growth Hormone Research*, edited by S. Raiti, p. 223. DHEW Publ. No. NIH 74–612, U.S. Government Printing Office, Washington, D.C., 1973.
16. Martin, J. B. Studies on the mechanism of pentobarbital-induced GH release in the rat. *Neuroendocrinology*, 13:339, 1973–74.
17. Halasz, B., Schalch, D., and Gorski, R. Growth hormone secretion in young rats after partial or total interruption of neural afferents to the medial hypothalamus. *Endocrinology*, 89:198, 1971.
18. Mitchell, J. A., Belsare, D., Hutchins, M., Schindler, W., and Critchlow, V. Increases in growth and plasma growth hormone levels following surgical isolation of medial basal hypothalamus in female rats. *Program, 53rd Annual Meeting, Endocrine Society*, p. A82, 1971.

DISCUSSION

Hayward: Have you studied the effects of morphine directly on pituitary cells with respect to growth hormone secretion?

Brazeau: Yes. We recently tried to stimulate growth hormone secretion in monolayers of anterior pituitary cells maintained *in vitro,* but were unable to do so.

Way: Have you used morphine antagonists in your studies in an attempt to stop the actions of the drug?

Brazeau: No.

Kokka: Have you studied the effects of pentobarbital on growth hormone secretion *in vitro?*

Brazeau: Yes, we tried this but found that pentobarbital caused damage to pituitary cells by a direct action and, thus, a high level of growth hormone in the cultures may be explained on the basis of tissue damage. Altering the pH does not eliminate this problem.

McCann: It seems to me that the lesion data you have presented could be explained on the basis that, whereas pentobarbital stimulates GRH and therefore growth hormone secretion, morphine may stimulate growth hormone secretion by an inhibition of growth hormone inhibiting factor. Based on our limited evidence regarding localization of these substances, the ventral medial hypothalamic lesions would be expected to eliminate growth hormone releasing hormone-producing neurons, but this would not impair growth hormone inhibiting factor secretion. If this is true, one would not expect to impair the response to morphine with the ventral medial hypothalamic nuclear lesions. This possible explanation is more appealing to me than the possibility that morphine acts directly on pituitary cells.

Mirsky: I am still puzzled that the rat shows a decrease in growth hormone secretion in response to noxious stimuli.

Brazeau: Yes, this is an interesting difference between rodents and various other species. We know that the growth hormone response to stress varies from one species to another. It is also true that growth hormone levels vary with time of day, there being several minor peaks in addition to a major peak. I would like to emphasize that all our studies were carried out at three o'clock in the afternoon when the rats are normally asleep since, under our laboratory conditions, the lights come on at seven in the morning.

Narcotics and the Hypothalamus, edited by
E. Zimmermann and R. George. Raven Press,
New York © 1974

Drug-Induced Alterations in Gonadotropin and Prolactin Release in the Rat

S. M. McCann, S. R. Ojeda, C. Libertun, P. G. Harms, and L. Krulich

Department of Physiology, University of Texas Health Science Center at Dallas, Southwestern Medical School, Dallas, Texas 75235

In the course of investigations designed to determine possible synaptic transmitters involved in control of gonadotropin and prolactin release, a variety of drugs, some of which are used in the treatment of psychotic conditions and one of which, morphine, is a drug of abuse, have been given to rats by either systemic, intraventricular, or intrapituitary injections. In this chapter we will outline the evidence for the role of various monoamines as possible synaptic transmitters involved in the control of pituitary hormone release. This information may serve as a vehicle for understanding the complex effects of various drugs on pituitary hormone release.

HYPOTHALAMIC GONADOTROPIN- AND PROLACTIN-CONTROLLING REGIONS

On the basis of both stimulation and lesion experiments, it is now quite clear that gonadotropin release is controlled by a region which extends from the medial preoptic area rostrally through the anterior hypothalamus to the arcuate-median eminence region caudally (1). The more rostral portions of this region, namely, the suprachiasmatic and anterior hypothalamic areas, appear to be involved in the preovulatory release of follicle-stimulating hormone (FSH) and luteinizing hormone (LH) and in mediating the stimulatory effects of gonadal steroids which provoke this preovulatory discharge. It appears that the region responsible for preovulatory FSH release is located slightly more caudally in the anterior hypothalamic area than that controlling preovulatory LH release, which is located primarily in the preoptic-suprachiasmatic region (2, 3). The more caudal portions of the gonadotropin-controlling region, that is, the median eminence-arcuate region, appear to be involved in mediating the negative feedback of gonadal steroids (1).

These feedback effects of gonadal steroids, both negative and positive, also appear to operate directly on the anterior pituitary as evidenced by recent studies showing that very small doses of these steroids can modify the pituitary responsiveness to synthetic LH-releasing factor (LRF) (4). We will not be concerned here with this aspect of the problem.

The hypothalamus exerts inhibitory control over prolactin release since median eminence lesions result in a marked elevation in plasma prolactin (5). The inhibition is mediated by hypothalamic prolactin-inhibiting factor (PIF) (6).

LOCALIZATION OF GONADOTROPIN-RELEASING FACTOR(S) AND MONOAMINES IN HYPOTHALAMUS

Bioassay of frozen hypothalamic sections has revealed that gonadotropin-releasing activity is found throughout the gonadotropin-controlling region from the medial preoptic area to the arcuate-median eminence region where the greatest activity is present. Extracts from this region preferentially provoke LH release from pituitaries incubated *in vitro,* but some FSH release is also stimulated (7). Since lesions in the suprachiasmatic region which blocked ovulation were associated with a 50% reduction in the content of LRF in the median eminence-arcuate region, we postulated that LRF was contained in secretory neurons and that some of these had cell bodies in the suprachiasmatic region. When the lesions destroyed these cell bodies, there was loss of LRF from the degenerating axon terminals which extended to the median eminence. Since some LRF was still present, we postulated that other LRF-secreting neurons had cell bodies located more caudally, perhaps in the arcuate nuclei and short axons extending to the median eminence, there to release LRF into hypophyseal portal vessels (8). Recent studies by Barry et al. (9) using fluorescent antibodies to synthetic LRF have confirmed our postulated localization of LRF neurons.

PIF, on the other hand, was not found in the median eminence but, surprisingly, activity was found in the lateral preoptic area (7). The suprachiasmatic region contained prolactin-releasing activity. Other workers have demonstrated a prolactin-releasing factor (PRF) under special circumstances, which suggests that prolactin may be under dual hypothalamic control by both PIF and PRF, with PIF predominating.

Recent histochemical fluorescence studies have given important clues to possible synaptic transmitters which may impinge on the gonadotropin-controlling centers. In the preoptic and anterior hypothalamic regions, for example, there are numerous terminals of noradrenergic neurons. Terminals of serotonergic neurons are located in the anterior hypothalamic area. The cell bodies of both the noradrenergic and serotonergic neurons appear to lie in the brainstem. On the other hand, cell bodies of the tuberoinfundibular dopaminergic neurons are located in the arcuate nucleus. Axons of these neurons appear to project to the external layer of the median eminence (10). It is also well known that the hypothalamus contains cholinergic synapses (11).

POSSIBLE SYNAPTIC TRANSMITTERS INVOLVED IN CONTROL OF GONADOTROPIN AND PROLACTIN RELEASE

We have made two approaches to the study of putative synaptic transmitters involved in anterior pituitary hormone release. The first of these was to employ an *in vitro* system in which pituitaries were incubated in the presence of various drugs, either alone or together with ventral hypothalamic fragments containing the arcuate-median eminence region. The second approach was to employ injection of various drugs systemically, into the third ventricle, or into the anterior pituitary, and to evaluate the effects of the drugs on gonadotropin and prolactin release.

In vitro Studies

Although very large doses of a number of drugs can influence the release of pituitary hormones *in vitro,* there was little effect with the addition of low doses of catecholamines, histamine, or serotonin on the release of FSH and LH. At high doses dopamine reduced the amounts of gonadotropins in the medium, but this was due to destruction of the hormones (12, 13). By contrast, dopamine in very small doses was effective in reducing prolactin release by pituitaries incubated *in vitro* (14). Norepinephrine was also effective, and the inhibition of release was dose-related not only in our studies but in those of others (15).

When hypothalami were incubated together with pituitaries, dopamine and, to a lesser extent, norepinephrine, were capable of releasing FSH and LH and inhibiting prolactin release in the coincubation system (12–14). These results were interpreted as indicating that dopamine released FSH-RF and LRF from the hypothalamic fragments since the catecholamine did not modify the response to added releasing factors. The release of gonadotropin-releasing factors by dopamine under these conditions appears to require rather precise conditions, because changing the number of hypothalamic fragments or the size of the fragments has resulted in a lack of response to dopamine (13, 14).

In the case of prolactin, the interpretation was complicated by the fact that dopamine alone inhibited prolactin release from the pituitaries. It was possible to block the response of the pituitary to dopamine with the drug haloperidol, which blocks dopaminergic receptors. In this situation, media from the incubation of ventral hypothalami in the presence of dopamine were still capable of inhibiting prolactin release. Consequently, we concluded that dopamine could cause a release of PIF from the ventral hypothalamic fragments (14).

In vivo Studies

Studies in living animals have involved the injection of putative transmitters into the third ventricle or into the anterior lobe of the pituitary and
the systemic or central injection of receptor-blocking drugs and drugs which
would alter the synthesis of the proposed transmitters.

Effects of Intraventricular Catecholamines on Gonadotropin and Prolactin Release

Injection of dopamine into the third ventricle of rats, which had been
previously ovariectomized and primed with a large dose of estrogen and
progesterone, provoked a release of LH as evidenced by an increase in plasma
titers of the hormone (16). In the absence of steroid priming, no effect was
observed in ovariectomized animals or in animals with intact ovaries on
estrus or on day 1 of diestrus. On day 2 of diestrus and on proestrus, a positive response was observed. It appears that the steroid background is
important in determining the response to dopamine, and estrogen sensitization
may be required in order to provoke LH release. In males, a relatively small
release of LH was observed with dopamine in our experiments. Porter et al.
(17, 18) obtained release of both FSH and LH in males; however, they have
not been able to confirm these results in later studies. In all of these experiments, norepinephrine was less active than dopamine and epinephrine was
the least active catecholamine. In contrast to these results, Rubinstein and
Sawyer (19) reported that epinephrine was the most effective catecholamine
in inducing ovulation on the afternoon of proestrus when injected into the
ventricle.

The third ventricular injection of the catecholamines appears to increase
release of FSH and LH by stimulating a discharge of gonadotropin-releasing
factors since dopamine increased FSH- and LH-releasing activity in portal
blood (17) and LH-releasing activity in peripheral blood of hypophysectomized rats (20).

The dopaminergic release of LRF in hypophysectomized rats was blocked
by the prior administration of estradiol into the third ventricle, suggesting
that negative feedback of estrogen might act to block the dopaminergic release of LRF (20). A similar effect of estrogen in blocking dopaminergic
release of LRF had been previously demonstrated in vitro (21). In that
situation the blockade could be reversed by incubation in the presence of
puromycin or cyclohexamide to inhibit protein synthesis, which suggested the
possibility that protein synthesis was required for the block to become effective. This led us to the concept that estrogen negative feedback might be
mediated at least partially by uptake of the steroid by hypothalamic cells and
its transport to the nucleus where RNA synthesis would be altered, leading

to the production of an inhibitory peptide or protein which then blocks the response to dopamine.

Similar injections of dopamine were capable of lowering plasma prolactin in normal male rats (17), lactating females (22), and ovariectomized estrogen-primed animals (23). In males this was accompanied by increased prolactin-inhibiting activity in portal blood. Norepinephrine, on the other hand, was ineffective.

Effects of Drugs Blocking Catecholamine Receptors or Altering Catecholamine Synthesis on Gonadotropin and Prolactin Release

Studies with these drugs have lent further support for the concept of a dopaminergic inhibitory control over prolactin release. For example, subcutaneous administration of the dopamine receptor blocker pimozide induced a dramatic elevation in plasma prolactin titers in ovariectomized rats (24), whereas the dopamine receptor stimulator apomorphine drastically lowered prolactin when injected into the third ventricle (23). Intraperitoneal administration of L-DOPA, which would be expected to elevate hypothalamic catecholamine stores, produced the expected decrease in prolactin (25). On the other hand, when catecholamine synthesis was blocked using α-methyl-p-tyrosine, there was a dramatic elevation in serum prolactin and this could be reversed by the administration of L-DOPA to reinitiate dopamine synthesis, but not by the administration of dihydroxyphenylserine (DOPS) to reinitiate only norepinephrine synthesis. In the latter instance there actually was a further rise in prolactin. The administration of DOPS alone also elevated prolactin, suggesting that an artificial elevation in norepinephrine could elevate release of prolactin. On the other hand, when diethyldithiocarbamate (DDC), an inhibitor of dopamine-β-oxidase, was given to block norepinephrine synthesis selectively, there was no effect on prolactin, which appears to indicate that norepinephrine does not have an essential role in the control of this hormone. Pargyline, to inhibit monoamine oxidase, led to a suppression of prolactin, as would be expected because of the increased amounts of central monoamines, including dopamine, whereas reserpine, to deplete monoamines such as catecholamines and serotonin, led to the expected increase. Thus there was an inverse correlation between the expected effects of the various drugs on brain dopamine levels and activity on the one hand, and plasma prolactin on the other (Table 1).

Further studies have been performed in an attempt to localize the site of the dopaminergic inhibitory control over prolactin. Rather surprisingly, when L-DOPA was administered to animals with median eminence lesions whose central nervous system control of prolactin was presumably eliminated, as indicated by high serum prolactin levels, there was a decrease in prolactin (26). This has also been observed in humans with stalk section (27). It is likely that in this situation, L-DOPA is taken up by the anterior pituitary cells

TABLE 1. *Effect of drugs altering monoamine activity on plasma prolactin*

Drug	Expected effect on monoamine activity			Effect on plasma prolactin
	DA	NE	5-HT	
Reserpine	$-^a$	−	−	+
α-MT	−	−	0	+
p-CPA	0	0	−	0
p-CPA + α-MT	−	−	−	+
Pargyline	+	+	+	−
α-MT + DOPA	0	0	0	0
DDC	0	−	0	0
DDC + DOPA	+	−	0	−
DDC + DOPS	0	$-,0^b$	0	0
DOPA	+	+	0	−
DOPS	0	+	0	+
Pimozide	−	0	0	+

^{a} − = decrease; + = increase; 0 = no change.
^{b} −.0 = decreased followed by return toward normal.
Modified from *Gonadotropins*, edited by B. Saxena, C. Beling, and H. Gandy, p. 49. Wiley-Interscience, New York, 1972.

and converted by DOPA decarboxylase into dopamine, which acts directly on the lactotrophs to decrease prolactin output. This is in keeping with the ability of dopamine to decrease prolactin release when incubated with pituitaries *in vitro*.

In recent studies pimozide has been implanted in either the hypothalamus or the anterior pituitary to determine its effects on plasma prolactin in ovariectomized rats (24). Implantation of the dopamine receptor blocker in the median eminence led to a rapid rise in plasma prolactin, whereas implants in the anterior hypothalamic area were ineffective. To our surprise, implants of the drug into the anterior pituitary itself were also associated with a small increase in plasma prolactin, which suggests that dopamine may in fact be released into portal vessels and pass down to the pituitary to inhibit prolactin release by a direct action on the gland. Since the effect of median eminence implants of pimozide was much greater than that of anterior pituitary implants of the drug, we believe that the median eminence implants of pimozide were blocking the release of PIF. Thus it would appear possible that dopamine has a dual action on prolactin release, the more important one stimulating PIF release from the median eminence, the less important one inhibiting prolactin release from the pituitary directly. The anatomic relationships are certainly consistent with a release of dopamine into portal vessels, since the dopaminergic terminals appear to end in the external layer of the median eminence in juxtaposition to the portal capillaries (10). So far, attempts to detect dopamine in portal vessel blood have failed (28), but this may be a reflection of the insensitivity of the methods used.

Studies with receptor blockers and drugs which modify catecholamine synthesis have also provided further support for a role of catecholamines in the regulation of gonadotropin release. We have evaluated the effects of these drugs in several situations. The first of these was to remove the gonads and measure the castration-induced increase in FSH and LH release as reflected in higher titers of circulating gonadotropins (29). In this experimental model, α-receptor blockers were effective in preventing the postcastration rise in gonadotropins (Table 2). The dopamine receptor blocker pimozide decreased the response of FSH but not LH to castration. Drugs which blocked catecholamine synthesis were effective in blocking the postcastration rise in gonadotropins, and there was partial reversal of the block when catecholamine synthesis was reinitiated with either DOPA or DOPS. Blockade of norepinephrine synthesis with DDC blocked the postcastration response of LH but not FSH; this blockade could be partially reversed by DOPS to reinitiate norepinephrine synthesis but not by DOPA, which would have increased only dopamine synthesis in this situation. These results are consistent with a role for both dopamine and norepinephrine in eliciting the postcastration rise in FSH and with a role for norepinephrine in the elevation in LH.

The effects of these drugs on the release of FSH and LH provoked by progesterone or estrogen were studied in ovariectomized, estrogen-primed rats. In these situations the evidence points clearly to a role for norepinephrine as a possible synaptic transmitter mediating the stimulatory effects of both steroids. The α-receptor blocker phentolamine blocked the stimulation of gonadotropin release induced by either progesterone or estrogen (30, 31). Blockade of catecholamine synthesis with α-methyl-p-tyrosine or of norepinephrine synthesis with DDC or U-14624, another dopamine oxidase inhibitor, also blocked progesterone- or estrogen-induced FSH and LH release. Reversal of the blockade of norepinephrine synthesis resulted in a reversal of the block of progesterone-induced gonadotropin release; however, in the case of estrogen, the reversal of the blockade when norepinephrine synthesis was reinitiated was not as striking. Furthermore, in this situation, there was some indication of inhibition by β-blocking drugs such as propranolol which had had no effect on the response to castration or on progesterone-induced gonadotropin release.

An attempt was then made to block the normal preovulatory discharge in adult rats with normal estrous cycles. Large doses of either α-methyl-p-tyrosine to block both dopamine and norepinephrine synthesis or DDC to block only norepinephrine synthesis were capable of blocking the preovulatory discharge of LH and ovulation; however, attempts to reverse the blockade with the administration of DOPA or DOPS were unsuccessful (32). Some success in reversing the block was obtained in these animals if they were also primed with progesterone to evoke a supernormal LH release on the afternoon of proestrus.

In order to localize the site of the presumed noradrenergic synapse in-

TABLE 2. Effect of drugs altering monoamine activity on the increase in gonadotropins in response to various stimuli

Drug	Expected effect on monoamine activity			EFFECT ON INCREASE IN GONADOTROPINS IN RESPONSE TO:							
				Castration (males)		Estrogen-primed				Preovulatory	Preoptic stimulation
						+ progesterone		+ estrogen			
	DA	NE	5-HT	FSH	LH	FSH	LH	FSH	LH	LH	LH
Phenoxybenzamine	0	−(α)	0	−	−	−	−	−	−	nt	nt
Haloperidol	−	−	0	nt	nt	−	−	−	−	nt	nt
Pronethalol or propranolol	0	−(β)	0	0	0	0	0	nt	−	nt	nt
Pimozide	−	0	0	−	0	nt	nt	nt	nt	nt	nt
α-MT	−	−	0	−	−	−	−	−	−	−	−
α-MT + DOPA	r	r	0	r	r	r	−	r	r	−	R
α-MT + DOPS	−	r	0	r	r	R	r	r	r	−	R
DDC	0	−	0	0	−	−	−	−	−	−	−
DDC + DOPA	+	−	0	0	−	R	R	−	−	−	−
DDC + DOPS	0	r	0	0	r	−	−	r	r	−	r
U-14624	0	−	0	nt	nt	R	R	r	−	nt	r
U-14624 + DOPS	0	r	0	nt	nt	R	R	r	r	nt	nt
p-CPA	0	0	−	0	0	0	0	nt	nt	nt	nt
Reserpine	−	−	−	nt	−	nt	nt	nt	nt	−	nt

R = complete restoration; r = partial restoration; 0 = no effect; − = decrease; nt = not tested.
Table modified from McCann, S. M., Ojeda, S. R., Fawcett, C. P., and Krulich, L. In: Advances in Neurology, Vol. 5; Second Canadian-American Conference on Parkinson's Disease, edited by F. McDowell and A. Barbeau, p. 441. Raven Press, New York, 1974.

volved in positive feedback of gonadal steroids, preoptic stimulation was performed and the effects of blockade of catecholamine synthesis on the discharge of LH was evaluated. In this situation either α-methyl-p-tyrosine to block catecholamine synthesis or DDC to block norepinephrine synthesis was capable of blocking the increase in plasma LH from preoptic stimulation; the blockade could be reversed in the case of α-methyl-p-tyrosine by either DOPA or DOPS, and in the case of DDC, only with DOPS to reinitiate norepinephrine synthesis (33). On the other hand, the blocking drugs did not alter the response to stimulation of the median eminence-arcuate region. In the latter instance we were presumably stimulating LRF-secreting neurons directly. These results were interpreted as indicating the presence of noradrenergic synapses in the preoptic-anterior hypothalamic region, a conclusion consistent with the demonstration of noradrenergic terminals in the region (10). Increased impulse traffic across these noradrenergic synapses is postulated to trigger increased LRF release from LRF neurons in response to estrogen or progesterone stimulation and, on the afternoon of proestrus, in response to the endogenous steroid environment.

Consistent with this concept is the increased turnover of norepinephrine in the anterior hypothalamus on the afternoon of proestrus (34). On the other hand, a dopaminergic synapse located in the arcuate-median eminence region may be involved in the discharge of gonadotropin-releasing factors as well. The evidence from the studies with the blocking drugs suggests that the noradrenergic synapse may be more important than the dopaminergic one with respect to gonadotropic release.

The Possible Role of Serotonin and Melatonin in the Regulation of Gonadotropin and Prolactin Release

Serotonin has been shown to inhibit gonadotropin and to stimulate prolactin release in several studies. In ovariectomized rats, for example, the intraventricular injection of serotonin caused a precipitous decline in plasma LH (16); however, no effects have been observed in our laboratory with p-chlorophenylalanine, the inhibitor of serotonin synthesis, thus casting doubt on the physiologic significance of serotonin in the control of the release of these hormones (25). In a recent paper, Kordon and Sawyer and associates (35) reported that p-chlorophenylalanine could block the suckling-induced rise of prolactin, which suggests that serotonin may be involved in mediating this increase in prolactin release.

The pineal hormone, melatonin, has an effect similar to serotonin. That is, it stimulates prolactin and inhibits gonadotropin release, apparently by hypothalamic action (17). We have recently observed that pinealectomy blocks the early morning discharge of prolactin which occurs in male rats (36) and in general leads to lower levels of the hormone than are found in intact animals, which suggests a role of the pineal in the control of prolactin release.

The effects of pinealectomy on gonadotropin release, by contrast, have been quite small.

The Possible Participation of Cholinergic Synapses in Gonadotropin and Prolactin Release

The early studies of Sawyer and collaborators (37) indicated that subcutaneous injections of atropine could block gonadotropin release. We have recently restudied this phenomenon and found that subcutaneous or intraventricular atropine can block the preovulatory discharge of gonadotropins and prolactin and can inhibit the postcastration rise of gonadotropins (38). Studies with cholinergic agonists such as pilocarpine and carbachol, on the other hand, have shown immediate inhibition of gonadotropin and prolactin release in estrogen-primed ovariectomized females (39). There is a discharge about 6 hr after this initial inhibition, at the time of the preovulatory release in intact rats. Thus the results are inconsistent and the role of acetylcholine remains to be elucidated.

The Possible Role of Prostaglandins in Mediating Gonadotropin and Prolactin Release

Inhibitors of prostaglandin synthesis can block ovulation, but there has been controversy as to the locus of action. In recent studies from our laboratory, it has been possible to show that injection of prostaglandins into the third ventricle can alter gonadotropin and prolactin release. Prostaglandin E_1 elevated prolactin release by inhibiting the release of prolactin-inhibiting factor (40) or, alternatively, perhaps by stimulating prolactin-releasing factor discharge. On the other hand, prostaglandin E_2 caused a discharge of LH, apparently by stimulating the release of LRF. There was a much smaller release of FSH. Prostaglandin F_{1a} and F_{2a} were without effect.

If the animals were primed with estrogen, prostaglandin E_2 was still the most potent in discharging LH, but a stimulatory effect of E_1 could also be demonstrated (41). This is in accord with the recent results obtained by Spies and Norman (42), who found that prostaglandin E_1 could increase LH release on the afternoon of proestrus, a situation in which the animal is under the influence of estrogen.

A small increase in plasma prolactin and LH has been found following the intrapituitary injection of prostaglandins E_1 and E_2, respectively. These responses were much smaller than those obtained from the intraventricular injection of the agents; consequently, in view of the limited distribution of intraventricularly injected substances to the pituitary, we believe that prostaglandins have two sites of action. They can provoke releasing factor discharge when administered into the ventricle, and they can also increase hormone release when administered into the pituitary. These results are in agreement with earlier *in vitro* studies showing that prostaglandins could markedly increase the cyclic AMP content in the anterior pituitary.

Possible Role of Cyclic Nucleotides in the Control of PIF Release

In other studies, third ventricle injections of cyclic AMP or dibutyryl cyclic AMP have been shown to result in a lowering of plasma prolactin levels, whereas similar injections in the pituitary were without effect (43). It appears that cyclic AMP may be involved as a second messenger to control the release of PIF, perhaps mediating the response to dopaminergic input. Only high doses of the cyclic nucleotide which were associated with behavioral changes discharged LH.

The Effect of Morphine on the Release of Gonadotropins and Prolactin

The early studies of Barraclough and Sawyer (44) demonstrated that morphine could block ovulation in the rat. To our surprise, the microinjection of morphine into the third ventricle of conscious, ovariectomized, estrogen-primed rats provoked a dramatic increase in prolactin release (23). This contrasted sharply with the decline induced by apomorphine at a similar dose. Even though morphine had a dramatic effect on prolactin release, it failed to modify the release of FSH and LH in these animals, presumably because it was already inhibited by estrogen. The rats injected with morphine exhibited rigidity and the Straub tail sign (45).

CONCLUSIONS

1. Prolactin appears to be under inhibitory dopaminergic control via the tuberoinfundibular dopaminergic pathway.

2. The inhibitory control appears to be mediated primarily by stimulation of PIF discharge, but dopamine released into portal vessels may directly inhibit pituitary prolactin release.

3. Elevation of hypothalamic norepinephrine may stimulate prolactin release.

4. Serotonin and melatonin can stimulate prolactin release.

5. Pineal ablation eliminates an early morning rise in prolactin in the male rat, which may be a reflection of melatonin deficiency.

6. Morphine injected into the third ventricle stimulates prolactin release.

7. Gonadotropin release appears to be under catecholaminergic control and there is evidence for a role for both dopamine and norepinephrine to release LRF.

8. The positive feedback of gonadal steroids may be mediated via increased impulse traffic across a noradrenergic synapse in the preoptic-anterior hypothalamic area which triggers LRF release.

9. Dopamine and norepinephrine may be involved in mediating negative feedback of gonadal steroids on gonadotropin release.

10. Indoles such as melatonin and serotonin can inhibit gonadotropin release by an action on the hypothalamus.

ACKNOWLEDGMENTS

This research was supported by grants from the National Institutes of Health (AM 10073 and HD 05151), Ford Foundation, and Texas Population Research Institute.

REFERENCES

1. McCann, S. M. Regulation of the secretion of follicle stimulating hormone (FSH) and luteinizing hormone (LH). In: *Handbook of Physiology,* edited by E. B. Astwood and R. O. Greep, American Physiological Society, Bethesda, Md. (*in press*).
2. Kalra, S. P., Ajika, K., Krulich, L., Fawcett, C. P., Quijada, M., and McCann, S. M. Effect of hypothalamic and preoptic electrochemical stimulation on gonadotropin and prolactin release in proestrous rats. *Endocrinology,* 88:1150–1158, 1971.
3. Bishop, W., Kalra, P. S. Fawcett, C. P., Krulich, L., and McCann, S. M. The effects of hypothalamic lesions on the release of gonadotropins and prolactin in response to estrogen and progesterone treatment in female rats. *Endocrinology,* 91:1404–1410, 1972.
4. Libertun, C., Orias, R., and McCann, S. M. Biphasic effect of estrogen on the sensitivity of the pituitary to luteinizing hormone releasing factor (LRF). *Endocrinology,* 94:1094–1100, 1974.
5. Bishop, W., Fawcett, C. P., Krulich, L., and McCann, S. M. Acute and chronic effects of hypothalamic lesions on the release of FSH, LH and prolactin in intact and castrated rats. *Endocrinology,* 91:643–656, 1972.
6. Meites, J., Lu, K. H., Wuttke, W., Welsch, C. W., Nagasawa, H., and Quadri, S. K. Recent studies on functions and control of prolactin secretion in rats. *Rec. Progr. Horm. Res.,* 28:471–526, 1972.
7. Krulich, L., Quijada, M., Illner, P., and McCann, S. M. The distribution of hypothalamic hypophysiotropic factors in the hypothalamus of the rat. *XXV Intl. Cong. Physiol. Sci.,* 9:326, 1971 (abstract).
8. Schneider, H. P. G., Crighton, D. B., and McCann, S. M. Suprachiasmatic LH-releasing factor. *Neuroendocrinology,* 5:271–280, 1969.
9. Barry, J., Dubois, M. P., Poulain, P., and Leonardelli, J. Caracterisation et topographie des neurones hypothalamiques immunoreactifs avec des anticorps anti-LRF de synthese. *C.R. Acad. Sci. D* (Paris) 276:3191–3193, 1973.
10. Fuxe, K., and Hokfelt, T. Catecholamines in the hypothalamus and the pituitary gland. In: *Frontiers in Neuroendocrinology,* edited by W. F. Ganong and L. Martini, p. 47. Oxford, New York, 1969.
11. Schute, C. C. D. Distribution of cholinesterase and cholinergic pathways. In: *The Hypothalamus,* edited by L. Martini, M. Motta, and F. Fraschini, pp. 167–179. Academic Press, New York, 1970.
12. Schneider, H. P. G., and McCann, S. M. Possible role of dopamine as transmitter to promote discharge of LH-releasing factor. *Endocrinology,* 85:121–132, 1969.

13. Kamberi, I. A., Schneider, H. P. G., and McCann, S. M. Action of dopamine to induce release of FSH-releasing factor (FRF) from hypothalamic tissue *in vitro. Endocrinology*, 86:278–284, 1970.
14. Quijada, M., Illner, P., Krulich, L., and McCann, S. M. The effect of catecholamines on hormone release from anterior pituitaries and ventral hypothalami incubated *in vitro. Neuroendocrinology*, 13:151–163, 1973/74.
15. MacLeod, R. M. Influence of norepinephrine and catecholamine-depleting agents on the synthesis and release of prolactin and growth hormone. *Endocrinology*, 85:916–923, 1969.
16. Schneider, H. P. G., and McCann, S. M. Mono- and indolamines and control of LH secretion. *Endocrinology*, 86:1127–1133, 1970.
17. Porter, J. C., Kamberi, I. A., and Ondo, J. G. Role of biogenic amines and cerebrospinal fluid in the neurovascular transmittal of hypophysiotropic substances. In: *Brain-Endocrine Interaction. Median Eminence: Structure and Function,* edited by K. M. Knigge, D. E. Scott, and A. Weindl, p. 245. Karger, Basel, 1972.
18. Cramer, O., and Porter, J. C. Input to releasing factor cells. In: *Progress in Brain Research,* Vol. 39: *Drug Effects on Neuroendocrine Regulation,* edited by E. Zimmermann, W H. Gispen, B. H. Marks, and D. de Wied, pp. 73–85. Elsevier, New York, 1973.
19. Rubenstein, L., and Sawyer, C. H. Role of catecholamines in stimulating the release of pituitary ovulating hormones in rat. *Endocrinology*, 86:980–995, 1970.
20. Schneider, H. P. G., and McCann, S. M. Release of LRF into the peripheral circulation of hypophysectomized rats by dopamine and its blockade by estradiol. *Endocrinology*, 87:249–253, 1970.
21. Schneider, H. P. G., and McCann, S. M. Estradiol and the neuroendocrine control of LH release *in vitro. Endocrinology*, 87:330–338, 1970.
22. Kuhn, E., Krulich, L., Quijada, M., Illner, P., Kalra, P. S., and McCann, S. M. Effect of oxytocin and adrenergic agents on prolactin release *in vivo* and *in vitro. Prog. 52nd Endo. Soc. Mtg.,* 1970, p. 126 (abstract).
23. Ojeda, S. R., Harms, P. G., and McCann, S. M. Possible role of cyclic AMP and prostaglandin E₁ in the dopaminergic control of prolactin release. *Endocrinology* (*in press*).
24. Ojeda, S. R., Harms, P. G., and McCann, S. M. Effect of blockade of dopaminergic receptors on prolactin and LH release: Median eminence and pituitary sites of action. *Endocrinology*, 94:1650, 1974.
25. Donoso, A. O., Bishop, W., Fawcett, C. P., and McCann, S. M. Effects of drugs that modify brain monoamine concentrations on plasma gonadotropin and prolactin levels in the rat. *Endocrinology*, 89:774–784, 1971.
26. Donoso, A. O., Bishop, W., and McCann, S. M. The effects of drugs which modify catecholamine synthesis on serum prolactin in rats with median eminence lesions. *Proc. Soc. Exp. Biol. Med.,* 143:360–363, 1973.
27. Frantz, A. G. Catecholamines and the control of prolactin secretion in humans. In: *Progress in Brain Research,* Vol. 39: *Drug Effects on Neuroendocrine Regulation,* edited by E. Zimmermann, W. H. Gispen, G. H. Marks, and D. de Wied, pp. 311–321. Elsevier, New York, 1973.
28. Ruf, K. B., Dreifuss, J. J., and Carr, P. J. Absence of measurable amounts of epinephrine, norepinephrine and dopamine in rat hypophysial portal blood during the various phases of the oestrous cycle. *J. Neuro-Visceral Rel.,* Suppl. X:65, 1971.
29. Ojeda, S. R., and McCann, S. M. Evidence for participation of a catecholaminergic mechanism in the post-castration rise in plasma gonadotropins. *Neuroendocrinology*, 12:295–315, 1973.
30. Kalra, P. S., Kalra, S. P., Krulich, L., Fawcett, C. P., and McCann, S. M. Involvement of norepinephrine in transmission of the stimulatory influence of progesterone on gonadotropin release. *Endocrinology*, 90:1168–1176, 1972.
31. Kalra, P. S., and McCann, S. M. Involvement of catecholamines in feedback mechanisms. In: *Progress in Brain Research,* Vol. 39: *Drug Effects on Neuroendocrine Regulation,* edited by E. Zimmermann, W. H. Gispen, B. H. Marks, and D. de Wied, pp. 185–198. Elsevier, New York, 1973.

32. Kalra, S. P., and McCann, S. M. Effects of drugs modifying catecholamine synthesis on plasma LH and ovulation in the rat. *Neuroendocrinology (in press)*.
33. Kalra, S. P., and McCann, S. M. Variations in the release of LH in response to electrochemical stimulation of preoptic area and of medial basal hypothalamus during the estrous cycle of the rat. *Endocrinology*, 93:665–669, 1973.
34. Donoso, A. O., and de Gutierrez Moyano, M. B. Adrenergic activity in hypothalamus and ovulation. *Proc. Soc. Exp. Biol. Med.*, 135:633–635, 1970.
35. Kordon, C., Blake, C. A., Terkel, J., and Sawyer, C. H. Participation of serotonin-containing neurons in the suckling-induced rise in plasma prolactin levels in lactating rats. *Neuroendocrinology*, 13:213–223, 1973/74.
36. Rønnekleiv, O., Krulich, L., and McCann, S. M. An early morning surge of prolactin in the male rat and its abolition by pinealectomy. *Endocrinology*, 92: 1339–1342, 1973.
37. Sawyer, C. H., Critchlow, B. V., and Barraclough, C. A. Mechanism of blockade of pituitary activation in the rat by morphine, atropine and barbiturates. *Endocrinology*, 57:345–354, 1955.
38. Libertun, C., and McCann, S. M. Blockade of the release of gonadotropins and prolactin by subcutaneous or intraventricular injection of atropine in male and female rats. *Endocrinology*, 92:1714–1724, 1973.
39. Libertun, C. Pharmacological evidence for a cholinergic mechanism controlling LH and prolactin secretion. *Program 55th Endo. Soc. Mtg.* 1973, 384(abs).
40. Harms, P. G., Ojeda, S. R., and McCann, S. M. Prostaglandin involvement in hypothalamic control of gonadotropin and prolactin release. *Science*, 181:760–761, 1973.
41. Harms, P. G., Ojeda, S. R. and McCann, S. M. Prostaglandin-induced release of pituitary gonadotropins: Central nervous system and pituitary sites of action. *Endocrinology*, 94:1459, 1974.
42. Spies, H. G., and Norman, R. L. *Prostaglandins*, 3:461, 1973.
43. Ojeda, S. R., Krulich, L., and McCann, S. M. Effect of intraventricular injection of cyclic AMP on plasma prolactin and LH levels of ovariectomized, estrogen-treated rats. *Neuroendocrinology (in press)*.
44. Barraclough, C. A., and Sawyer, C. H. Induction of pseudopregnancy in the rat by reserpine and chlorpromazine. *Endocrinology*, 65:563–571, 1959.
45. Kerr, F. W. L., and Pozuelo, J. Suppression of physical dependence and induction of hypersensitivity to morphine by stereotaxic hypothalamic lesions in addicted rats. *Mayo Clin. Proc.*, 46:653–665, 1971.

REMARKS: C. H. SAWYER*

Dr. McCann has mentioned our work published nearly 20 years ago with Barraclough (1) in which we blocked ovulation in the cyclic rat by treating the proestrous animal with morphine sulfate (20 to 50 mg/kg, s.c.) prior to its 2 to 4 p.m. "critical period" (during which "spontaneous" neurogenous stimulation of release of an ovulating surge of gonadotropin occurs). By withholding injection until 4 p.m. we found that even the larger dose was completely ineffective in blocking the ovulation that was to occur early the next morning. We observed that ovulation-blocking dosages of morphine as well as atropine and pentobarbital induced high-amplitude slow waves in the hypothalamic EEG record (2), and that the threshold of EEG arousal was elevated by these drugs. We proposed, therefore, that the critical site of blockade might lie in the reticular formation (2). We later noted with Khazan (3)

---

* Department of Anatomy, UCLA School of Medicine, Los Angeles, California 90024

that in the rabbit these three drugs delayed transmission of evoked potentials between midbrain and cerebral cortex, apparently confirming our proposal. However, we found that ovulation-inducing electrical stimulation of the medial amygdala or even the basal hypothalamus was blocked in the rabbit by atropine, pentobarbital, or morphine unless the stimulating electrode impinged on the median eminence itself, suggesting that the critical blocking site lay in basal hypothalamic synapses (4). Later, in rabbit electrical stimulation and recording experiments, we found that a rhinencephalic-hypothalamic "EEG-afterreaction" threshold was even more sensitive to these drugs than was the reticular system's "EEG-arousal" threshold (5, 6). The EEG afterreaction includes a phase of paradoxical sleep, and Dr. Kawakami, who collaborated in the rabbit-recording experiments, later reported with his Japanese colleagues (7) that morphine blocks paradoxical sleep at a dosage which does not affect EEG arousal. Our results have confirmed the wide diversity in sites of drug action on the brain, but suggest that neuroendocrine effects may be exerted most critically at basal hypothalamic-median eminence synapses of rhinencephalic and/or hypothalamic neurons.

1. Barraclough, C. A., and Sawyer, C. H. Inhibition of the release of pituitary ovulatory hormone in the rat by morphine. *Endocrinology*, 57:329–337, 1955.
2. Sawyer, C. H., Critchlow, B. V., and Barraclough, C. A. Mechanism of blockade of pituitary activation in the rat by morphine, atropine and barbiturates. *Endocrinology*, 57:345–354, 1955.
3. Khazan, N., and Sawyer, C. H. Mechanisms of paradoxical sleep as revealed by neurophysiologic and pharmacologic approaches in the rabbit. *Psychopharmacologia*, 5:457–466, 1964.
4. Sawyer, C. H. Neuroendocrine blocking agents and gonadotropin release. In: *Advances in Neuroendocrinology*, edited by A. V. Nalbandov, pp. 444–459. University of Illinois Press, Urbana, 1963.
5. Sawyer, C. H. Blockade of the release of gonadotrophic hormones by pharmacologic agents. *Proceedings of the Second International Congress of Endocrinology*, Int. Congr. Ser. No. 83, pp. 629–634. Excerpta Medica, 1964.
6. Sawyer, C. H., Kawakami, M., and Kanematsu, S. Neuroendocrine aspects of reproduction. In: *Endocrines and the Central Nervous System, Res. Publ. Assn. Res. Nerv. Ment. Dis.*, 43:59–85, 1966.
7. Kawakami, M., Negoro, H., and Takahashi, T. Neuropharmacological studies on the mechanisms of paradoxical sleep. *Japan. J. Physiol.*, 16:667–683, 1966.

DISCUSSION

Brazeau: In your localization studies did you find TRF activity in the same region in which you found prolactin-releasing activity?

McCann: That is a very interesting question since we know that TRF has some prolactin-releasing activity as, for example, in the estrogen-primed rat. In our localization studies we assayed various activities using hemipituitaries from male rats, and under these conditions there is no correlation between TRF activity and prolactin-releasing activity.

de Wied: Regarding the effects of DOPS, that is, dihydroxyphenylserine, do you see any effects in non-pretreated animals?

McCann: In his initial studies, Dr. Donoso in our laboratory observed an increase in prolactin secretion following systemic administration of DOPS.

de Wied: Dr. Ganong, would you comment on the effects of DOPS on ACTH secretion? In other words, does increasing the norepinephrine pool increase the noradrenergic inhibition of ACTH secretion?

Ganong: We find that administration of DOPS alone has very little effect. I would remind you that DOPS, like L-Dopa, is an amino acid and has many complex effects, as well as direct effects on norepinephrine.

Marks: I don't think we can say that the norephinephrine-secreting neurons are the only ones which convert the DOPS to norepinephrine.

McCann: I certainly agree. It is known that L-Dopa is taken up by capillaries in the hypothalamus and is converted right there into dopamine. In view of this effect, what, in fact, is the meaning of the measurement of hypothalamic levels of dopamine? Certainly the available methodology is full of pitfalls.

Zimmermann: We recently obtained evidence that rather large doses of morphine in the neighborhood of 40 to 60 mg/kg intraperitoneally will suppress the preovulatory surge in plasma LH and FSH levels in the female rat. Also, administration of 40 mg/kg of morphine intraperitoneally stimulated plasma prolactin levels in the male rat. Thus, under appropriate circumstances, systemic administration of large doses of morphine will inhibit LH and FSH secretion and stimulate prolactin secretion.

Narcotics and the Hypothalamus, edited by
E. Zimmermann and R. George. Raven Press,
New York © 1974

Effects of Narcotic Analgesics, Anesthetics, and Hypothalamic Lesions on Growth Hormone and Adrenocorticotropic Hormone Secretion in Rats

Norio Kokka and Robert George

Department of Medical Pharmacology and Therapeutics, California College of Medicine, University of California, Irvine 92664, and Department of Pharmacology, Center for Health Sciences and Brain Research Institute, University of California, Los Angeles, California 90024

Numerous studies in man and subhuman primates have shown that several regulatory systems enhance growth hormone (GH) secretion in response to stress, exercise, hypoglycemia, administration of arginine, and during slow-wave sleep. Many of the procedures that cause an increase in plasma GH concentration also stimulate ACTH secretion, but in comparison with the considerable data on regulation of ACTH secretion by the central nervous system (CNS), relatively little information is available regarding CNS control of GH secretion.

In contrast to the findings in man, radioimmunoassay data from this and other laboratories have shown that various procedures which cause a rise in concentration of plasma corticosterone simultaneously produce a fall of plasma GH in rats (1–4). Elevation of plasma GH concentrations is reported to occur following gentling (1), administration of pentobarbital (3, 6) or morphine (4–7), and electrical stimulation of the ventromedial nucleus (VMN) of the hypothalamus (8–11). Our results with gentling and CNS depressants suggested that GH secretion in rats may be stimulated by a mechanism similar to the one responsible for the rise in plasma GH concentration in man during deep sleep, and that increased or decreased GH secretion could be due to suppression or activation of a central inhibitory mechanism (1). However, the rise of plasma GH concentration following electrical stimulation of the VMN region reported by Bernardis and Frohman (9), and later confirmed and extended by Martin and associates (10, 11), suggested that GH secretion was augmented by increased secretion of a GH-releasing factor (GRF). Krulich et al. (12) assayed extracts prepared from hypothalamic sections and found that GRF activity was located in the VMN or its immediate vicinity while GH inhibiting factor (GIF) was distributed mainly in the median eminence, with a small amount in the rostral hypothalamus.

Hypothalamic extracts which produced marked increases in plasma GH concentration in monkeys were reported to lack similar effects in rats (2). However, Malacara et al. (13) recently reported increases of plasma GH concentrations after injection of hypothalamic extract in rats sensitized with estrogen, and attributed the failure to stimulate GH secretion in other experiments to the use of inadequate doses of hypothalamic extract. Also, Frohman et al. (14) reported that hypothalamic extract injected directly into the pituitary had similar effects on plasma GH. On the other hand, the recent purification, characterization, and synthesis of a hypothalamic peptide, somatostatin (15), that inhibits GH secretion lend strong support to the hypothesis that an inhibitory mechanism plays an important role in the regulation of GH secretion (16).

Current evidence indicates that GH secretion is under dual hypothalamic control. Numerous studies have shown that ACTH secretion also is governed by excitatory and inhibitory systems (17, 18), and neurochemical findings have in addition led to the proposal of adrenergic-inhibitory and/or cholinergic-stimulatory regulation of ACTH secretion (19–21). Morphine is known to have a dual action on the nervous system that is mainly dose-dependent. Acute administration of morphine in rats stimulates both ACTH (22–24) and GH secretion (4). Chronic administration of morphine is reported to produce inhibition or tolerance to its effects on ACTH secretion (25), but not to its stimulant action on GH secretion (7). Most of the available evidence indicates that morphine activation of ACTH secretion is mediated via a direct action on the rostral regions of the hypothalamus and median eminence (26–28), although extrahypothalamic sites and peripheral mechanisms cannot be excluded. The central sites involved in the morphine-induced rise in plasma GH concentration are not known, and therefore a direct stimulant action on the pituitary remains a possibility at this time.

This paper describes experiments that were performed to determine whether the stimulant effects of morphine on GH and ACTH secretion could be dissociated with hypothalamic lesions. The effects of pentobarbital were also determined because this anesthetic is known to stimulate GH secretion (3–5) and to inhibit the ACTH response to mild stress (29). The effects of acute and chronic administration of morphine on GH and ACTH secretion are also described, as well as the effects of stress in rats chronically treated with morphine.

MATERIALS AND METHODS

Only male Sprague-Dawley rats weighing 200 to 300 g were used in these studies. To minimize variations of plasma corticosterone associated with room transfer or circadian rhythm, the rats were kept in the laboratory overnight to adapt to their new surroundings, and all experiments were performed between 8:00 and 12:00 A.M. Rats were fasted 16 to 18 hr but were allowed water ad libitum prior to use in this study.

Drugs were administered intraperitoneally in doses calculated as the free base. Except as noted otherwise (see Results and Discussion), blood was collected after decapitation with a guillotine in heparinized beakers at 30, 60, and 120 min postinjection. One-tenth milliliter was removed for determination of blood glucose (30), the remainder was centrifuged in tubes, and plasma separated immediately and stored at $-15°C$. Plasma GH was measured as described previously with a double antibody radioimmunoassay system (2). ACTH secretion was determined indirectly by fluorometric measurement of plasma corticosterone (31). For the chronic studies, rats were injected subcutaneously twice daily at 8:00 to 8:30 A.M. and 4:30 to 5:00 P.M.

Bilateral electrolytic lesions were placed stereotactically in the anterior (A-L), ventromedial nucleus (V-L), and posterior (P-L) regions of the hypothalamus. The de Groot coordinates (mm) used for electrode placement were the following: A-L (A-P, 6.6–6.8; L, 1.0; H, −2.0), V-L (A-P, 5.6–5.8; L, 0.7; H, −3.5), and P-L (A-P, 4.4–4.6; L, 0.7; H, −3.0). The electrode was made from 26-gauge, 90% platinum-10% iridium wire insulated to within 0.7 mm of the tip. The lesions were produced with an anodal current of 2 mA applied for 15 sec under sodium pentobarbital anesthesia. Sham-operated animals were treated identically except for the passage of current. In all cases the animals were not used for a postoperative period of 5 days.

The lesion sites were determined in serial sections of hypothalamus stained by the Nissl method after fixation in formalin. Localization and size of lesions for each rat were marked on individual diagrams and later plotted on a schematic sagittal diagram from the atlas of König and Klippel (32). This study was performed in two phases separated by 3 months. The second group of experiments was done after confirming accuracy of lesion placement in the initial group, but data from both groups were pooled for statistical analysis by Student's T test. A p value < 0.05 was considered statistically significant.

RESULTS AND DISCUSSION

Plasma GH and Corticosterone Concentrations of Normal and Stressed Rats

Experiments were performed initially to determine plasma GH and corticosterone concentrations in a control group of fasted, unstressed rats injected with saline i.p. The results in Fig. 1 show that plasma GH levels vary widely in unstressed rats. Plasma corticosterone concentrations, in contrast, were distributed more uniformly within the lower range of values. Figure 1 also shows that a small increase of plasma corticosterone ($p < 0.05$) and a decrease of GH that was not statistically significant occurred 30 min after injection of saline. These changes in hormone levels have been attributed to the mild stress of the i.p. injection procedure and disappear after 30 min because plasma GH and corticosterone concentrations were not significantly different from the noninjected controls at 60 and 120 min.

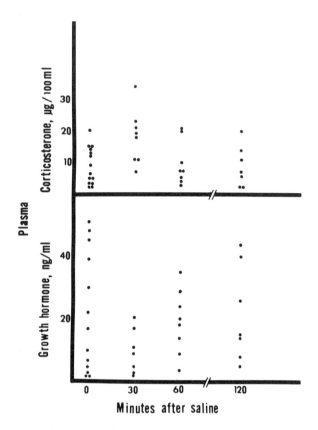

FIG. 1. Time course of plasma GH and corticosterone concentrations of normal rats injected with saline. Blood was collected by decapitation.

Although resting plasma GH concentrations of rats fluctuate widely, stress causes a reduction in GH secretion that results in less scatter and lower plasma GH values. In agreement with the findings of Takahashi et al. (3), stressful stimuli that produce a rise in plasma corticosterone concentration were shown to cause a significant fall of plasma GH. Figure 2 is an expansion of an earlier study (4) and shows plasma GH and corticosterone concentrations of individual rats ($N = 185$) that were unstressed or subjected to insulin hypoglycemia, cold exposure, ether inhalation, noise and vibration stress, and administration of pentylenetetrazol or 2-D-deoxyglucose. The scattergram shows that "nonspecific" activation by stress results in enhanced ACTH secretion and decreased GH secretion. A nonparametric test of correlation showed a highly significant inverse relationship between plasma corticosterone and GH concentrations ($p < 0.001$).

The only exceptions to this inverse relationship between GH and ACTH secretion were found after administration of morphine and other narcotic analgesics (4, 7). As shown in Fig. 3, i.p. injection of 20 mg/kg morphine

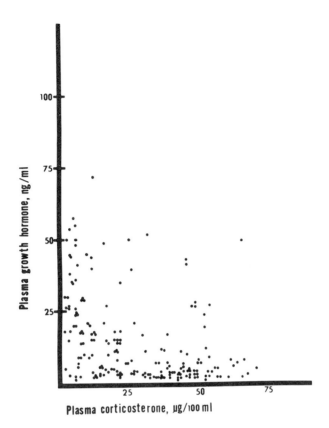

FIG. 2. Scattergram showing plasma GH and corticosterone concentrations of stressed and non-stressed rats (N = 185).

produced a marked increase in plasma concentration of corticosterone and GH. A comparison of Fig. 3 with Fig. 2 shows a significant difference in the distribution of GH values of rats treated with morphine. The results in Fig. 3 also confirm earlier work that pentobarbital, 50 mg/kg, causes a rise of plasma GH but has no effect on resting corticosterone levels of unstressed rats (4). In previous work we have shown that dexamethasone blocks the morphine-induced rise of corticosterone but not of GH, thus producing plasma concentrations of GH and corticosterone similar to those observed after injection of pentobarbital (4). Dexamethasone blockade of the rise in plasma corticosterone produced by morphine has also been reported by Zimmerman and Critchlow in female rats (28).

EFFECTS OF PENTOBARBITAL AND URETHANE

All the blood samples for corticosterone and GH shown in Fig. 1 were obtained by decapitation. Because of the large scatter in resting GH concentra-

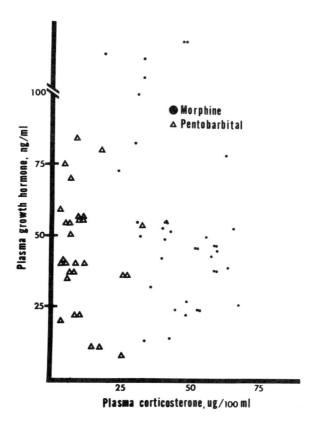

FIG. 3. Scattergram showing plasma GH and corticosterone concentrations of rats injected with morphine, 20 mg/kg, or pentobarbital, 50 mg/kg. Blood was collected by decapitation 30 min after drug injection.

tions, a method for obtaining serial samples of blood without stressing the rats would be of advantage since plasma GH changes could be determined in each animal. Several laboratories have reported increases of plasma GH following electrical stimulation of discrete brain areas in pentobarbital-anesthetized rats (8–10) or administration of various pharmacologic agents in urethane-treated rats (33, 34). The possibility of utilizing one of these approaches to study GH and ACTH secretion was examined in the next series of rats.

Data obtained with pentobarbital and urethane are summarized in Fig. 4 and compared with the mean plasma GH and corticosterone values of the saline controls from Fig. 1. Rats injected with 50 mg/kg of pentobarbital i.p. and sacrificed by decapitation at 30 and 60 min showed significant increases of plasma GH with no change in corticosterone concentration. Figure 4 also shows that corticosterone rose within 30 min and remained elevated for at least 2 hr after i.p. administration of 1.5 g/kg of urethane. Plasma GH levels declined, but the difference from the controls was not statistically significant.

In contrast to pentobarbital, urethane has opposite effects on plasma GH and corticosterone and thus resembles diethyl ether in its effects on endocrine activity. From data obtained in urethane-anesthetized rats, Collu et al. (33) postulated the rat GH secretion is under dual control of a beta-dopaminergic inhibitory and tryptaminergic stimulatory mechanism, whereas Kato et al. (34) proposed that GH secretion is stimulated through a beta-adrenergic receptor and inhibited through an alpha-adrenergic receptor.

As reported by Takahashi et al. (3), the rise in plasma GH did not occur when blood was drawn from a polyethylene cannula placed in the external jugular vein 6 to 12 min after administration of the same dose of pentobarbital (Fig. 5). Instead, an increase of plasma corticosterone occurred concomitantly with blockade of the pentobarbital effects on GH, indicating that cannulation stress can override the inhibitory and stimulatory effects of pentobarbital on ACTH and GH secretion, respectively.

Pentobarbital in combination with morphine produces inhibition of pituitary-adrenal activation by stress (25), and since both drugs cause marked increases of plasma GH, experiments were performed to determine whether

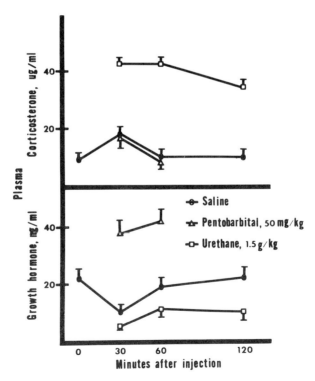

FIG. 4. Comparison of plasma GH and corticosterone concentrations of rats injected with saline, pentobarbital, or urethane. Saline-treated animals are from Fig. 1. Each point for the pentobarbital- and urethane-treated rats represents the mean ± SEM of five to seven animals.

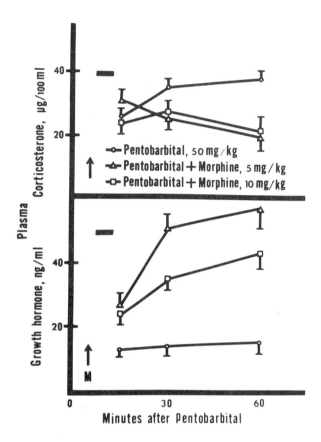

FIG. 5. Pentobarbital-morphine inhibition of cannulation stress-induced decrease of GH and increase of corticosterone in plasma. Each point represents the mean and SEM of six to nine rats. Arrow indicates time of morphine injection; shaded area represents cannulation period.

this drug combination would block the inhibitory effects of cannulation stress on GH secretion. When 5 or 10 mg/kg of morphine was administered 1 to 2 min prior to jugular vein cannulation, the rise of plasma corticosterone and fall of GH were diminished, showing that GH secretion augmented by pentobarbital-morphine was not suppressed by cannulation stress. The data in Fig. 5 also indicate that rats treated with pentobarbital-morphine would be useful for GIF assay in the same manner that the pentobarbital-morphine-dexamethasone treated rat is used in corticotropin-releasing factor (CRF) assays.

Effects of Morphine, Methadone, Nalorphine, and Naloxone

The results of dose–response studies with morphine are summarized in Fig. 6. The lowest dose, 5 mg/kg, produced sedation, and plasma GH and corti-

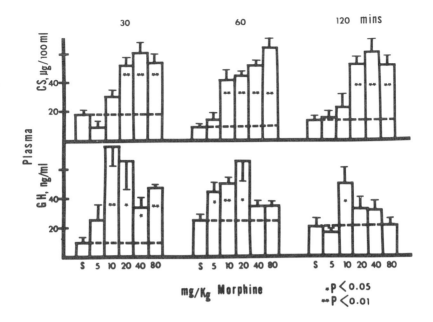

FIG. 6. Dose–response effects of morphine on plasma GH and corticosterone concentrations of rats. Values represent the mean and SEM of four to eight rats.

costerone concentrations were not significantly different from the controls except for an increase of GH at 60 min. With 10 mg/kg of morphine, plasma GH concentration was elevated at all three sampling intervals but plasma corticosterone showed an increase only at 60 min. The results show that 20 mg/kg of morphine was required to produce consistent elevation of both plasma corticosterone concentration and plasma GH. Doses of 40 and 80 mg/kg also produced a marked increase in plasma corticosterone concentration but were less effective than the 10 mg/kg dose in stimulating GH secretion. The results in Fig. 6 show that the effects of morphine on GH and ACTH secretion are dose-dependent. Lower doses produce mainly sedation, elevation of plasma GH concentration, and minimal stimulation of ACTH secretion. The higher doses have a long stimulant effect on ACTH secretion and a shorter effect on GH secretion. The decreased effectiveness of high doses of morphine on GH secretion may be due to the stressful effects that may abolish or reduce its stimulant effects.

The effects of 5, 10, and 20 mg/kg doses of methadone are shown in Fig. 7. The 5 mg/kg dose produced a significant rise of GH at 30 min. Plasma GH and corticosterone concentrations were not significantly altered at the other time intervals. The 10 and 20 mg/kg doses produced an elevation in concentration of both plasma corticosterone and GH. The effects on corticosterone lasted 120 min whereas plasma GH was not significantly different from the controls after 30 min. It was necessary to use low doses of methadone in

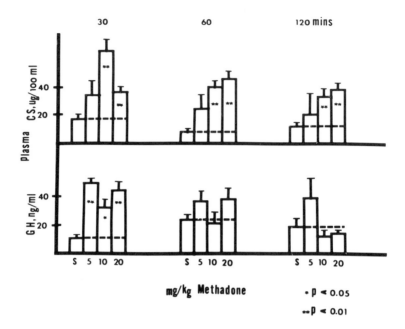

FIG. 7. Dose—response effects of methadone on plasma GH and corticosterone concentrations of rats. Values represent the mean and SEM of four to six rats.

these experiments because of its high potency and toxicity compared with morphine. The gross behavioral effects of 10 and 20 mg/kg of methadone as well as the effects on GH and ACTH secretion correlate well with those produced by 40 and 80 mg/kg doses of morphine.

The effects of narcotic antagonists on GH and ACTH secretion are summarized in Figs. 8 and 9. Nalorphine, which has many of the agonist properties of morphine, in doses equimolar to 10, 20, and 40 mg/kg of morphine produced increases in plasma concentration of GH and corticosterone at 30 min but not at 60 and 120 min. Fig. 9 shows that naloxone, a pure antagonist, had no effects on GH but produced a small, statistically significant elevation in plasma corticosterone concentration at 30 and 60 min with 23 and 46 mg/kg, respectively.

The results obtained with the narcotic agonists morphine and methadone, with the partial agonist-antagonist nalorphine, and with the pure antagonist naloxone suggested a relationship between agonist activity of narcotic analgesics and their effects on GH and ACTH secretion. Whether the acute stimulant effects of morphine on these two pituitary hormones are mediated by different pharmacologic actions was examined by determining the effects of morphine on GH and ACTH secretion in rats pretreated with naloxone to provide high antagonist:agonist ratios of 1:2 and 1:4. The results (Fig. 10) show that the effects of 20 and 40 mg/kg morphine on plasma corticosterone were

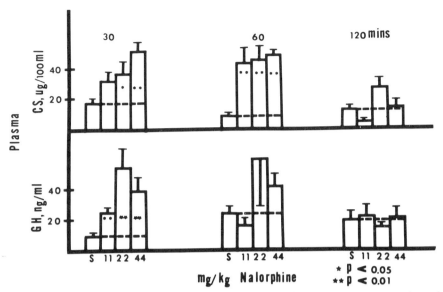

FIG. 8. Dose–response effects of nalorphine on plasma GH and corticosterone concentrations of rats. Values represent the mean and SEM of four to five rats.

completely blocked by 11 mg/kg of naloxone. The increase in plasma GH concentration, in contrast, was not blocked by naloxone, indicating that the mechanisms regulating the secretion of these hormones are activated by different pharmacologic actions of morphine. The structurally related compound apomorphine produces a rise of corticosterone and a fall of GH concentration in plasma, in contrast to the elevation of plasma GH produced by morphine

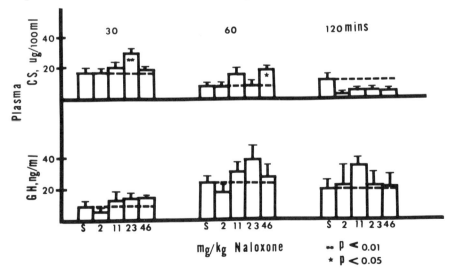

FIG. 9. Dose–response effects of naloxone on plasma GH and corticosterone concentrations of rats. Values represent the mean and SEM of four to nine rats.

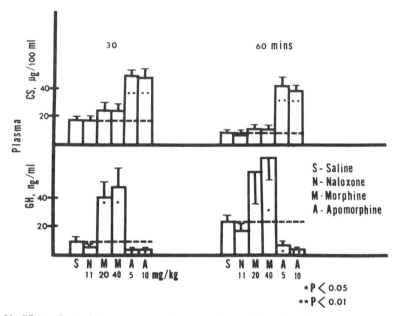

FIG. 10. Effects of morphine and apomorphine on plasma GH and corticosterone concentrations of naloxone-pretreated rats. Values represent the mean and SEM of five to six rats.

(7). Fig. 10 also shows that naloxone pretreatment did not alter the effects of apomorphine. Although both morphine and apomorphine produce an increase in plasma corticosterone concentration, the data obtained with naloxone indicate that these two drugs produce their effects by different mechanisms.

Effects of Chronic Administration of Morphine and Methadone

Since tolerance to the depressant effects of narcotics is reportedly acquired more readily than to the stimulant effects, GH and ACTH secretion were studied in rats chronically treated with morphine and methadone. The results of these experiments are summarized in Figs. 11 and 12, respectively. The results in Fig. 11 show that tolerance to the stimulant effect on ACTH secretion developed rapidly in rats injected twice daily with 20 or 40 mg/kg of morphine. In these experiments the last dose of morphine was administered i.p. and plasma GH and corticosterone were measured 30 min after injection. Morphine stimulation of GH secretion was not diminished but seemed to be enhanced as the rats developed tolerance to the toxic, stressful effects of morphine. Fig. 12 shows that chronic administration of methadone, 10 mg/kg twice daily, produced behavioral and endocrine effects that were comparable to 40 mg/kg of morphine. Marked tolerance to the stimulant effect of methadone on ACTH secretion was evident after 4 days, as well as an augmentation of GH secretion with chronic treatment.

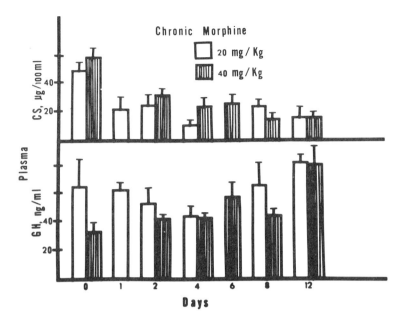

FIG. 11. Effects of chronic morphine treatment on plasma GH and corticosterone concentrations of rats. Values represent the mean and SEM of five to eight rats.

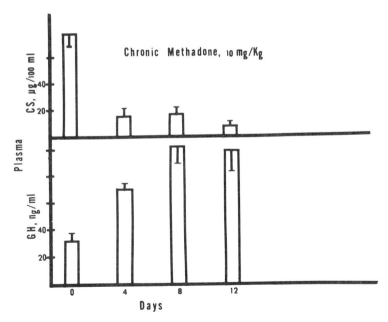

FIG. 12. Effects of chronic methadone treatment on plasma GH and corticosterone of rats. Values represent the mean and SEM of four to five rats.

Chronic injection of morphine in rats has been reported to inhibit adrenal ascorbic acid depletion in response to stress (22), and to block the increased urinary excretion of steroids that normally occurs during cold exposure (35). Since exogenous ACTH produced a normal response in chronically-morphinized rats, the inhibition cannot be attributed to refractory adrenals. From these data and the results in Figs. 11 and 12, it may be concluded that chronic morphine administration reduces pituitary-adrenal activity and that this effect is not due to a direct suppressive action on the adrenal cortex.

In the next series of rats, experiments were performed to determine whether the GH and ACTH secretory responses to various stimuli were altered after chronic administration of morphine. In this series, 40 mg/kg of morphine was administered twice daily for 12 days; the rats were then subjected to the stress procedures summarized in Fig. 13. Since plasma GH and corticosterone concentrations show an inverse relationship in stressed rats (Fig. 2), the data in Fig. 13 show that chronic administration of morphine did not alter the normal ACTH and GH secretory response to stress. In contrast to earlier reports of inhibition of stress activation of ACTH secretion (25), marked increases of plasma corticosterone as well as significant decreases of plasma GH occurred with naloxone-precipitated withdrawal and with the other procedures described in Fig. 13. In agreement with the findings of Briggs and Munson (22), the adrenal-cortical response to ACTH was not

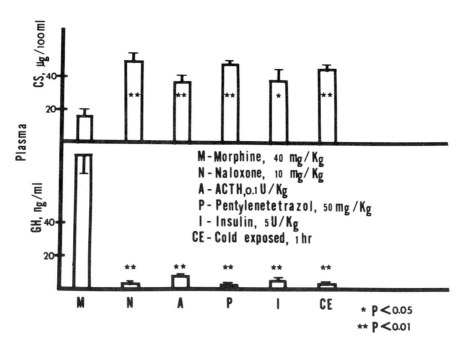

FIG. 13. Effects of naloxone and stress on plasma GH and corticosterone of rats chronically treated with morphine. Values represent the mean and SEM of four to six rats.

impaired in these morphine-tolerant rats. From these results it would seem clear that GH and ACTH secretion in response to stress is not altered in tolerant rats even though chronic administration of morphine produces tolerance to its acute stimulant effect on ACTH secretion and seems to enhance its effects on GH secretion.

Effects of Hypothalamic Lesions

The next series of experiments were done to determine whether hypothalamic lesions modify the effects of morphine on GH and ACTH secretion. Since there is evidence that GH secretion in rats is regulated by the VMN region of the hypothalamus via release of GRF (8–11), it was the purpose of these experiments to selectively destroy this area of the hypothalamus and to compare the effects of lesions placed ventral and caudal to this area on GH and ACTH secretion. Figure 14 is a composite diagram of the lesion sites. The VMN lesions involved 80 to 100% destruction of the VMN region with partial destruction of the adjacent anterior or caudal regions. Rats with anterior hypothalamic lesions as a group had lesions extending caudally from the preoptic area to the rostral portion of the VMN. The posterior lesions involved partial destruction of the VMN and most of the mammillary bodies. Data from rats with nonsymmetrical bilateral lesions were not included in this study.

The mean plasma GH and corticosterone values of rats with hypothalamic lesions and the sham-lesioned controls after i.p. injection of saline are shown in Fig. 15. Our results show that plasma corticosterone and GH concentrations were not significantly changed by hypothalamic lesions. Many lesioned rats exhibited rage behavior during injection with saline but, as shown in Fig. 15, plasma corticosterone levels of the three groups of rats with lesions were not significantly different from the controls at all four sampling intervals. Also, initial plasma GH levels of rats with lesions in the anterior, VMN, or posterior hypothalamus were slightly higher than the controls, but the increases were not statistically significant.

From the dose–response results shown in Fig. 6, a 20 mg/kg dose was selected to examine the effects of morphine in rats with hypothalamic lesions. These results are summarized in Fig. 16. Morphine in sham-lesioned rats produced marked increases of plasma corticosterone at all postinjection sampling intervals as well as significant increases of GH at 30 and 60 min. The data also show that morphine stimulation of ACTH secretion was suppressed in A-L rats. Plasma corticosterone concentrations were significantly lower than those of the sham-operated animals and a delayed increase was not observed. In contrast, mean plasma GH values of A-L rats were higher than their controls at 30 and 60 min, but only the latter were statistically significant.

The data also show that morphine stimulation of GH secretion was not

COMPOSITE MORPHINE

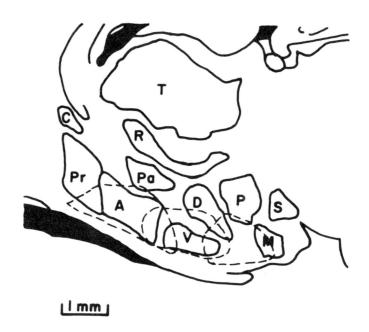

FIG. 14. Composite diagram of electrolytic lesions in anterior, VMN, and posterior hypothalamic sites. A: anterior hypothalamic nucleus; C: anterior commissure; D: dorsal medial nucleus; M: mammillary bdy; P: posterior nucleus; Pa: paraventricular nucleus; Pr: preoptic area; R: reuniens nucleus; S: supramammillary nucleus; T: thalamus; V: ventral medial nucleus.

impaired in V-L or P-L rats. Mean plasma GH concentration of P-L rats was higher at 30 min and lower at 60 min than that of the controls but neither difference was statistically significant. Also, the increase of plasma corticosterone following injection of morphine was reduced in both V-L and P-L rats. These lesions produced partial inhibition of the ACTH response to morphine since plasma corticosterone concentrations still were significantly higher than those of the saline-treated rats in Fig. 15.

Our results with morphine show that all three lesion sites produce partial blockade of morphine stimulation of ACTH secretion with the anterior lesions being the most effective and VMN lesions least effective. However, since none of these lesions blocked GH secretion in response to morphine, the question remains as to how or where morphine acts to stimulate GH secretion. Frohman et al. (8) have postulated that GH secretion may be regulated via GRF secretion by the VMN region, but our data from lesioned animals show that morphine stimulation of GH secretion cannot be due to this mechanism.

Martin and associates recently reported that morphine acts directly at the

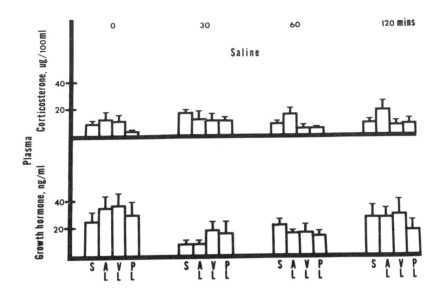

FIG. 15. Effects of saline on plasma GH and corticosterone concentrations of rats with hypo-thalamic lesions. Values represent mean and SEM of four to seven rats.

pituitary level because large VMN lesions did not modify morphine stimulation of GH secretion (36), whereas similar lesions blocked the pentobarbital-induced rise of plasma GH (37), suggesting that morphine and pentobarbital act by different mechanisms to enhance GH secretion. Unpublished data from this laboratory, however, are not in complete accord with those of Martin et al., since plasma GH and corticosterone concentrations of rats with VMN lesions were not significantly different from the controls 30 min after injection of 50 mg/kg of pentobarbital. This dose of pentobarbital produces a rapid and sustained rise in mean plasma GH concentration of rats when blood is collected by decapitation (3, 4). When blood is drawn from an indwelling venous cannula implanted 2 or 3 days before study, the same 50 mg/kg dose of pentobarbital i.p. is reported by Martin to produce an acute rise of plasma GH with peak values at 10 min, followed by a return to baseline levels 20 to 30 min after injection (37). Although VMN lesions may block the acute stimulant effects of pentobarbital on GH secretion as reported by Martin, our preliminary findings using decapitation suggest that the sustained increases of plasma GH observed 30 to 60 min after injection are not VMN-mediated.

Since enhanced GH secretion produced by morphine (Fig. 16) or pento-barbital (*unpublished data*) was not decreased by hypothalamic lesions, it may be inferred that these pharmacologic agents act directly on the anterior pituitary. Another possible explanation for the stimulant action of morphine and pentobarbital on GH secretion should be considered at this time. Insulin hypoglycemia and cannulation stress have been shown to block stimulation of

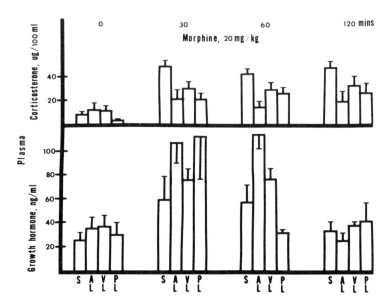

FIG. 16. Effects of morphine, 20 mg/kg, on plasma GH and corticosterone concentrations of rats with hypothalamic lesions. Values represent the mean and SEM of four to eight rats.

GH induced by morphine (4) and pentobarbital (3). If these drugs exert their effects at the pituitary level, it could be assumed that hypoglycemia and cannulation stress act directly on the pituitary to inhibit GH secretion. An alternative and more probable explanation is that hypoglycemia and cannulation stress activate central inhibitory mechanisms that override the stimulant effects of morphine and pentobarbital on GH secretion. Conversely, it was shown in Fig. 5 that pentobarbital-morphine blocks the inhibition of GH secretion produced by cannulation stress. Whether pentobarbital-morphine stimulates GRF or inhibits GIF secretion in cannulated rats remains to be determined.

The data of Krulich et al. (12) offer another explanation for the failure of hypothalamic lesions to alter the GH response to morphine. These investigators reported that GIF is diffusely distributed throughout the median eminence. In our experiments hypothalamic lesions caused little or no damage of the median eminence, so it is possible that morphine, and perhaps pentobarbital as well, may increase GH secretion by inhibiting the release of GIF. If morphine acts in this manner to stimulate GH secretion, lesions of the median eminence should block morphine stimulation of GH secretion. In addition, it would be expected that the reduction of the GH response to morphine would be related to the size of the lesion as reported by Brodish for CRF-ACTH (38). This possibility is currently under investigation.

SUMMARY

Plasma growth hormone (GH) and corticosterone measurements show that GH and ACTH secretion in response to stressful stimuli are inversely related in rats. Stimulation of both GH and ACTH secretion was observed only after administration of narcotic analgesics. These effects were dose-related, lower doses of morphine or methadone producing mainly a rise in plasma GH and higher doses causing greater plasma increases of corticosterone than of GH. Chronic administration of morphine or methadone resulted in tolerance to the stimulant effects of ACTH secretion; tolerance did not develop to the stimulant effect on GH secretion. Naloxone blocked the stimulant effects of morphine on ACTH but not on GH secretion. Although chronic administration of morphine resulted in tolerance to its stimulant effects on ACTH secretion, stressful stimuli caused a marked increase of plasma corticosterone and a fall of plasma GH in tolerant rats, showing that tolerance to morphine did not impair the endocrine response to stress.

The endocrine effects of urethane were similar to those of ether, causing a rise in concentration of corticosterone and a fall of GH in plasma. The inhibition of GH and stimulation of ACTH secretion by cannulation stress in pentobarbital-anesthetized animals was blocked by morphine, 5 and 10 mg/kg, injected 2 to 3 min before surgery. It is suggested that the pentobarbital-morphine anesthetized rat would be a useful preparation for assay of growth hormone-inhibiting factor. (GIF).

Bilateral electrolytic lesions of the ventromedial nucleus (VMN) partially blocked morphine-induced stimulation of ACTH secretion but not of GH secretion. Similar results were obtained in rats with hypothalamic lesions rostral or caudal to the VMN region. These results suggest that morphine stimulation of ACTH secretion is mediated via the ventral-medial region of the hypothalamus. Stimulation of GH secretion may be due to a direct effect of morphine on the anterior pituitary, but the possibility that morphine acts at the level of the median eminence to inhibit release of GIF (somatostatin) is not excluded.

ACKNOWLEDGMENTS

This work was supported in part by grants from the University of California at Irvine, California College of Medicine Research and Education Foundation, and U.S. Public Health Service (MH 20787).

REFERENCES

1. Schalch, D. S., and Reichlin, S. Stress and growth hormone release. In: *Growth Hormone,* edited by A. Pecile and E. E. Müller, pp. 211–225. Exerpta Medica, Amsterdam, 1968.

2. Garcia, J. F., and Geschwind, I. I. Investigation of growth hormone secretion in selected mammalian species. In: *Growth Hormone,* edited by A. Pecile and E. E. Müller, pp. 267–291. Excerpta Medica, Amsterdam, 1968.

3. Takahashi, K., Daughaday, W. H., and Kipnis, D. M. Regulation of immunoreactive growth hormone secretion in male rats. *Endocrinology,* 88:909–917, 1971.

4. Kokka, N., Garcia, J. F., George, R., and Elliott, H. W. Growth hormone and ACTH secretion: Evidence for an inverse relationship in rats. *Endocrinology,* 90: 735–743, 1972.

5. Howard, N., and Martin, J. M. A stimulatory test for growth hormone release in the rat. *Endocrinology,* 88:497–500, 1971.

6. Wakabayashi, I., Arimura, A., and Schally, A. V. Effects of dexamethasone and pentobarbital on plasma growth hormone levels in rats. *Neuroendocrinology,* 8:340–346, 1971.

7. Kokka, N., Garcia, J. F., and Elliott, H. W. Effects of acute and chronic administration of narcotic analgesics on growth hormone and corticotrophin (ACTH) secretion in rats. *Prog. Brain Res.,* 39:347–360, 1973.

8. Frohman, L. A., Bernardis, L. L., and Kant, K. J. Effect of hypothalamic stimulation on pituitary and plasma growth hormone levels in rats. *Science,* 162:580–582, 1968.

9. Bernardis, L. L., and Frohman, L. A. Plasma growth hormone responses to electrical stimulation of the hypothalamus in the rat. *Neuroendocrinology,* 7:193–201, 1971.

10. Martin, J. B. Plasma growth hormone (GH) response to hypothalamic or extra-hypothalamic electrical stimulation. *Endocrinology,* 91:107–115, 1972.

11. Martin, J. B., Kontor, J., and Mead, P. Plasma GH responses to hypothalamic, hippocampal and amygdaloid electrical stimulation: Effects of variation in stimulus parameters and treatment with α-methyl-p-tyrosine. *Endocrinology,* 92:1354–1361, 1973.

12. Krulich, L., Illner, P., Fawcett, C. P., Quijada, M., and McCann, S. M. Dual hypothalamic regulation of growth hormone secretion. In: *Growth and Growth Hormone,* International Congress Series, No. 244, edited by A. Pecile and E. E. Müller, pp. 306–316. Excerpta Medica, Amsterdam, 1972.

13. Malacara, J. M., Valverde-R., C., Reichlin, S., and Bollinger, J. Elevation of plasma radioimmunoassayable growth hormone in the rat induced by porcine hypothalamic extract. *Endocrinology,* 91:1189–1198, 1972.

14. Frohman, L. A., Maran, J. W., and Dhariwal, A. P. S. Plasma growth hormone responses to intrapituitary injections of growth hormone releasing factor (GRF) in the rat. *Endocrinology,* 88:1483–1488, 1971.

15. Brazeau, P., Vale, W., Burgus, R., Ling, N., Butcher, M., Rivier, J., and Guillemin, R. Hypothalamic polypeptide that inhibits the secretion of immunoreactive pituitary growth hormone. *Science,* 179:77–79, 1973.

16. Brazeau, P., Rivier, J., Vale, W., and Guillemin, R. Inhibition of growth hormone secretion in the rat by synthetic somatostatin. *Endocrinology,* 94:184–187, 1974.

17. Fortier, C. Nervous control of ACTH secretion. In: *The Pituitary Gland,* Vol. II, edited by G. W. Harris and B. T. Donovan, pp. 195–234. Butterworth, London, 1966.

18. Mangili, G., Motta, M., and Martini, L. Control of adrenocorticotropic hormone secretion. In: *Neuroendocrinology,* Vol. I, edited by L. Martini and W. F. Ganong, pp. 297–370. Academic Press, New York, 1966.

19. Ganong, W. F. Evidence for a central noradrenergic system that inhibits ACTH secretion. In: *Brain—Endocrine Interaction,* edited by K. M. Knigge, D. E. Scott, and A. Weindl, pp. 254–266. Karger, Basel, 1972.

20. de Wied, D., and de Jong, W. Drug effects and hypothalamic anterior pituitary function. *Ann. Rev. Pharmacol,* 14:389–412, 1974.

21. Marks, B. H., Hall, M. M., and Bhattacharya, A. N. Psychopharmacological effects and pituitary-adrenal activity. *Prog. Brain Res.,* 32:57–70, 1970.

22. Briggs, F. N., and Munson, P. L. Studies on the mechanism of stimulation of ACTH secretion with the aid of morphine as a blocking agent. *Endocrinology,* 57:205–219, 1955.

23. George, R., and Way, E. L. Studies on the mechanism of pituitary-adrenal activation by morphine. *Brit. J. Pharmacol.,* 10:260–264, 1955.
24. Nikidijevic, O., and Maickel, R. P. Some effects of morphine on pituitary-adrenocortical function in the rat. *Biochem. Pharmacol.,* 16:2137–2142, 1967.
25. George, R. Hypothalamus: Anterior pituitary gland. In: *Narcotic Drugs, Biochemical Pharmacology,* edited by D. Clouet, pp. 283–299. Plenum Press, New York, 1971.
26. George, R., and Way, E. L. The role of the hypothalamus in pituitary-adrenal activation and antidiuresis by morphine. *J. Pharmacol. Exp. Ther.,* 125:111–115, 1959.
27. Lotti, V., Kokka, N., and George, R. Pituitary-adrenal activation following intrahypothalamic microinjection of morphine. *Neuroendocrinology,* 4:326–332, 1969.
28. Zimmermann, E., and Critchlow, V. Inhibition of morphine-induced pituitary-adrenal activation by dexamethasone in the female rat. *Proc. Soc. Exp. Biol. Med.,* 143:1224–1226, 1973.
29. Gold, E. M., and Ganong, W. F. Effects of drugs on neuroendocrine processes. In: *Neuroendocrinology,* Vol. II, edited by L. Martini and W. F. Ganong, pp. 377–437. Academic Press, New York, 1967.
30. Washko, M. E., and Rice, E. W. Determination of glucose by an improved enzymatic procedure. *Clin. Chem.,* 7:542–545, 1961.
31. Guillemin, R., Clayton, G. W., Lipscomb, H. S., and Smith, J. D. Fluorometric measurement of rat plasma and adrenal corticosterone concentration. *J. Lab. Clin. Med.,* 53:830–832, 1959.
32. König, J. F. R., and Klippel, R. A. The Rat Brain. A stereotaxic atlas of the forebrain and lower parts of the brain stem. Krieger, New York, 1970.
33. Collu, R., Visconti, P., Fraschini, F., and Martini, L. Adrenergic and serotoninergic control of growth hormone secretion in adult male rats. *Endocrinology,* 90:1231–1237, 1972.
34. Kato, Y., Dupre, J., and Beck, J. C. Plasma growth hormone in the anesthetized rat: Effects of dibutyryl cyclic AMP, prostaglandin E₁, adrenergic agents, vasopressin, chlorpromazine, amphetamine and L-DOPA. *Endocrinology,* 93:135–146, 1973.
35. Paroli, E., and Melchiorri, P. Urinary excretion of hydroxysteroids, 17-ketosteroids and aldosterone in rats during a cycle of treatment with morphine. *Biochem. Pharmacol.,* 6:1–17, 1961.
36. Martin, J. B. The role of hypothalamic and extrahypothalamic structures in the control of GH secretion. (*In press.*).
37. Martin, J. B. Studies on the mechanism of pentobarbital-induced GH release in the rat. *Neuroendocrinology,* 13:339–350, 1974.
38. Brodish, A. Diffuse hypothalamic system for the regulation of ACTH secretion. *Endocrinology,* 73:727–735, 1963.

DISCUSSION

Weiner: Since there are no cell bodies in the median eminence and since you had lesions in the anterior, middle, and posterior hypothalamus, where do you picture the GIF-secreting cells as being located?

Kokka: As Dr. Brazeau indicated yesterday, they could be located in the arcuate nucleus or they might be situated more laterally in the hypothalamus.

Ganong: These are very interesting results, although I think we should remember that there are marked species differences in response to apomorphine. Brown has reported that apomorphine stimulates growth hormone secretion in the monkey, but he thinks this might be due to the stress effect of the drug. He finds that this effect of apomorphine does not occur in the absence of a concomitant rise in corticosteroid levels in blood. On the other hand, several reports now indicate that apomorphine in subemetic doses causes growth hormone secretion in humans, and it has even been suggested as a provocative test for growth hormone secretion for clinical purposes. We have been working with dogs and find that small doses given intraventricularly do not stimulate ACTH secretion. I must point out, however, that our dogs were anesthetized and this would be expected to influence their response to apomorphine.

Kokka: Thank you for these interesting comments. I should point out, by way of preface to Dr. Cushman's presentation, that growth hormone levels and cortisol levels in man appear to vary directly with each other as opposed to our findings in the rat of an inverse relation between these two hormones under most circumstances.

Zimmermann: It is interesting that growth hormone elevation in response to morphine is a response which does not disappear upon repeated injections of the drug, that is, tolerance to this effect of morphine does not develop. How do you explain this?

Kokka: This may be due to a direct effect of morphine on the pituitary.

Lomax: In our studies on thyroid activity, we found that small doses of morphine, 5 mg/kg, which do not produce behavioral depression, did depress thyroid activity when given repeatedly, and tolerance did not develop to this effect of the drug.

Narcotics and the Hypothalamus, edited by
E. Zimmermann and R. George. Raven Press,
New York © 1974

Some Endocrinologic Observations in Narcotic Addicts

Paul Cushman, Jr., and Mary Jeanne Kreek

*Department of Medicine, St. Luke's Hospital and Columbia University, New York, New York 10025,
and Rockefeller University, New York, New York 10021*

INTRODUCTION

Psychically active drugs frequently abused by man have been shown to exert a variety of endocrine disturbances. Controlled pharmacologic experiments in the laboratory animal have shown morphine to release antidiuretic hormone (1) and to activate the pituitary-adrenal axis (2, 3), while there has also been evidence suggesting the inhibition of corticotrophin-releasing factor and of ACTH release (4–6). There is considerable clinical and pharmacologic interest in neuroendrocrine functions in human drug abuse.

In man there are formidable legal and ethical difficulties which have hampered the compilation of controlled endocrinologic observations. Studies that closely parallel the animal data were carried out in Lexington, Kentucky, in a small group of confined, volunteer ex-addicts who received morphine and oral methadone under controlled conditions.

We approached the problem through the study of the narcotic addict directly. He has the advantage of having consumed appreciable amounts of the drug in question; however, it was usually difficult to control rigorously the conditions of the study. Not only were the quantities of morphine administered beyond control, but it was also difficult to ascertain to what degree other substances, possibly active in the central nervous system, may have been consumed as well. Nevertheless, it was reasoned that a study of a reasonably large sample of narcotic addicts should reveal whatever disruptive effect chronic morphine administration could produce in the endocrine system.

PATIENTS AND METHODS

Five patient populations were studied:

(a) Male "heroin" addicts who were so classified on the basis of history, cutaneous evidence of drug abuse, and a single urine which contained morphine and/or quinine only when examined for dangerous drugs.

(b) Male methadone-maintained patients who were attending the St. Luke's Hospital Center methadone maintenance clinic. There was no urinary or historical evidence of other drug use for at least 3 months before the study.

(c) Drug-free and methadone-maintained patients admitted to the Rockefeller University Hospital for inpatient study.

(d) Male ex-addicts from Exodus House, a therapeutic community, where they have been considered drug-free on the basis of history, behavior, and serial negative urines for at least 1 year.

(e) Controls were hospital employees and local volunteers.

Physical examinations performed on all patients disclosed no clinical suggestions of hypothyroidism, hypogonadism, or hypopituitarism except in a few chronic alcoholics who exhibited the expected changes such as spider angiomata and small testes.

The pituitary polypeptides were measured by radioimmunoassay. Cortisol was determined by the Porter-Silber reaction or by competitive binding, testosterone by competitive protein binding, and methadone by gas-liquid chromatography. Thyroxine (T-4) was measured by column chromatography and competitive protein binding. Triiodothyronine (T-3), T-3 resin uptake, and thyroid-binding globulin (TBG) binding capacities were measured by standard techniques. The 24-hr urine corticoids were determined using the 17-ketogenic method of Norymberski and the Peterson modification of the Porter-Silber reaction. Spot urines were surveyed for drug content by thin-layer chromatography (7).

RESULTS

Table 1 lists some endocrinologic measurements in cross-sectional studies of heroin addicts, methadone-treated patients, and detoxified patients. Thyroid function tests were normal except in some heroin addicts, 85% male, who had a tendency to increased T-4 levels, reduced T-3 resin uptakes, and increase in TBG binding capacities (8). They were clinically euthyroid and had normal free T-4 levels as laboratory confirmation.

Cortisol levels in the addicts were normal. Several other studies had similar results except one which showed reduced plasma cortisol and urinary 17-hydroxycorticosteroids (17-OHCS) during morphine addiction (9). However, a later study by the same group showed no significant change in the urinary 17-OHCS (10) during a cycle of morphine addiction. Serum insulin levels tended to be somewhat high in the heroin addict (11), unlike the normal or methadone-maintained patient, but it was difficult to be sure that they were really in the fasting state.

Pituitary test results are listed in Table 2. Fasting growth hormone (GH) values were normal in male heroin addicts. Their response to insulin hypoglycemia was subnormal in 35% and to arginine infusions also in a small sample. On the other hand, luteinizing hormone (LH) levels were within the range of normal. Some methadone-maintained patients also showed a reduced GH response to insulin.

Regarding ACTH function, untreated and methadone-maintained patients

TABLE 1. Some endocrine measurements in heroin addicts and methadone-maintained patients

Endocrine measurement	Heroin addicts	Methadone-maintained patients	Detoxified patients
I. 24-hr urinary			
17-ketosteroids	—	N	N
17-ketogenic steroids	—	N	N
II. Serum			
T-4	N (↑ in 22%)	N (↑ in 3%)	N
T-3 resin uptake	N (↓ in 25%)	N (↓ in 2%)	N
TBG binding capacity	high normal	normal	not done
T-3	N[a]	N[a]	not done
free T-4	N[a]	N[a]	not done
fasting insulin	N or high	N	not done
III. Plasma			
cortisol	N	N	N

N = Normal; TBG = thyroid-binding globulin.
[a] Based on limited number of observations (5).

had normal resting plasma cortisol and most responded normally to insulin hypoglycemia (11). Oral metapirone testing produced normal results in stable, chronic methadone-maintained patients (12). A detailed examination of serial metapirone testing is instructive. Eight chronic addicts were studied in the metabolic unit of the Rockefeller University. After being detoxified from all drugs they were started on oral methadone. Before reaching full

TABLE 2. Pituitary function in narcotic addicts—plasma pituitary polypeptides and cortisol levels in heroin addicts early and late in the course of methadone maintenance treatment

Hormone measured	Normal	Heroin addict	Methadone-maintained patient	
			early 1st 3 months	stabilized >3 months
Growth hormone (ng/ml)				
resting[a]	1.7 ± 1	1.8 ± 1 (22)	—	1.5 ± 1 (41)
stimulated[b]	>8	65% N (14)	—	75% N (21)
Cortisol (as an indirect measurement of ACTH) (ng/dl)				
resting[a]	13 ± 7	13.4 ± 8 (32)	N	10.1 ± 7 (17)
stimulated[b]	≥9	77% N (14)	N	90% N (21)
LH (mIU/ml)				
male[a]	9 ± 3	10 (34)	10 (21)	11 (66)
FSH (mIU/ml)				
male[a]	4–25	12 (6)	—	10 (17)

N = Normal or within range of normal. Numbers in parentheses are the number of individual observations.
[a] Based on single measurement or aggregates of single measurements.
[b] With insulin hypoglycemia arginine infusions.

TABLE 3. Abnormal results of oral metapirone testing during the first 2 months of methadone maintenance treatment in eight addicts

	17-OHCS excretion (mg/24 hr) in urine		
Case no.	Day 1: control	Day 2: metapirone, 750 mg q 4 hr × 6	Day 3: day following metapirone
1	4.0	7.7	11.4
2	3.6	5.2	6.9
3	3.2	5.6	5.7
4	4.8	8.7	13.2
5	12.4	20.6	29.5
6	4.3	6.3	10.5
7	2.9	4.3	6.1
8	4.8	9.5	11.5
Normal	3–10 mg/24 hr	2 × control	3 × control

treatment doses they underwent oral metapirone testing. If the criteria of Liddle (13) are used, i.e., doubling of the 17-OHCS (Porter-Silber technique) the day the metapirone is given and tripling the next day in serial 24-hr urines, then all eight were abnormal. The results are given in Table 3 (case no. 5 undoubtedly was a normal responder but started from an unusually high baseline; cases 2, 3, and 7 showed especially poor responses).

TABLE 4. Metapirone test results in two male former heroin addicts studied in drug-free state and repeatedly during induction and stabilization on methadone maintenance treatment

		Metapirone test: 17-OHCS, mg/24 hr		
Case no.		Day 1: control	Day 2: metapirone	Day 3: metapirone
1. Pretreatment with methadone		6.7	15.3	16.0
months	mg			
0.5	30	4.0	7.7	11.4
1.5	40	6.4	11.6	11.8
2.0	70	5.0	10.2	18.0
2.5	100	6.0	9.3	19.9
3.0	100	7.6	14.4	26.1
2. Pretreatment with methadone		4.4	11.9	17.2
months	mg			
0.5	30	3.6	5.2	6.9
1.5	70	3.2	4.7	11.6
2.0	80	2.2	3.9	8.5
2.5	100	2.4	4.8	11.6
3.0	100	3.1	7.0	14.4

Serial oral metapirone testing was performed in two of these patients (cases 1 and 2) before and at frequent intervals during the methadone buildup. The data in Table 4 indicate that normal metapirone responsiveness was evident by 2 or 2.5 months and suggest that there may be a transient phase of hypothalamic-pituitary-adrenal dysfunction during the early part of treatment, before tolerance to the effects of methadone has been fully developed. These patients may have become tolerant to some endocrine effect of methadone as well.

Although the plasma gonadotropins were within the range of normal in the chronic methadone-treated patients, Martin et al. (14) have recently reported that a cycle of oral methadone addiction resulted in spotty reductions in the levels of plasma LH and follicle-stimulating hormone (FSH) during addiction but that absolute levels remained within normal limits. Another study of daily LH and FSH levels found that some female methadone-maintained patients had reduced serum levels early in the course of treatment (15). Our laboratory has looked at thyroid-stimulating hormone (TSH) levels in a small number of methadone-treated and untreated heroin addicts. In all instances their TSH levels were below the lower limit of the method, the usual finding in the normal. Schenckman et al. (16) found normal TSH levels together with T-3 before and after thyroid-releasing hormone administration in eight methadone-treated patients. Prolactin levels in a few methadone-treated males showed no abnormal values in our limited experience.

MENSTRUAL CYCLES IN ADDICTS

Symptoms of sexual dysfunction are common in male heroin addicts (17). When they undergo methadone maintenance, most patients report that their erectional insufficiency, reduced libido, and delayed time for ejaculation improve at various rates. A few patients report a worsening of their sexual performance and desire during the early stages of methadone maintenance, which usually abates with time or reduction in methadone dose or both (18). In the female narcotic addict in her reproductive years, oligo- and amenorrhea are commonly encountered (19). In our experience, 98% of 41 unselected patients, ages 33 ± 7 yr (21–41), reported normal patterns of menstrual bleeding before they became addicted (i.e., more or less monthly menses). During addiction 54% reported amenorrhea (5 or more months of absent menses) and an additional 2% reported oligomenorrhea as well (i.e., menses every 2 to 3 months). When surveyed 2.7 ± 6 yr after their entry into methadone treatment (range 3 to 72 months), 83% reported they were menstruating monthly. Of the nine patients whose amenorrhea disappeared during methadone treatment, six reported regaining normal menses during the first 2 to 4 months, but the mean was 6.1 ± 8 (range 2 to 25 months). Two of the remaining amenorrheic patients appeared to be postmenopausal by usual clinical criteria.

Since a more normal pattern of menstrual bleeding commonly and rapidly followed methadone treatment in these patients, it appears that there must have been some adverse factor associated with illicit narcotic abuse. Whether menses returned because the patients regained a more tranquil state of mind as a result of having their narcotic problems alleviated to some degree, or because their narcotic status was stabilized to a more or less continuous level of tolerant addiction, or for some other reason, cannot be differentiated. The contrast between the narcotic stability of the methadone patient and the alternating cycles of pulses of narcotics followed by abstinence in the usual street addict is impressive.

TESTOSTERONE AND GONADOTROPINS

Our laboratory previously reported that mean plasma testosterone levels were not significantly different from the norm in male untreated heroin addicts, methadone-maintained patients, ex-addicts, and former methadone-maintained patients (18). A prospective study of 21 male heroin addicts showed no change in mean testosterone levels during treatment and no correlation between testosterone values and the presence or absence of symptoms of sexual disturbances.

However, some addicts had testosterone values below the lower limit of normal for the time of day. Since patients receiving methadone in doses of 40 mg or more per day had lower testosterone levels than those receiving less than 40 mg per day, it is possible that methadone exerted some effect on the patients' testosterone values. It should be recalled that there were significant correlations found between quantitation of liver diseases as reflected by the SGOT value and a history of alcohol consumption, but the detection of illicit drug abuse in the methadone-maintained patients did not correlate with the level of plasma testosterone.

A detailed study was therefore performed in eight selected stable methadone-maintained patients. Correlations between plasma methadone, testosterone, LH, and FSH levels were sought in these normal males who claimed normal sexual functions and who had been addicted for 7.9 ± 3 yr before entry into methadone treatment, which had been carried out for 3.4 ± 0.9 yr at doses of 30 to 100 mg (Table 5).

The patients were examined at 11 A.M. or 24 hr after their last methadone dose and had serial plasmas obtained at 0, 2, 4, 24, 26, and 28 hr—intended to minimize the effect of any diurnal variation and also to examine the patient during rapidly increasing and slowly descending phases of plasma methadone concentration. Liver functions, immunoglobulins and urinary drug excretion were typical of the methadone-maintained patient (all had SGOT values over 40 mIU/ml), six of the eight had high alkaline phosphatase levels, but none were hyperbilirubinemic or had abnormal levels of plasma proteins. Only methadone was detected in their urine; morphine, quinine, etc. were not found.

TABLE 5. Some clinical features of 8 selected methadone-maintained patients

Case no.	Age (years)	Methadone dose mg/day	Methadone years of RX	SGOT mIU/ml	Alkaline phosphatase mIU/ml	Bilirubin mg/dl	Urinary drug excretion methadone	Urinary drug excretion morphine	Urinary drug excretion other drug
1	42	100	2	41	74	1.0	++	—	—
2	28	30	3	113	93	0.9	+++	—	—
3	24	80	2.5	81	92	0.9	+++	—	—
4	25	100	2	60	120	0.8	++++	—	—
5	33	80	1.5	15	224	0.7	+++	—	—
6	26	80	6	58	103	0.6	+++	—	—
7	35	70	2	141	145	0.9	++	—	—
8	41	100	5	31	61	0.4	+	—	—

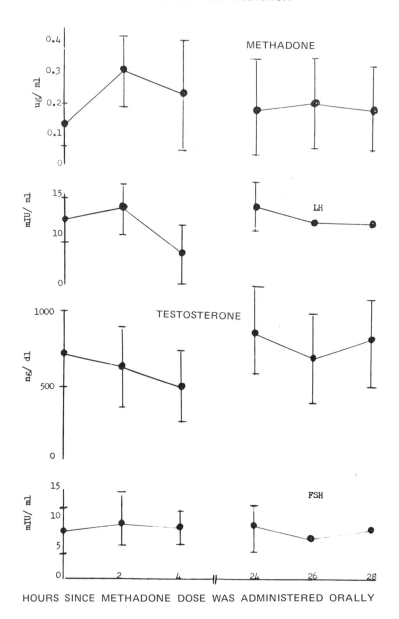

HOURS SINCE METHADONE DOSE WAS ADMINISTERED ORALLY

FIG. 1. Methadone, LH, testosterone, and FSH levels in methadone-maintained patients. Connected points on the left are before and after methadone dose. The points on the right are at the same time of day but with methadone withheld.

In Fig. 1 are plotted the methadone, LH, FSH, and testosterone values. The rise in methadone from 0 to 4 hr was not repeated the next day when methadone was withheld until the end of the study. No change in FSH and no significant change in LH were seen. Testosterone levels fell somewhat shortly after methadone administration. The relationship between plasma methadone versus testosterone concentrations are plotted in Fig. 2. A broad scatter of values was evident but no simple relationship was found.

This study showed that oral methadone given to stabilized, selected "normal" methadone-maintained patients did not produce a change in LH or FSH. The testosterone values probably did not change significantly either,

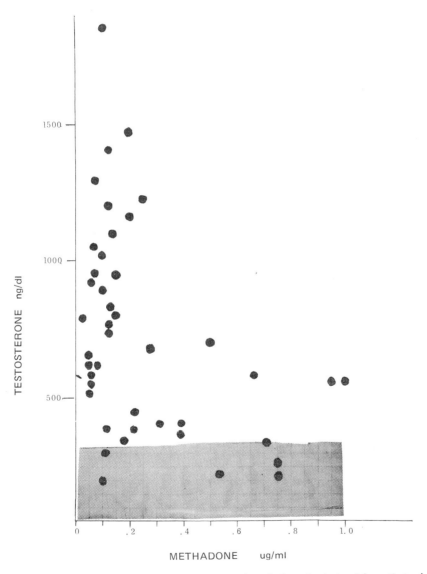

FIG. 2. Relationship between plasma, testosterone, and methadone levels in eight patients determined from 11 A.M. to 3 P.M. The shaded area constitutes values considered to be abnormally low.

although lower values were seen at 3 P.M. than at 11 A.M., a finding which has been often but not invariably reported. It is recognized that the interpretation of single values of LH or testosterone can be difficult in view of the wide, almost pulsatile fluctuations that these hormones normally undergo. Possibly the fewer secretory bursts of testosterone shortly after the methadone dose were directly related, but there was a similar reduction in testosterone levels on the control day in some of the patients.

The plasma methadone sampled the plasma pool only. Although highly precise, these values are difficult to interpret regarding tissue methadone levels. Since methadone has a long half time and a large extravascular pool size, the plasma levels may not be a good measure of the levels of methadone occupying tissue effector sites.

CONCLUSIONS

1. A number of hormones obtained from both chronic heroin addicts and methadone-maintained patients were studied. Plasma cortisol, GH, LH, and FSH levels were normal. Plasma testosterone and thyroid function tests were generally within normal limits except for a tendency for increase in TBG binding capacities in the untreated heroin addict and related changes in T-4 and T-3 resin uptakes.

2. Patients did not manifest any apparent clinical stigma of endocrine disturbance. The major clinical endocrine findings were amenorrhea in the heroin-addicted female and reduction in sexual performance and desire in both sexes. The mechanisms of these disturbances are unknown; however, the pituitary gonadotropins and testosterone levels in plasma are normal or near normal.

3. Some laboratory abnormalities were found: (a) Some heroin addicts and methadone-maintained patients had poor GH responses to stimulatory procedures such as insulin hypoglycemia and arginine. (b) A few heroin addicts and a very few methadone-treated patients had subnormal cortisol responses to insulin hypoglycemia. (c) Some patients, starting from a detoxified baseline, had transient reduction in hypothalamic-pituitary-adrenal function in association with initiation of methadone maintenance treatment.

4. Patients appear to develop tolerance to some endocrine effects of methadone treatment. This phase of addiction should be more carefully studied and patients should be studied serially.

5. Plasma narcotic concentrations should be obtained routinely in future studies. This will avoid problems in the interpretation of possible effects of absorption and degradation rates, narcotic pool size, idiosyncratic metabolic pathways, etc., that necessarily arise when only the dose and route of administration are given. It will also add to the precision by which the narcotic status of the patient can be studied.

ACKNOWLEDGMENTS

This work was supported in part by grants from the National Institute of Mental Health (DA 00335); Special Action Office for Drug Abuse Prevention; the Health Research Council of New York City; General Clinical Research Centers Program of the Division of Research Resources, National Institutes of Health (RR-102); and the New York State Narcotic Addiction Control Commission (conclusions stated herein are not necessarily those of the Commission).

The expert technical services of Mrs. Huang, Mrs. Chen, Mrs. Rupners, Mrs. Gutjahr were much appreciated. The cheerful cooperation of the Exodus House staff and patients was also invaluable. Some of the assays were performed by Bioscience Laboratories, Van Nuys, California.

REFERENCES

1. de Bodo, R. C. Antidiuretic action of morphine and its mechanism. *J. Pharmacol. Exp. Ther.,* 82:74, 1944.
2. Zimmermann, E., and Critchlow, V. Inhibition of morphine-induced pituitary-adrenal activation by dexamethasone in the female rat. *Proc. Soc. Exp. Biol. Med.,* 143:1224, 1973.
3. Briggs, F. N., and Munson, P. L. Studies on the mechanism of stimulation of ACTH secretion with the aid of morphine as a blocking agent. *Endocrinology,* 57:205, 1955.
4. McDonald, R. K., Evans, F. T., Weise, V. K., and Patrick, R. W. Effect of morphine and nalorphine on plasma hydrocortisone levels in man. *J. Pharmacol. Exper. Ther.,* 126:241, 1959.
5. Nakao, T., Hiraga, K., Inaba, M., and Urata, Y. Influence of morphine on corticoid production. In: *Steroid Dynamics,* edited by G. Pincus, T. Nakao, and J. F. Tait, pp. 179–213. Academic Press, New York, 1966.
6. Arimura, A., Saito, T., and Schally, A. V. Assays for corticotropin-releasing factor (CRF) using rats treated with morphine, chlorpromazine, dexamethasone and nembutal. *J. Clin. Endocrinol. Metab.,* 81:235, 1967.
7. Dole, V. P., Kim, W. K., and Eglitis, I. Detection of narcotic drugs, tranquilizers, amphetamines, and barbiturates in urine. *JAMA* 198:349, 1966.
8. Webster, B. J., Coupal, J. J., and Cushman, P. Increased serum thyroxine levels in euthyroid narcotic addicts *J. Clin. Endocrinol. Metab.,* 37:928, 1973.
9. Eisenman, A. J., Fraser, H. E., and Brooks, J. W. Urinary excretion and plasma levels of 17-hydroxycorticosteroids during a cycle of addiction to morphine. *J. Pharmacol. Exper. Ther.,* 132:226, 1961.
10. Eisenman, A. J., Martin, W. R., Jasinski, D. R., and Brooks, J. W. Catecholamine and 17-hydroxycorticosteroid excretion during a cycle of morphine dependence in man. *J. Psychiatr. Res.,* 7:19, 1969.
11. Cushman, P. Growth hormone in narcotic addiction. *J. Clin. Endocrinol. Metab.,* 35:352, 1972.
12. Cushman, P., Bordier, B., and Hilton, J. G. Hypothalamic-pituitary-adrenal axis in methadone-treated heroin addicts. *J. Clin. Endocrinol. Metab.,* 30:24, 1970.
13. Liddle, G. L., Estep, H. L., Kendall, J. W., Williams, W. C., and Townes, A. W. Clinical application of a new test of pituitary reserve. *J. Clin. Endocrinol. Metab.,* 19:875, 1959.
14. Martin, W. R., Jasinski, D. R., Haertzen, C. A., Kay, D. C., Jones, B. E., Mansky,

P. A., and Carpenter, R. W. Methadone—A reevaluation. *Arch. Gen. Psychiat.,* 28:286, 1973.
15. Santen, R. J., and Bilic, N. Evaluation of the pituitary-gonadal axis in women with amenorrhea associated with narcotic addiction. *Endo. Soc. Abstr.,* A-112, June 1973.
16. Schenkman, L., Massie, B., Mitsuma, T., and Hollander, C. S. Effects of chronic methadone administration on the hypothalamic-pituitary-thyroid axis. *J. Clin. Endocrinol. Metab.,* 35:169, 1972.
17. Cushman, P. Methadone maintenance in hard-core criminal addicts. *N.Y.S. J. Med.,* 71:1768, 1971.
18. Cushman, P. Plasma testosterone in narcotic addiction. *Amer. J. Med.,* 55:452, 1973.
19. Kreek, M. J. Medical safety and side effects of methadone in tolerant individuals. *JAMA,* 223:665, 1973.

DISCUSSION

Lomax: Is epilepsy prevalent among your addict population? That is, do you see much seizure activity in this group?

Cushman: We have seen seizures in our patients, but it is difficult to know the cause of them. These individuals frequently abuse other drugs, such as alcohol and barbiturates, and seizures may be caused by abstinence from these agents.

Wikler: In general, the incidence of genuine epilepsy among narcotic addicts is comparable to that of the general population.

Oldendorf: Dr. Wikler, is there any evidence that electroconvulsive therapy modifies morphine withdrawal syndrome?

Wikler: In the old literature there are several reports that the effects of electroconvulsive therapy are very beneficial during withdrawal, but these studies were uncontrolled and no measurements were made and, to my knowledge, they have not been repeated using proper techniques.

Narcotics and the Hypothalamus, edited by
E. Zimmermann and R. George. Raven Press,
New York © 1974

Effect of Central Acting Drugs on the Onset of Puberty

Richard I. Weiner and Umberto Scapagnini

Department of Anatomy, University of Southern California School of Medicine, Los Angeles, California 90033, and Institute of Pharmacology, Faculty of Medicine, University of Naples, Naples, Italy

INTRODUCTION

The mechanisms controlling the onset of puberty in the female are still incompletely understood. The majority of research in this area has been done using the rat, since the onset of puberty is clearly marked by the occurrence of vaginal opening. This occurs at approximately 40 days of age and is accompanied by a fertile ovulation. Early workers demonstrated that both the ovary and the anterior pituitary were capable of adult function well before vaginal opening (1, 2). Clinical observations in children and lesion experiments in rats suggest that the central nervous system inhibits activation of the pituitary-gonadal axis before the onset of puberty. Electrolytic lesions in the anterior and posterior hypothalamus advance the time of vaginal opening (3, 4). Numerous reports have correlated the occurrence of precocious puberty in children with hypothalamic and pineal tumors (5). Pharmacologic agents affecting activity of the central nervous system also affect the onset of puberty (6, 7). The following studies were performed to study further the effects of central acting drugs on the onset of puberty.

EFFECT OF RESERPINE AND α-METHYL-*p*-TYROSINE ON THE ONSET OF PUBERTY

Khazan et al. (6) reported that the daily administration of reserpine to immature rats delayed the time of vaginal opening. Reserpine is known to cause a depletion of brain catecholamines. In adult animals, brain catecholamines appear to play an important role in the regulation of luteinizing hormone and prolactin secretion. Therefore, it was of interest to attempt to relate the inhibitory action of reserpine on the onset of puberty to its action on brain catecholamines.

In our initial study we confirmed the finding that the daily administration of 0.2 mg/kg of reserpine delayed the occurrence of vaginal opening. However, this treatment also significantly inhibited the rate of growth of the animals (8). Kennedy and Mitra (9) clearly demonstrated that the time of vaginal opening correlates closely with the rate of growth of the animal, as well as with chronological age. Chronic underfeeding decreased the rate of body growth and delayed the sexual development of female rats. The decrease in growth rate associated with reserpine has been linked to its action as an anorexic. Therefore, in the next study, reserpine-treated animals were pair-fed with their controls. Pair-feeding resulted in identical rates of body growth in the two groups (Fig. 1). The mean age at vaginal opening was

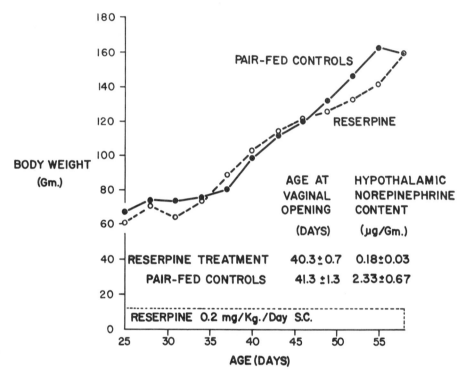

FIG. 1. Effect of reserpine treatment (0.2 mg/kg/day s.c.) on body growth, vaginal opening, and norepinephrine content. Values for the time of vaginal opening and norepinephrine content are expressed as the mean ± SEM. From Weiner and Ganong, Neuroendocrinology, 8:125–135, 1971.

also identical in both groups but was significantly delayed in both when compared with ad libitum fed controls. The ability of reserpine to delay puberty thus could be explained through its action as an anorexic. At the time of sacrifice at 60 days of age, the hypothalamic norepinephrine content of the reserpine-treated animals was 8% of that of the pair-fed controls. Therefore, catecholamine depletion did not add to the delay of onset of puberty due to the anorexic action of reserpine.

Treatment at two separate dosages with α-methyl-p-tyrosine, a catecholamine synthesis inhibitor, did not delay the onset of puberty (8). Treatment with this drug also did not decrease the rate of body growth. Chronic treatment with 200 mg/kg per day of α-methyl-*p*-tyrosine caused a 46% depletion of hypothalamic norepinephrine content approximately 16 hr following the last injection. In these experiments, depletion of hypothalamic catecholamines in the absence of a decreased rate of body growth did not affect the time of the onset of puberty. Once vaginal opening had occurred, the reserpine- and α-methyl-*p*-tyrosine-treated animals showed prolonged periods of diestrus and apparent pseudopregnancy. Barraclough and Sawyer (10) first reported that reserpine treatment caused the induction of pseudopregnancy in adult rats. Chronic treatment of animals with reserpine and α-methyl-*p*-tyrosine starting at 22 days of age did not interfere with the ability of these drugs to cause pseudopregnancy following vaginal opening.

EFFECT OF MORPHINE AND NALORPHINE ON THE ONSET OF PUBERTY

Morphine has been demonstrated to cause changes in the secretion of a number of anterior pituitary hormones (11, 12). The site of action of these effects appears to be in the central nervous system (11). A great deal of evidence supports the concept that the onset of puberty is controlled by the central nervous system. It was therefore of interest to test whether morphine treatment could affect the occurrence of vaginal opening.

Female Sprague-Dawley rats were injected intraperitoneally with 2 mg/kg per day of morphine, nalorphine, or morphine plus nalorphine starting at 20 days of age. Low doses of the drugs were used in an attempt to prevent effects on the rate of body growth. In Study I, no change in the rate of body growth was observed following treatment with morphine, nalorphine, or a combination of these agents (Fig. 2). In Study II there was a statistically significant decrease in body weight at the time of sacrifice in the morphine, nalorphine, and morphine plus nalorphine groups (controls, 130.3 g ± 3.3; morphine, 114.5 g ± 3.5; nalorphine, 121.1 g ± 2.6; morphine plus nalorphine, 119.4 g ± 2.9). In both studies morphine treatment caused an advancement of the mean age at vaginal opening (Table 1). However, only in Study II was this difference statistically significant ($p < 0.01$). Nalorphine treatment had no statistically significant effect in either study on the time of occurrence of puberty. Nalorphine, when given in conjunction with morphine, did not block the ability of morphine to cause precocious puberty. In Study II, morphine plus nalorphine caused a significant advancement of vaginal opening. None of the drug treatments had any effect on the estrous cycle once vaginal opening occurred (Fig. 3). No difference in the mean cycle length was observed.

The advancement of vaginal opening by morphine can best be explained by an action on the central nervous system. Lesions in the anterior and posterior hypothalamus have been found to cause precocious puberty (3, 4). Lesions of the amygdala were found to cause early vaginal opening, whereas stimulation of the amygdala prevents vaginal opening (13, 14). These findings can

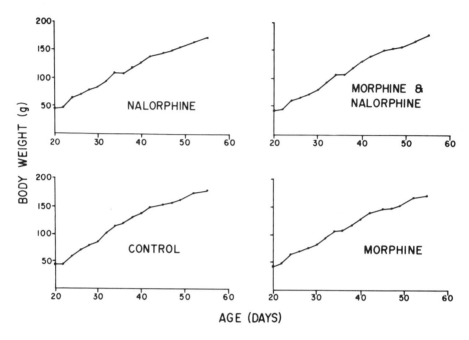

FIG. 2. Body growth rate in control morphine-, nalorphine-, and morphine plus nalorphine-treated rats from Study I.

best be explained by an inhibition of the previously matured pituitary-gonadal axis. The most widely held hypothesis for the control of the onset of puberty by the central nervous system is that the threshold of the central nervous system to negative feedback increases at the onset of puberty. A

TABLE 1. Mean age at vaginal opening ± SEM for control, morphine-, nalorphine-, and morphine plus nalorphine-treated animals

Treatment	Study I		Study II	
	n	age vaginal opening (days)	n	age vaginal opening (days)
Control	8	36.1 ± 1.1	16	36.4 ± 0.7
Morphine (2 mg/kg/day)	8	34.9 ± 1.6	18	33.6 ± 0.7[a]
Nalorphine (2 mg/kg/day)	7	37.0 ± 1.7	16	38.5 ± 0.9
Morphine + nalophrine (2 mg/kg/day)	6	33.7 ± 1.4	14	33.9 ± 0.7[b]

[a] $p < 0.01$.
[b] $p < 0.05$.

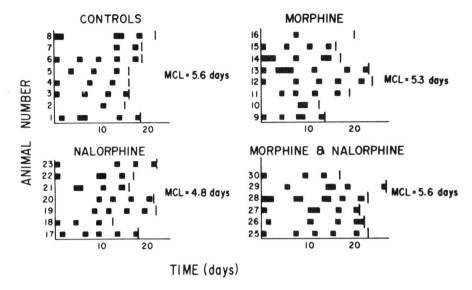

FIG. 3. Effect of morphine, nalorphine, and morphine plus nalorphine treatment on vaginal cyclicity in animals from Study I. From the day of vaginal opening until the time of sacrifice, vaginal smears were examined daily. Day 1 on the figure represents the smear obtained on the day of vaginal opening. Each darkened block indicates that an estrous smear was obtained on that day. The vertical line indicates the last day on which a vaginal smear was obtained. MCL = mean cycle length.

lower dose of estrogen is capable of inhibiting the postcastration rise in luteinizing hormone in immature animals when compared with mature animals (15). Implantation of a small amount of estrogen in the hypothalamus of immature female rats caused a significant decrease in ovarian weight (16). The same size implant in the adult female had no effect on ovarian weight. The mechanism by which neurons in the hypothalamus change their sensitivity to the negative feedback of steroids is a key question in understanding the control of the onset of puberty. Morphine is known to have both excitatory and inhibitory actions on the central nervous system. Therefore, it is impossible at this time to speculate further as to the role of morphine in inducing precocious puberty. At present we are studying whether morphine treatment in prepubertal animals causes an increased threshold to the negative feedback effects of estrogen.

SUMMARY

The occurrence of the onset of puberty appears to be under the control of the central nervous system. Reserpine was found to be capable of delaying the time of vaginal opening. This action of reserpine appeared to be related to its influence on body growth rather than to its ability to affect brain catecholamines. The catecholamine synthesis inhibitor α-methyl-p-tyrosine had no effect on body growth or on the time of vaginal opening. Morphine treatment caused precocious puberty, an effect not blocked by nalorphine. The ability of morphine to cause precocious vaginal opening could be explained by the removal of an inhibitory action of the brain on previously matured components of the pituitary-gonadal axis.

REFERENCES

1. Long, G. A., and Evans, H. M. The estrous cycle in the rat and its associated phenomena. *Mem. Univ. Calif.*, 6:1–148, 1922.
2. Harris, G. W., and Jacobsohn, D. Functional grafts of the anterior pituitary gland. *Proc. R. Soc. Lond.*, B139:263–276, 1952.
3. Donovan, B. T., and Van der Werff ten Bosch, J. J. The hypothalamus and sexual maturation in the rat. *J. Physiol.*, 147:78–92, 1959.
4. Gellert, R. J., and Ganong, W. F. Precocious puberty in rats with hypothalamic lesions. *Acta Endocrinol.*, 33:569–576, 1960.
5. Lowrey, G. H., and Brown, E. F. Precocious sexual development. A study of thirty cases. *J. Pediat.*, 38:325–340, 1939.
6. Khazan, N., Sulman, F., and Winik, H. Effect of reserpine on pituitary-gonadal axis. *Proc. Soc. Exp. Biol. Med.*, 105:201–204, 1960.
7. Setnikar, I., Murmann, W., and Magistretti, M. J. Retardation of sexual development in female rats due to iproniazid treatment. *Endocrinology*, 67:511–520, 1960.
8. Weiner, R. I., and Ganong, W. F. Effect of the depletion of brain catecholamines on puberty and the estrous cycle in the rat. *Neuroendocrinology*, 8:125–135, 1971.
9. Kennedy, G. C., and Mitra, J. Body weight and food intake as initiating factors for puberty in the rat. *J. Physiol.*, 166:408–418, 1963.
10. Barraclough, C. A., and Sawyer, C. H. Induction of pseudopregnancy in the rat by reserpine and chlorpromazine. *Endocrinology*, 65:563–571, 1959.
11. George, R. Effects of narcotic analgesics on hypothalamo-pituitary-thyroid function. In: *Progress in Brain Research, Vol. 39: Drug Effects on Neuroendocrine Regulation,* edited by E. Zimmermann, W. H. Gispen, B. H. Marks, and D. de Weid, pp. 339–345. Elsevier, Amsterdam, 1973.
12. Sloan, J. W. Corticosteroid hormones. In: *Narcotic Drugs, Biochemistry and Pharmacology,* edited by D. H. Clovet, pp. 262–282. Plenum, New York, 1971.
13. Elwers, M., and Critchlow, V. Precocious ovarian stimulation following hypothalamic and amygdaloid lesions in rats. *Amer. J. Physiol.*, 198:381–385, 1960.
14. Bar-Sela, M. E., and Critchlow, V. Delayed puberty following electrical stimulation of amygdala in female rats. *Amer. J. Physiol.*, 211:1103–1107, 1966.
15. Ramirez, V. D., and McCann, S. M. Comparison of regulation of luteinizing hormone (LH) secretion in immature and adult rats. *Endocrinology*, 72:452–464, 1963.
16. Smith, E. R., and Davidson, J. M. Role of estrogen in the cerebral control of puberty in female rats. *Endocrinology*, 82:100–108, 1968.

DISCUSSION

Lomax: How did you decide on the dose of morphine used in your study and what did your animals look like?

Weiner: Dose was selected which would not impair growth rate in these animals since from previous work, particularly with reserpine, we learned that agents which depress growth almost invariably tend to delay the onset of vaginal opening. Thus, we wanted a dose which would not affect growth rate. The animals appeared normal in every respect; they were healthy and well groomed. We tried 0.5, 1, and 2 mg/kg of morphine and at 2 mg/kg we thought we first saw a body weight effect.

Lomax: This could be important because with this dose of morphine one does not get analgesia and, in fact, the animals become hyperactive in the hot-plate test. Also, this dose produces a hyperthermia, as opposed to the hypothermia seen with larger doses. Moreover, none of these effects can be blocked by nalorphine. Rather, they are thought to be the stimulant effects of morphine.

Kerr: Why did you wait until day 20 to begin your injections?

Weiner: For two reasons. First, we did not want to treat our rats prior to weaning, which was carried out at 21 days of age, and secondly, the pituitary-gonadal axis in the rat is not mature until approximately 20 days of age. In avoiding the effects of earlier injections, we thought the interpretation would be cleaner if we started drug administration following complete maturation of this system.

Mirsky: In view of the correlation between body weight and onset of puberty, have you ever tried to force-feed your animals to study the effect of this on puberty?

Weiner: No.

McCann: Do you know the exact weight of your animals at the time of vaginal opening? I ask this because we have reason to believe that it is the actual weight, rather than the age, of the animal which correlates best with the time of the vaginal opening. We found that when rats reached 110 g body weight vaginal opening occurred in most cases.

Weiner: I do not have the exact figures on body weight at the time of vaginal opening.

Sawyer: You will remember that Ramirez advanced vaginal opening without affecting body weight in rats treated from day 26 through 30 with a small dose of estrogen. I'm wondering if your stimulatory dose of morphine might not be causing the small amount of estrogen secretion and thereby be acting by a similar mechanism?

Weiner: I think that is definitely a possibility. It is also possible that the morphine modifies the sensitivity of the pituitary to the feedback action of estrogen.

Zimmermann: In relation to Dr. Kerr's question earlier, I would like to point out that we have treated rats from day 1 through 21 of life with morphine, using a dose (8 mg/kg, b.i.d.) somewhat larger than that used by Dr. Weiner. This treatment did result in significant decrease in body weight during the time of administration and this deficit persisted long afterwards. Despite the diminished body weight, however, morphine-treated animals showed vaginal opening at the same time as did the saline-injected controls, at about 36 days of age.

Ford: We have obtained similar results in rats treated prenatally during the last 4 days of pregnancy—their mothers received 40 mg/kg of morphine daily. Although this dose resulted in a slight decrease in body weight at the time of birth, these animals proceeded subsequently to grow normally and vaginal opening occurred coincident with that of the saline-injected control animals.

Narcotics and the Hypothalamus, edited by
E. Zimmermann and R. George. Raven Press,
New York © 1974

Long-Lasting Effects of Prepuberal Administration of Morphine in Adult Rats

E. Zimmermann, B. Branch, A. Newman Taylor, J. Young, and C. N. Pang

Department of Anatomy and Brain Research Institute, UCLA School of Medicine, Los Angeles, California 90024

In recent years, experimental evidence has accumulated which indicates that morphine exerts effects which far outlast the presence of the drug or its metabolites in the body. Cochin and Kornetsky (1) obtained evidence of tolerance to morphine more than 1 year following a single injection of the drug. Martin et al. (2) demonstrated physiologic signs of "protracted abstinence" in rats several months following cessation of repeated administration of morphine. The basis for these persistent drug effects is not known, although some alteration in protein synthesis has been implicated in the development of tolerance to morphine (3) and such biochemical alteration might be involved in protracted tolerance and dependence.

It is now well established that various adult patterns of neural regulation depend upon appropriate maturation of protein synthetic processes in the hypothalamus of the newborn rat. Pharmacologic or endocrinologic disturbance of these maturational events at critical periods of development result in prolonged or permanent alteration of neuroendocrine and behavioral functioning (4–6). We reasoned that the developing animal may be particularly sensitive to the long-lasting effects of morphine and provide a potentially useful model for the study of protracted tolerance and physical dependence. Therefore we undertook the following study to determine if treatment of the immature rat with morphine results in prolonged tolerance as evidenced by altered pituitary-adrenal and behavioral responses to the drug in adulthood.

Pregnant Sprague-Dawley rats (Simonsen) were maintained under standardized conditions of illumination (lighting from 4 A.M. to 6 P.M. alternating with darkness 6 P.M. to 4 A.M.) and temperature ($24 \pm 1°C$). Purina lab chow and tap water were available at all times. Following birth (day 0), each litter size was adjusted to eight pups (four male and four female). Two pups of each sex were given two daily subcutaneous injections of morphine sulfate or 0.9% saline, which served as control for the morphine vehicle and for the effect of handling and injection. The initial dose of morphine (0.5 mg/kg, free base) was doubled every other day during the first week of life and then maintained at 8 mg/kg from days 8 to 18. The dose was tapered rapidly on days 19 to 21 and then discontinued. This dosage schedule was chosen on the basis of preliminary experience indicating that it produces minimal mortality and is well tolerated by most pups; the maximum dose was maintained until, at the end of the first week, it became clear that significant growth retardation had occurred as a result of morphine administration. We chose to begin injections postnatally to avoid problems associated with the placental barrier to morphine (7) and with the interpretation of drug-induced modification of maternal factors (behavior, milk production, etc.). All pups were weaned at 21 days of age and thereafter housed two or three per cage according to sex and maintained under the conditions noted above.

During the subsequent 13 weeks, a series of studies was performed on these animals and the results obtained in morphine- and saline-treated rats of the

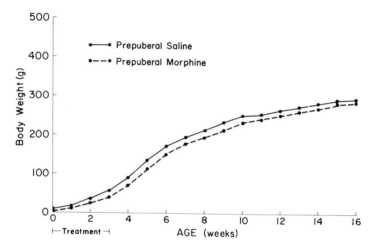

FIG. 1. Effects of prepuberal administration of morphine (8 mg/kg twice daily) on body weight in female rats. Each point represents the mean weight of 31 (saline group) or 29 (morphine group) animals. Weights of the two groups differed significantly ($p < 0.05$) at weeks 1 to 15.

same sex were compared. Each study conformed to a randomized statistical design. The t-test was used to compare group means and a probability value of less than 0.05 was considered significant.

Body weight was determined on day 1 and at weekly intervals thereafter during the 16-week period of observation (Fig. 1). Early administration of morphine resulted in slight depression ($p < 0.05$) in body weight in female rats by the end of the first week of life, and this growth retardation appeared to increase slightly by the end of the third week of drug administration. Following cessation of daily injection of morphine, the rate of body weight increase appeared to be similar in morphine- and saline-treated animals; however, the depression in weight of morphine-treated rats persisted until 105 days of age, after which the deficit was no longer significant ($p > 0.05$). A similar pattern of ponderal changes was observed in male rats (Fig.

2), except that body weights in morphine-treated animals remained lower ($p < 0.05$) than those of the controls throughout the 4-month period of observation.

Beginning on day 34, all animals were inspected daily for evidence of the onset of puberty (vaginal or prepucial opening). Under conditions of these experiments, prepuberal administration of morphine had no apparent effect on the onset of puberty. The time of vaginal opening occurring in morphine-treated females (36.2 ± 0.3) was indistinguishable from that of the controls (35.9 ± 0.3 days of age). Similarly, prepucial opening occurred in morphine- and saline-treated male rats at approximately the same age (40.9 ± 0.3 and 40.7 ± 0.2 days, respectively).

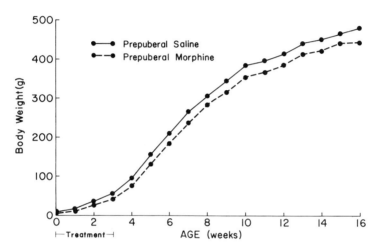

FIG. 2. Effect of prepuberal administration of morphine (8 mg/kg twice daily) on body weight in male rats. Each point represents the mean weight of 33 (saline group) or 24 (morphine group) animals. Weights of the two groups differed significantly ($p < 0.05$) at weeks 1 to 16.

At 56 days of age, the effects of early administration of morphine on the normal diurnal variation in resting pituitary-adrenal function was studied with the use of standardized procedures developed previously (8, 9). Approximately equal numbers of morphine- and saline-treated rats of each sex were subjected to ether anesthesia and rapid jugular venipuncture (< 3 min) at either 9 A.M. or 4 P.M. that day. Blood samples were collected at these times to correspond with the expected trough and peak concentrations of corticosterone in the circulation of rats maintained under the conditions used in this study (8, 9). Plasma was frozen for subsequent fluorometric determination of concentrations of corticosterone (10).

The typical marked diurnal increase in plasma levels of corticosterone was observed in female rats treated prepuberally with either morphine or saline; steroid concentrations in the two groups were comparable at each time of day

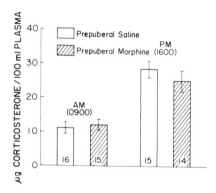

FIG. 3. Effect of prepuberal administration of morphine on the diurnal rise in plasma non-stress levels of corticosterone in 56-day-old female rats. In this and in subsequent figures, vertical lines represent ± SE and figures in columns denote number of animals.

(Fig. 3). Similar results were obtained in male rats (Fig. 4), except that the absolute levels of corticosterone in each treatment group were lower than those of the females. The latter observation is consistent with the well-known sex difference in resting levels of plasma corticosterone which appears following puberty in the rat (8).

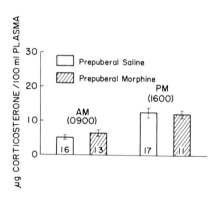

FIG. 4. Effect of prepuberal administration of morphine on the diurnal rise in plasma non-stress levels of corticosterone in 56-day-old male rats.

At 78 days of age, stress-induced pituitary-adrenal function was tested. At 9 A.M., male and female rats of either prepuberal treatment group were exposed to ether vapor for 3 min or injected intraperitoneally with saline or morphine (20 or 40 mg/kg). Thirty min later, each rat was rapidly anesthetized with ether and a sample of jugular venous blood was obtained. In contrast to low morning resting levels observed in a group of uninjected animals, female rats of both prepuberal treatment groups showed similar marked elevation of corticosterone levels in response to 3-min ether stress (Fig. 5). Injection of saline had no apparent stressful effect; corticosterone levels in both prepuberal treatment groups were comparable to those of the uninjected untreated controls. Females treated prepuberally with saline showed a slight but insignificant rise in steroid levels in response to 20 mg/kg morphine and a marked ($p < 0.01$) increase in response to 40 mg/kg morphine. These findings are consistent with the known initial excitatory effect of

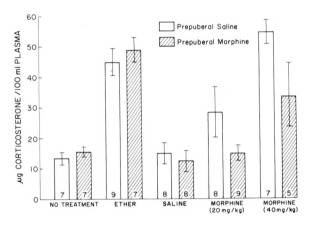

FIG. 5. Effects of prepuberal administration of morphine on plasma corticosterone responses 30 min after administration of ether (3 min) or morphine in 72-day-old female rats.

morphine on pituitary-adrenal activity in naive rats (11, 12). In contrast, females treated prepuberally with morphine showed no corticosterone response to the challenge dose of 20 mg/kg and evidenced a diminished ($p < 0.05$) response to 40 mg/kg morphine. Like the females, male rats of either prepuberal treatment group showed similar marked increases in corticosterone levels in response to 3-min ether and failure to respond to saline injection (Fig. 6). Unlike females, however, male rats of either prepuberal treatment group showed comparable significant increases in corticosterone levels in response to 20 or 40 mg/kg morphine.

At 80 days of age, the influence of prepuberal administration of morphine on the analgesic response to morphine in adulthood was tested with the hot-plate technique (13). Rats which received morphine in the preceding study were excluded from this and subsequent studies. The response latency on the hot plate (54.5°C) was determined at consecutive 30-min intervals. Immediately after the third control test, morphine (10 mg/kg) or saline was injected intraperitoneally. The hot-plate test was repeated 30, 60, 90, and 120 min after injection. The average preinjection latency was calculated for each animal and subtracted from each postinjection latency. The results obtained in female rats are shown in Fig. 7. Compared with saline-injected controls, rats treated prepuberally with saline showed a typical marked increase

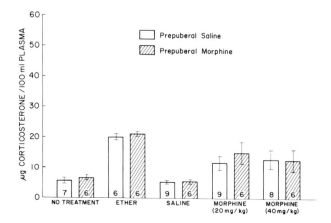

FIG. 6. Effects of prepuberal administration of morphine on plasma corticosterone responses 30 min after administration of ether (3 min) or morphine in 72-day-old male rats.

in response latency 30 ($p < 0.05$), 60 ($p < 0.01$)), and 90 min ($p < 0.01$) after injection of the test dose of morphine. By 120 min after injection this effect had disappeared. In contrast, rats treated prepuberally with morphine showed a slight increase in response latency only at 30 min after injection of the test dose of morphine; however, at each time after injection the response in this group was less than that of rats treated prepuberally with saline and given morphine for the first time as adults in this study. Injection of saline produced no appreciable change in response to the hot plate in female rats of either prepuberal treatment group.

The same protocol described above for females was used to study effects of prepuberal administration of morphine on the analgesic action of morphine in adult male rats. The results are presented in Fig. 8. Compared with effects of

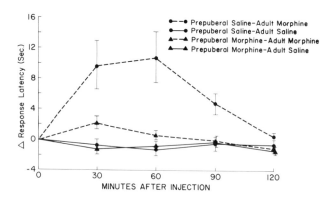

FIG. 7. Effect of prepuberal administration of morphine on the analgesic response to morphine (10 mg/kg, i.p.) in 80-day-old female rats tested with the hot-plate technique (13). Each group contained six to nine animals. (See text for details.)

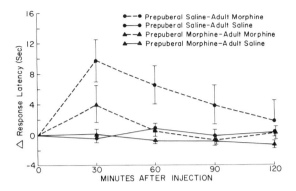

FIG. 8. Effect of prepuberal administration of morphine on the analgesic response to morphine (10 mg/kg, i.p.) in 80-day-old male rats tested with the hot-plate technique (13). Each group contained six to ten animals. (See text for details.)

saline injection, morphine (10 mg/kg) given to rats treated prepuberally with saline caused a significant increase in the response latency in the hot-plate test at 30, 60, and 90 min after injection. On the other hand, rats injected prepuberally with morphine showed only a minimal analgesic response 30 min after the adult challenge dose of morphine. Because of the large variation in responses of individual rats to morphine, the differences in response latencies of the two groups injected with the narcotic were not significantly different when compared with the t-test. However, an analysis of variance performed on the data revealed significant difference between the adult morphine-treated groups 60 min after injection.

At 92 days of age, the male and female control animals injected with saline in the preceding study were used to study effects of prepuberal morphine administration on the pituitary-adrenal response to naloxone in adulthood. This specific narcotic antagonist lacks agonistic action in the pituitary-adrenal system of adult rats (11). However, in rats made dependent on morphine by subcutaneous implantation of a morphine pellet (14), naloxone causes a prompt and dramatic increase in circulating levels of corticosterone (*unpublished observations*). At 8:30 A.M., rats treated prepuberally with either morphine or saline were given naloxone (5 mg/kg) intraperitoneally. Thirty min later, each animal was quickly anesthetized with ether and a sample of jugular venous blood was obtained for subsequent determination of corticosterone concentration. The results obtained in female rats are presented in Fig. 9 (Exp. 1). Female animals treated prepuberally with saline showed typical low morning resting levels of plasma corticosterone. In contrast, rats exposed to morphine early in life showed a significant increase in corticosterone in response to naloxone. Similar results were obtained (Fig. 9, Exp. 2) when this study was repeated with the same animals at 108 days of age. Prepuberal administration of morphine was not associated with any

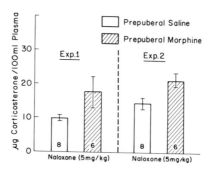

FIG. 9. Effect of naloxone on plasma levels of corticosterone in adult female rats treated prepuberally with morphine or saline. Exp. 1 was performed at 92 and Exp. 2 at 108 days of age.

change in corticosterone levels following adult challenge with naloxone in male rats at 92 or at 108 days of age, even though the dose of naloxone was increased to 10 mg/kg in the second study.

DISCUSSION

The main findings of this study are that prepuberal administration of morphine results in persistent reduction in body weight, long-lasting tolerance to pituitary-adrenal stimulating and antinociceptive effects of morphine, and pituitary-adrenal stimulation by naloxone. These effects, seen clearly in adult female rats, were only partially evident or absent in males. The bases for these findings and for the sex differences are not known, but presumably involve effects of morphine on development of neuroendocrine (presumably hypothalamic) mechanisms responsible for regulation of growth, pituitary-ovarian, and pituitary-adrenal activities.

Several factors must be considered as possible causes of the growth inhibition induced by morphine. Reduced food intake might account for the initial retardation of growth, but would not explain the continued deficit in weight beyond the period of drug treatment. It is interesting that tolerance to the growth-inhibiting effect of morphine apparently did not develop during treatment as might be expected if a gastrointestinal or brain mechanism were involved. Moreover, following cessation of drug administration, the animals did not undergo rapid catch-up growth as might occur if their reduced weight were due to simple undernutrition (15). The observed effect of morphine on body weight agrees with the recent findings of Bakke et al. (16), who reported diminished body weights at 21 and 108 days of age in male and female rats treated neonatally with morphine. This finding is also consistent with that of Crofford and Smith (17), who observed a weight deficit in mice for at least 6 weeks following cessation of neonatal administration of methadone. Persistence of a weight deficit following early exposure to morphine is not likely due to stressful or nutritive effects of the drug, but suggests that morphine may exert a relatively specific action on the immature hypothalamus, which results in a permanent alteration of homeostatic mechanisms responsible for growth regulation.

Despite its prolonged somatic effect, early administration of morphine did not disrupt sexual maturation as judged by the onset of vaginal or prepucial opening. This finding agrees with that of Bakke et al. (16), who found that vaginal opening occurred simultaneously in rats treated neonatally with morphine or saline. However, depending on the dose of morphine administered, these investigators observed diminished weights of the pituitary, gonads, and accessory sex organs in their animals at 108 days of age. Their findings thus indicate that exposure to morphine early in life is associated with prolonged changes in pituitary-gonadal systems.

Early exposure to morphine does not prevent appearance of normal adult patterns of pituitary-adrenal function. A comparable diurnal rise in non-stress levels of corticosterone was observed in morphine- and saline-treated rats at 56 days of age, and the observed sex difference in the magnitude of the A.M.–P.M. levels of corticosterone are consistent with that reported by others in mature male and female rats (8). Because the circadian rhythm of circulating levels of corticosterone is fully developed well before 56 days of age, our findings do not exclude the possibility that early administration of morphine altered the onset of the normal cyclic pattern of adult non-stress pituitary-adrenal activity. The results obtained with ether stress at 72 days of age indicate that early administration of morphine does not disrupt the response of the pituitary-adrenal axis to nonspecific stress. However, the diminished corticosterone response to morphine observed in female rats treated prepuberally with morphine indicates that mechanisms subserving this response remain tolerant to morphine for at least 51 days after cessation of drug administration. The intact response to ether indicates that the pituitary-adrenal axis is not functionally impaired by treatment with morphine early in life, and suggests that central mechanisms involved in the responses to ether and morphine may be differentiated on the basis of morphine-specific tolerance. This suggestion is consistent with evidence that morphine acts at the level of the hypothalamus to cause ACTH release (18), and that dexamethasone blockade of this action of morphine does not block the pituitary-adrenal response to ether (12). Finally, the steroid results of this study provide neuroendocrine evidence of protracted tolerance to morphine in the rat.

Huidobro and Huidobro (19) recently reported development of tolerance to the analgesic action of morphine in rats treated neonatally with morphine, and Johannesson and Becker (20) obtained similar results in rats exposed to morphine just prior to birth. These investigators observed diminished analgesic responses to a test dose of morphine approximately 2 weeks after a single injection of the drug. The results of the present study indicate that tolerance to this action of morphine in the immature rat is particularly long-lasting, and may be demonstrated with the hot-plate test at least 11 weeks after termination of neonatal drug treatment.

It is difficult to explain the pituitary-adrenal response to naloxone observed in 92-day-old female rats 71 days after cessation of prepuberal morphine treatment. Because of the long interval between administration of this antagonist and the last injection of the agonist, it seems unlikely that the corticosterone response involves competition at the morphine receptor. Naloxone itself does not stimulate corticosterone release in naive rats (11) but causes a prompt increase in corticosterone levels in morphine-dependent rats (*unpublished observation*). It is also unlikely that the corticosterone response to naloxone represents a sign of conditioned abstinence since naloxone had not been administered previously. Another plausible explanation for the response might be derived from the observations of Himmelsbach (21) and of Martin et al. (2) that protracted abstinence is associated with hyperresponsivity to stress. Accordingly, the corticosterone response to naloxone seen in rats treated neonatally with morphine might simply be attributed to the stress of injection. This explanation, however, is not supported by the results obtained at 72 days of age which showed that both prepuberal-saline and prepuberal-morphine treated animals failed to respond to stress of injection with an increase in corticosterone levels. Similar reasoning might apply to explaining the response to naloxone at 108 days of age, except that the animals had previously received one injection of naloxone. Injection of naloxone at either 92 or 108 days of age was not associated with gross behavioral signs of precipitated abstinence (e.g., wet-dog shakes). Thus, the results of this study suggest that neuroendocrine responses to naloxone challenge, such as pituitary-adrenal activation, may be useful and particularly sensitive parameters of protracted abstinence. At this time, however, the basis for such responses is obscure and further studies are required to determine if the brain of the post-addict can recognize and respond to a "pure" antagonist in the absence of the agonist or its metabolites.

Finally, the reason for the absence of clear-cut prolonged effects of prepuberal morphine on the pituitary-adrenal system in male rats in the present study is not known. It is possible that the dose schedule used in this study was inadequate to produce protracted tolerance and dependence in this system in males. Sex differences in the metabolism of narcotic drugs have been reported (22), and such differences may relate to the outcome of this study. At any rate, the existence of a sex difference in the results suggests that endocrine factors are important in determining the body's long-term responses to morphine administration.

SUMMARY

To study effects of prepuberal administration of morphine on body growth and pituitary-adrenal function, newborn Sprague-Dawley male and female rats were given subcutaneous saline or morphine (to 8 mg/kg twice daily) from 1 to 21 days of age. Compared with controls, body weights of morphine-treated animals were reduced ($p < 0.01$) by day 7 and remained significantly depressed for 105 days in females, and for at least 120 days in males. Puberty (vaginal or prepucial opening) occurred simultaneously in morphine- and saline-treated rats of each sex. On day 56, all groups showed normal diurnal patterns of non-stress levels of plasma corticosterone. Compared with non-stressed controls on day 72, morphine-treated male and female rats showed intact corticosterone responses to ether stress. However, female but not male rats showed reduced ($p < 0.05$) corticosterone responses to morphine (20 or 40 mg/kg). Similarly, on day 80, morphine-treated females showed reduced ($p < 0.05$) analgesic response to morphine (10 mg/kg), tested using the hot-plate technique, while the males showed an equivocal response. Finally, on day 92, morphine-treated females but not female controls or males showed increased ($p < 0.05$) plasma corticosterone levels 30 min after injection of naloxone (5 mg/kg). The persistence of growth deficit, tolerance to morphine, and sensitivity to naloxone suggests that exposure of the immature female rat to morphine results in prolonged, possibly permanent, morphine-specific alteration of neuroendocrine and nociceptive brain mechanisms.

ACKNOWLEDGMENTS

This research was supported in part by grant DA-514 from the National Institutes of Health and by the Ford Foundation.

REFERENCES

1. Cochin, J., and Kornetsky, C. Development and loss of tolerance to morphine in rat after single and multiple injections. *J. Pharmacol. Exp. Ther.*, 145:1–10, 1964.
2. Martin, W. R., Wikler, A., Eades, C. G., and Pescor, F. T. Tolerance to and physical dependence on morphine in rats. *Psychopharmacologia*, 4:247–260, 1963.
3. Cohen, M., Keats, A. S., Krivoy, W., and Ungar, G. Effect of actinomycin D on morphine tolerance. *Proc. Soc. Exp. Biol. Med.*, 119:381–384, 1965.
4. Kobayashi, F., and Gorski, R. A. Effects of antibiotics on androgenization of the neonatal female rat. *Endocrinology*, 86:285–289, 1970.
5. Werboff, J., and Gottlieb, J. S. Drugs in pregnancy: Behavioral teratology *Obstet. Gynecol. Surv.*, 18:420–423, 1963.
6. Tonge, S. R. Neurochemical teratology: 5 Hydroxyindole concentrations in discrete areas of rat brain after the pre- and neonatal administration of phencyclidine and imipramine. *Life Sci.*, 12:481–486, 1973.
7. Johannesson, T., Steele, W. J., and Becker, B. A. Infusion of morphine in maternal rats at near-term: Maternal and foetal distribution and effects on analgesia, brain DNA, RNA and protein. *Acta Pharmacol. Toxicol.*, 31:353–368, 1972.
8. Critchlow, V., Liebelt, R. A., Bar-Sela, M., Mountcastle, W., and Lipscomb, H. S. Sex difference in resting pituitary-adrenal function in the rat. *Am. J. Physiol.*, 205:807–815, 1963.
9. Zimmermann, E., and Critchlow, V. Effects of diurnal variation in plasma corticosterone levels on adrenocortical response to stress. *Proc. Soc. Exp. Biol. Med.*, 125:658–663, 1967.
10. Glick, D., von Redlich, D., and Levine, S. Fluorometric determination of corti-

costerone and cortisol in 0.02–0.05 milliliters of plasma or submilligram samples of adrenal tissue. *Endocrinology,* 74:652–655, 1964.

11. Kokka, N., Garcia, J. F., and Elliott, H. W. Effects of acute and chronic administration of narcotic analgesics on growth hormone and corticotrophin (ACTH) secretion in rats. *Prog. Brain Res.,* 39:347–360, 1973.

12. Zimmermann, E., and Critchlow, V. Inhibition of morphine-induced pituitary-adrenal activation by dexamethasone in the female rat. *Proc. Soc. Exp. Biol. Med.,* 143:1224–1226, 1973.

13. Eddy, N. B., and Leimbach, D. Synthetic analgesics. II. Dithienylbutenyl and dithienylbutylamines. *J. Pharmacol. Exp. Ther.,* 107:385–393, 1953.

14. Way, E. L., Loh, H. H., and Shen, F. H. Simultaneous quantitative assessment of morphine tolerance and physical dependence. *J. Pharmacol. Exp. Ther.,* 167:1–8, 1969.

15. Sinha, Y. N., Wilkins, J. N., Selby, F., and VanderLaan, W. P. Pituitary and serum growth hormone during undernutrition and catch-up growth in young rats. *Endocrinology,* 92:1768–1771, 1973.

16. Bakke, J. L., Lawrence, N. L., and Bennett, J. Late effects of perinatal morphine administration on pituitary-thyroidal and gonadal function. *Biol. Neonate,* 23:59–77, 1973.

17. Crofford, M., and Smith, A. A. Growth retardation in young mice, treated with DL-methadone. *Science,* 181:947–949, 1973.

18. Lotti, V. J., Kokka, N., and George, R. Pituitary-adrenal activation following intrahypothalamic microinjection of morphine. *Neuroendocrinology,* 4:326–332, 1969.

19. Huidobro, D. P., and Huidobro, F. Acute morphine tolerance in new born and young rats. *Psychopharmacologia,* 28:27–34, 1973.

20. Johannesson, T., and Becker, B. A. The effects of maternally-administered morphine on rat foetal development and resultant tolerance to the analgesic effect of morphine. *Acta Pharmacol. Toxicol.* 31:305–313, 1972.

21. Himmelsbach, C. K. Studies on the relation of drug addiction to the autonomic nervous system: Results of cold pressor tests. *J. Pharmacol. Exp. Ther.,* 73:91–98, 1941.

22. Axelrod, J. The enzymatic N-demethylation of narcotic drugs. *J. Pharmacol. Exp. Ther.,* 117:322–330, 1956.

DISCUSSION

Kerr: I am concerned about the large dose of naloxone used in your last studies. We obtain antagonistic responses against morphine with much lower doses. Isn't it possible that this dose somehow stressed your animals?

Zimmermann: I agree that this dose of naloxone is quite large, but we learned from Dr. Kokka this morning that doses of naloxone several times as large as that used here failed to cause an increase in steroid levels in the rat. Thus, I am not concerned about the stressful effect of naloxone in this study.

Way: Protracted signs of abstinence and tolerance have been observed in other systems. Thus, I cannot conclude that this is necessarily an endocrine abnormality.

Zimmermann: I fully agree. In fact, the endocrine function in these animals was quite normal—that is, resting and stress-induced pituitary adrenal function was intact in our animals exposed to morphine throughout the pre-weaning period. The only responses that were abnormal in our animals were those which appeared or failed to appear on challenge with morphine or on administration of naloxone. We do not conclude that these abnormal responses are due to a disturbance in neuroendocrine function, rather that neuroendocrine systems reflect some underlying long-lasting effect of the drug, just as we have seen in other systems, as you indicate. I must add, however, that our effects were most clearly seen in females and the fact that some responses were absent in the males suggests that there may be an important endocrine factor involved in these results.

Ganong: How long does tolerance last in the human?

Zimmermann: Perhaps Dr. Way would like to answer that.

Way: For the most part, tolerance disappears rapidly during the first week following morphine administration. However, this depends in part upon what indices you are measuring in following tolerance and there are signs of residual tolerance which may persist for months.

Wikler: There is also evidence of Jasinski and Martin, which appeared in the minutes of the Drug Abuse Committee last year, indicating that post-addicts when treated with a single dose of morphine or methadone and subsequently challenged with a single dose of naloxone a week later did show measurable signs of abstinence.

Ganong: I'm still concerned about the possible sites of action of these drugs on pituitary-adrenal function. Is it known where they act?

Zimmermann: There is good evidence that morphine acts at the hypothalamic level to cause ACTH secretion. Earlier work by George and Way showed that hypothalamic lesions blocked this response and, more recently, Kokka et al. have shown that morphine injected into the middle hypothalamus causes ACTH secretion. In addition, work done in Dr. Critchlow's laboratory has demonstrated significant pituitary adrenal activation in response to acute morphine administration in animals following complete deafferentation of the hypothalamus. I'm not aware that this response has been tested in animals following brain removal. With regard to the development of tolerance and/or dependence on morphine, the location of these events is not known. However, evidence we have heard discussed these past few days would suggest that the hypothalamus, and certainly the brain, is a logical place to look for the origin of pituitary-adrenal responses to the drug.

Narcotics and the Hypothalamus, edited by
E. Zimmermann and R. George. Raven Press,
New York © 1974

Barbiturates and Sexual Differentiation of the Brain

Roger A. Gorski

Department of Anatomy and Brain Research Institute, UCLA School of Medicine, Los Angeles,
California 90024

It is generally accepted that the neural (presumably hypothalamic) regulation of pituitary activity and the neural control of sexual behavior undergo sexual differentiation. In experiments designed to investigate the possible mechanism of action of testosterone in masculinizing the developing brain of the rat, we demonstrated that two barbiturates, pentobarbital (PB) and phenobarbital (PhB), could inhibit the action of exogenous androgen in the female. This observation is of particular importance to our present consideration of the effects of drugs of abuse on hypothalamic function, since it suggests the possibility that certain drugs, if abused by the pregnant woman, might have permanent and far-reaching effects on the offspring of that pregnancy. The purpose of this discussion is to review that possibility rather than to elucidate the mechanisms of sexual differentiation. However, to accomplish this goal, it will be necessary to review the fundamental concept of the sexual differentiation of the brain in the rat, and to consider how this concept may apply to the human. Against this background, I will then review our experimental data.

SEXUAL DIFFERENTIATION OF THE BRAIN IN THE RAT

Figure 1 schematically illustrates the various events of the estrous cycle of the rat. Although these include vaginal, behavioral, and hormonal cycles, the key event appears to be the cyclic release of luteinizing hormone-releasing factor (LH-RF), presumably from neurons of the medial basal hypothalamus. This event in turn is apparently the product of the integration of plasma estrogen titers and a central cyclic stimulus. (For reviews of the justification for Fig. 1, see references 1–5.) In contrast, reproductive activity of the male rat is characterized by a marked constancy in terms of both hormonal secretion and sexual behavior. What is the source of this sex difference in reproductive activity? There are three possible explanations:

1. Since the pattern of gonadotropin (GTH) secretion reflects the feedback action of gonadal hormones, the characteristic sex differences could be due to functional differences between the ovaries and testes.

2. It is also possible that the pituitary gland itself is functionally sexually dimorphic.

3. It is possible that the brain is functionally sexually dimorphic.

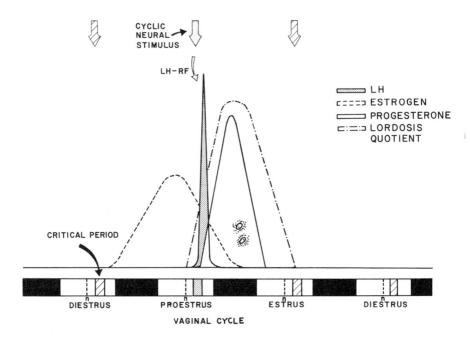

FIG. 1. Highly schematic representation of the neural and behavioral events throughout the estrous cycle of the female rat. Note that the discharge of luteinizing hormone (LH) which results in ovulation shortly after midnight (at ova) is the result of an estrogen-triggered cyclic neural stimulus which activates the release of LH-releasing factor (LH-RF) during the critical period beginning approximately 2 hr after noon (n) on the day of vaginal proestrus. Reproduced with permission from Gorski (5).

Transplantation studies have ruled out the first two alternatives. When adult male and female rats are gonadectomized and provided with sub-cutaneous or intraocular grafts of ovarian tissue, the morphology of the ovarian grafts is predictably sexually dimorphic (6, 7). In the female, as the grafts vascularize and respond to plasma GTH, they secrete estrogen which ultimately triggers the ovulatory surge of LH-RF. In fact, ovarian grafts in the otherwise ovariectomized rat luteinize cyclically and maintain normal cyclic reproductive activity. In contrast, ovarian grafts in the gona-dectomized male become polyfollicular and do not form corpora lutea (CL). Thus, the pituitary and/or brain of the male cannot support normal ovarian function. This sex difference does not reside in the pituitary gland, however, since the pituitary of the male rat, when transplanted into the vacant sella of the hypophysectomized female, supports normal ovarian function (8). The sexual dimorphism in reproductive function, therefore, appears to reside chiefly in the brain.

The sex difference in brain function is not an expression of neuronal genetics. On the contrary, the male rat is born with the potential to support cyclic ovarian function (6, 7, 9, 10). The male rat, if castrated at 6 days of age or beyond, develops in adulthood the typical masculine pattern of tonic GTH secretion as measured by the morphology of ovarian grafts. However, a male rat castrated within the first 3 days of life can, as an adult, support cyclic CL formation in ovarian grafts as well as the female pattern of cyclic fluctuations in running activity. We have called the neonatally castrated or feminine male, the fale (11). In contrast, if the fale or female rat is given a single subcutaneous injection of as little as 10 μg of testosterone propionate (TP), spontaneous ovulation is permanently abolished (9, 12). The masculinized or androgenized female exhibits persistent vaginal estrus rather than vaginal cycles, and the ovaries become polyfollicular and never form CL spontaneously.

It is generally accepted that neonatal androgen exposure in some way permanently masculinizes the preoptic-anterior hypothalamic area (POA-AHA), which in turn is thought to regulate ovulation in the normal female or the fale with ovarian grafts (Fig. 2). Although presentation of the experimen-

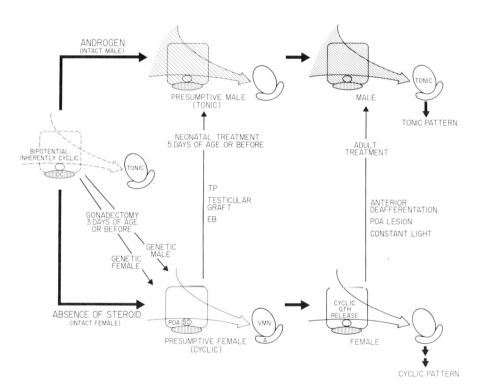

FIG. 2. Schematic summary of the concept of the sexual differentiation of the neural control of gonadotropin (GTH) secretion in the rat. For a review of the experimental evidence for this concept see references 9 and 10. Abbreviations: A, arcuate nucleus; EB, estradiol benzoate; OC, optic chiasm; POA, preoptic area; SC, suprachiasmatic nucleus; TP, testosterone propionate; VMN, ventromedial nucleus. Reproduced with permission from Gorski (45).

tal evidence in support of Fig. 2 is beyond the scope of this chapter, the concept of sexual differentiation of the neural control of GTH secretion assumes that the "POA-AHA system" is undifferentiated or inherently female in the newborn rat of either sex. If postnatal development occurs in the absence of androgen, this system attains full development and can support CL formation. On the other hand, if the animal is exposed to gonadal steroids (endogenous testicular androgen in the male, or exogenous TP or estradiol benzoate in the female or fale), the cyclic function of the POA-AHA is permanently abolished. The fact that neonatal exposure to estrogen also induces permanent sterility might appear surprising. However, the fetal and neonatal rat brain contains high quantities of an estrogen-binding macromolecule (13) which may block the action of endogenous estrogen. On the other hand, it has been suggested that the conversion of testosterone to estrogen at its site of action is necessary for masculinization (14). It is sufficient for the present discussion to conclude simply that exposure of the developing brain of the newborn rat to gonadal steroids permanently masculinizes neuroendocrine regulatory mechanisms.

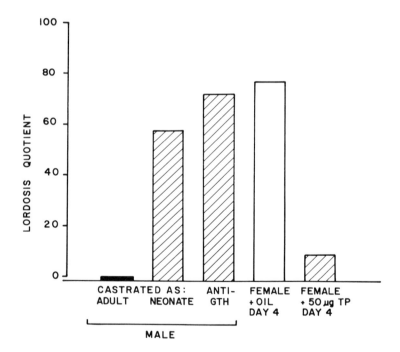

FIG. 3. Experimental evidence for the concept of hormone-induced sexual differentiation of the neural control of female sexual behavior in the rat. The lordosis quotients presented were obtained in adult gonadectomized animals following priming with estradiol benzoate and progesterone and after different postnatal treatment. The classic sex difference in lordosis behavior (compare first and fourth columns) is reversed by testosterone propionate (TP) injection in the neonatal female and castration or treatment with antigonadotropin (anti-GTH) serum in the neonatal male. Reproduced with permission from Gorski (5).

The concept of sexual differentiation also applies to the regulation of sexual behavior (5). Figure 3 illustrates the marked sex difference in the behavioral response of the adult rat to estradiol benzoate-progesterone (EB-P) treatment. The ovariectomized rat, when treated with EB-P, becomes sexually receptive as measured by a high lordosis quotient (number of lordoses by the test animal per number of mounts by a stud male × 100). In contrast, the male gonadectomized as an adult or as early as 6 days of age rarely displays lordosis behavior following EB-P priming and exposure to a stud male. This obvious sex difference is not determined by neuronal genetics. Once again, exposure of the female to a single subcutaneous injection of TP within the first 5 days of life permanently suppresses lordosis behavior (15, 16, and see

TABLE 1. A summary of sexual differentiation in the rat

Process	Dimorphic form	
Sex determination (at fertilization)	female: XX	male: XY
Differentiation of gonad (prenatal)	ovary	testis
Gonadal secretion (prenatal)	none	androgen (critical)
Differentiation of internal reproductive organs (prenatal)	Mullerian Duct (uterus, vagina)	Wolffian Duct (vas deferens)
Differentiation of genitalia (prenatal)	clitoris, labia	penis, scrotum
Differentiation of brain (postnatal) Pattern of gonadotropin control	cyclic	tonic
Behavioral response to: female hormones	female behavior	none[a]
male hormones	none[a]	male behavior

[a] The behavioral response to gonadal hormones is much more complex than indicated here. For a more complete review see Gorski (5).

5), whereas the genetic male, if castrated within the first 3 days of life (fale; 17, 18, and see 5) or treated neonatally with GTH-antiserum (19), exhibits lordosis behavior upon EB-P priming as frequently as the normal female (Fig. 3).

The ability of the male rat to exhibit masculine sexual behavior also appears to depend upon early exposure to androgen, but in the rat this may take place prenatally (see 5). Because masculine sexual behavior is measured experimentally in terms of intromission and ejaculation, the lack of normal phallic development in the female or the fale precludes a clear demonstration of the sexual differentiation of the central mechanisms which regulate masculine behavior. Nevertheless, the dramatic effect of the postnatal hormone environment on the development of the neural regulation of lordosis behavior clearly illustrates the fact that behavioral mechanisms in the rat also undergo sexual differentiation. Table 1 presents an overall scheme of sexual differentiation in the rat. Although the identity of the gonad is determined genetically, the appearance of subsequent sex differences in the accessory ducts, genitalia, and neural regulation of GTH secretion, lordosis behavior, and possibly masculine behavior depends on the presence (male) or absence (female) of the testes and their presumed secretion of testosterone.

SEXUAL DIFFERENTIATION OF THE HUMAN BRAIN

Although we have considered the process of sexual differentiation of the brain in the rat, and in fact will consider the action of barbiturates only in this species, I want to reemphasize that my main purpose is to consider the possible relevance of this information to the human. The question, Can we consider the rat as an animal model of sexual differentiation in the human?, is difficult to answer. Although sexual differentiation of the brain has been demonstrated in several species including the rat, hamster (20), guinea pig (21), and rhesus monkey (22), several differences have been reported. For example, in the guinea pig and monkey, sexual differentiation is already complete at birth. Moreover, although administration of androgen to the pregnant monkey masculinizes the genitalia and the social and sexual behavior of the female offspring, these females ovulate and menstruate regularly although via the penile urethra (22). In the human there is a complex syndrome of functional amenorrhea (23) in which the ovarian condition is similar to that of the androgenized female rat; however, no correlation has yet been demonstrated between functional amenorrhea and prenatal hormonal alterations in neural development. Sufficient clinical evidence does exist to support the possibility that the prenatal hormone environment can contribute to the development of human behavior. Two human syndromes in particular illustrate the potential value of the rat experimental models of the androgenized female and the fale. These are, respectively, the congenital adrenogenital syndrome and the feminizing testis syndrome. For our consideration of these conditions, we must introduce the concept of psychosexual identity. Money and Ehrhardt (24) have proposed the following definitions:

Gender Identity: One's individuality as male, female, or ambivalent, especially as it is experienced in self-awareness and behavior. Gender identity is the private experience of gender role.

Gender Role: "Everything that a person says and does, to indicate to others or to the self the degree that one is either male, or female, or ambivalent; it includes but is not restricted to sexual arousal and response; gender role is the public expression of gender identity."

It is obvious that the analysis of an individual's gender identity and gender role, i.e., his or her psychosexual identity, is difficult and must depend on psychological tests and the evaluation of family, friends, and trained observers. For a review of these techniques, the interested reader should consult Money and Ehrhardt (24). As this particularly informative book indicates, human psychosexual identity is particularly sensitive to cultural and environmental factors, yet it is likely that the perinatal hormone environment may be significant as well.

In the adrenogenital syndrome there is an enzymatic defect in the adrenal cortex. This leads to a deficit in glucocorticoid secretion and consequently to a marked stimulation of the adrenals by adrenocorticotropic hormone, so that adrenal androgen secretion is greatly increased (25). The female, as a result of this congenital condition, is born with masculinized genitalia, possibly to such an extent that the baby may be erroneously determined to be male. In spite of the error in clinical sex assignment, if the child is raised unambiguously as a boy, psychosexual identity may develop as in the normal male (24). Since the hypersecretion of adrenal androgens can be inhibited by cortisone therapy, females correctly diagnosed and treated can develop normally as females reproductively and can have children. However, Money and Ehrhardt (24) report that such girls exhibit certain behavioral traits that can be labeled tomboyism much more frequently than normal girls. Moreover, in those cases where rearing has been rather ambiguous, such genetic females may report (although not exclusively) a fundamentally masculine psychosexual identity.

In the feminizing testis syndrome, the genetic male is insensitive to androgen, again because of a metabolic defect (25). These genetic males develop phenotypically and psychosexually as females (24). From these two examples it is evident that, in the human, genetic sex does not determine psychosexual development. In this brief presentation these complex clinical syndromes have been grossly oversimplified. Because of the profound influence of the experience of an individual throughout rearing, it is difficult to confirm or deny significant effects of the hormone environment. Although it is most likely erroneous to make comparisons in detail, the androgenized female rat and the human female with the adrenogenital syndrome, or the fale and the human with the feminizing testis syndrome, may represent analogous examples of similar phenomena in diverse species. To conclude from this that the androgenized rat or fale are animal models of homosexuality (26), or more appropriately, of transsexualism, would be unfounded speculation. On the other hand, consideration of the possibility that barbiturates could permanently disturb the differentiation of the fetal brain if abused by the pregnant woman should not be ignored.

BARBITURATES AND ANDROGENIZATION IN THE RAT

Our studies of the interaction between barbiturates and androgen in the neonatal rat were not performed with the problem of drug abuse in mind.

Rather, we were interested in elucidating the mechanism of action of androgen in inducing masculine differentiation of the brain. We believed, as we still do, that if we could identify specific inhibitors of androgenization we would learn a great deal about the possible mode of action of this steroid. We chose to study the action of exogenous TP in the female rat. Although we plan eventually to study the action of testicular hormones in normal development of the male, we do not know precisely when or how much androgen is secreted by the neonatal testes. By studying the female the experimenter can control both the dose of exogenous androgen and the onset of its action. Initially we attempted to inhibit androgenization in the female with progesterone, chlorpromazine, or reserpine (27). Although these agents at-

TABLE 2. *The inhibition of androgenization by simultaneous barbiturate injection*

Injection(s) at day 5 of age	Incidence of sterility (IS) (no. anovulatory/no. injected)			
	at 45 days of age		at 90 days of age	
	IS	%	IS	%
30 μg TP + saline	32/37	86.5	15/16	93.8
30 μg TP + pentobarbital [a]	2/30	6.5	4/15	26.7
30 μg TP + pentobarbital [a] + pentylenetetrazol [b]	18/25	72.0	7/10	70.0
30 μg TP + phenobarbital [c]	4/31	12.9	4/17	23.5
Pentobarbital [a]	0/12	0	0/12	0
Phenobarbital [c]	0/9	0	0/9	0

[a] Two injections of 0.3 mg per rat given 4 to 5 hr apart.
[b] Injections of 2 mg per rat given with pentobarbital.
[c] Single injection of 0.5 mg per rat.
Data from Arai and Gorski, *Endocrinology*, 82:1005–1009 and 1010–1014, 1968.

tenuate androgen action, we were not able to inhibit androgenization completely. We next turned to the barbiturates, primarily because these drugs have been particularly useful in neuroendocrine studies.

As seen in Table 2, the simultaneous subcutaneous injection of either PB or PhB with TP markedly inhibits the action of androgen (27). We chose doses of barbiturate (0.3 mg per rat for PB; 0.5 mg per rat for PhB) which approached those that have been used to block spontaneous ovulation in the normal adult female (28). We assumed initially that the action of TP would be prolonged beyond the usual duration of anesthesia following PB injection. Therefore, two injections of PB were administered 4 to 5 hr apart, although PhB was given as a single injection. In a subsequent study (29), two injections of PB were invariably fatal but we were able to confirm the observation that PB, even given as a single injection, can significantly inhibit androgenization. The injection of barbiturates alone in the neonatal female had no apparent effect on ovulation in the adult. The simultaneous injection of pentylenetetrazol (Metrazol®, Knoll) and PB blocked the effect of the barbiturate on androgenization (Table 2).

Given the effectiveness of PB or PhB against androgenization of GTH regulating mechanisms, we next attempted to define the minimal exposure of the brain to androgen required for masculinization (30). As illustrated in Fig. 4, the effectiveness of these barbiturates against androgenization fell

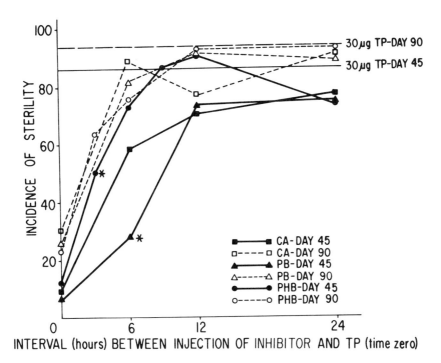

FIG. 4. Incidence of sterility (IS; number anovulatory per number injected) at 45 and 90 days of age following the injection of 30 μg testosterone propionate (TP) alone (horizontal lines), simultaneously with, or at various times prior to pentobarbital (PB), phenobarbital (PhB), or cyproterone acetate (CA) injection in 5-day-old female rats. Asterisk indicates a significantly decreased IS in comparison to the injection of TP only. All three drugs significantly reduced the IS at both 45 and 90 days of age when administered simultaneously with TP. Reproduced with permission from Gorski (10).

dramatically as the TP was permitted more time to act prior to PB or PhB administration. If the injection of barbiturate was delayed just 6 hr from the time of TP administration, the ability of PhB to antagonize androgen was virtually eliminated, although PB administered after this delay still suppressed the incidence of sterility in the early postpubertal period (day 45). Even in these animals, however, subsequent development of the delayed anovulation syndrome (31) eliminated any significant effect of PB treatment. On the basis of this evidence we concluded that permanent anovulatory sterility could result in the female rat following a rather brief exposure to androgen, perhaps for only approximately 6 hr (30).

Unfortunately, no clear explanation of barbiturate antagonism of androgenization can be offered. As illustrated in Fig. 4, an antiandrogenic drug, cyproterone acetate, also blocks the perinatal action of androgen on sexual differentiation (32), and its time course of action is comparable to that of the barbiturates (33). Cyproterone presumably acts by inhibiting androgen uptake (34); do barbiturates act similarly?

It is likely that androgen acts at a fundamental neurochemical level in the developing brain, and in fact permanent changes in RNA metabolism (35, 36), amino acid incorporation (37, 38), and oxidative metabolism (39) have been reported in the androgenized female. The intracerebral implantation of cycloheximide also attenuates androgen action (40). Is it possible that barbiturates act at the neurochemical level either by a nonspecific inhibition of nerve cell metabolism or by a more specific inhibition? In the latter regard, Baserga and Weiss (41) report that PB can inhibit DNA synthesis in the mouse. Although a PB-induced inhibition of thymidine incorporation was shown only for rapidly dividing non-neural cells, neurons under the influence of androgen could be in a state of active biochemical synthesis. It is obvious from these speculations that the mechanism of interaction between barbiturates, androgen, and the developing central nervous system is unknown.

In fact, is there conclusive evidence that this interaction actually takes place at the level of the nervous system? Although the ability of pentylenetetrazol to antagonize both the anesthetic action of PB and its effect on androgenization is consistent with an interaction at the level of the brain, we failed to block the action of subcutaneous TP by the intrahypothalamic infusion of PB (29). Since the precise intracerebral site(s) of action of androgen is unknown, this negative study cannot be considered decisive. Table 3 presents data from our final study with PB which suggest that the effect of PB can be

TABLE 3. Effect of daily subcutaneous treatment with 0.2 mg pentobarbital (PB) on the incidence of sterility resulting from an injection of 30 μg testosterone propionate (TP) at 5 days of age in the female rat

Days of PB treatment	Day of TP injection	Incidence of sterility (IS) (no. anovulatory/no. injected)			
		at 45 days of age		at 90 days of age	
		IS	%	IS	%
None	5	12/24	50.0	23/24	95.8
2, 3, and 4	5	9/22	40.9	20/22	90.9
2, 3, 4, and 5	5[a]	10/23	43.5	16/23[b]	69.6

[a] TP administered after recovery from anesthesia.
[b] p < 0.02 compared with TP only.
Data from Sutherland and Gorski, Neuroendocrinology, 10:94–108, 1972.

mediated *centrally* or by a *peripheral* action, presumably on the liver. It is the latter observation which may be most relevant to our consideration of the potential effect of barbiturate abuse by the pregnant woman on the prenatal development of the fetal brain.

It is well-known that barbiturates induce the formation of liver microsomal enzymes which inactivate both barbiturates and steroid hormones (see 42). Although unable to measure enzyme activity, we designed an indirect experiment to test the possibility that PB is effective against androgenization by virtue of a stimulation of liver enzymes (29). In one group of rats 0.2 mg of PB was injected on days 2, 3, and 4 of life, and TP on day 5. The TP was as effective in blocking ovulation as in rats not given PB (Table 3). If treatment of the neonatal rat for 3 days is not sufficient to induce adequate liver enzymatic activity to interfere with androgenization, it is difficult to suggest that a single injection of PB blocks the action of a simultaneous injection of TP by an action on the liver.

In a second group of animals PB was administered on days 2 to 5 of age. TP was injected on day 5 after the females had fully recovered from the anesthesia induced by PB. Note that the incidence of sterility at 90 days of age was significantly reduced in this group. From these results we concluded that it is possible to interfere with androgenization by an action of PB at the liver, but that repetitive administration of the barbiturate for at least 4 days is required.

Earlier in this discussion we considered the possibility that sexual differentiation occurs in the human. We concluded that there is a distinct possibility that the prenatal hormone environment can be a significant, but certainly not exclusive, factor in the differentiation of psychosexual identity. As in the rat, it appears that exposure of the brain to adequate levels of androgen at the appropriate time in development is necessary for normal masculine development, although experiential factors may be more decisive. Studies of the effect of barbiturates on sexual differentiation have been limited to the rat and to the response of the female to exogenous androgen. Nevertheless, it is intriguing to ask what effect chronic barbiturate ingestion by the pregnant woman might have on the action of testicular androgen on the sexual differentiation of the male fetus.

Although the period of sexual differentiation of the human brain is unknown, it is likely to take place in temporal association with the differentiation of the genital ducts and genitalia, perhaps early in the second trimester of pregnancy. The woman who repeatedly ingests barbiturates, therefore, could potentially alter the future psychosexual development of her male child even before she realizes that she is pregnant. Although our studies with the rat suggest that barbiturates may inhibit androgen action directly on the brain, it must be stressed that these studies were performed using the rather artificial system of exposing the female to exogenous TP for a brief pulse. If one considers the human situation, it is more likely that barbiturate use would be chronic and, therefore, also able to stimulate enzyme activity in the fetal liver, perhaps to such an extent that the action of endogenous testicular hormones would be inhibited or attenuated. There is considerable clinical evidence to suggest that PhB treatment of the pregnant woman does stimulate fetal liver activity. In fact, treatment of the mother late in pregnancy has been used as prophylactic therapy in cases of expected fetal hyperbilirubinemia (43, 44). Based on this observation and the experimental studies in the rat, it can be concluded that there is reason to believe that chronic barbiturate abuse, as well as the abuse of other drugs, may disrupt the process of psychosexual differentiation in man.

In summary, we have reviewed briefly the concept of sexual differentiation of the neural control of GTH secretion and of sexual behavior in the rat, and the data which suggest that barbiturates can interfere with this process. Although it is hazardous to apply these concepts to the human, current clinical evidence does suggest that the action of testicular hormones during fetal life is a significant factor in masculine psychosexual development. The fact that experiential influences are of paramount importance makes it difficult to evaluate hormonal influences. On the tenuous basis of experimental studies in the rat, chronic misuse of barbiturates and perhaps other drugs by the pregnant woman could be predicted to alter permanently masculine development of the male fetus. I have presented this discussion not because I am convinced that the children of a chronic barbiturate abuser are necessarily abnormal, but because I am convinced that it is important to consider the general principle that the chronic prenatal exposure to drugs *could* have permanent effects on the development of adult neuroendocrine or behavioral mechanisms. In addition, we should be aware of the possibility that exposure to various drugs may have dramatic effects depending on the state of neural development at the time of drug exposure.

ACKNOWLEDGMENT

Research in the author's laboratory was supported by grant HD-01182 from the National Institutes of Health, and by the Ford Foundation.

REFERENCES

1. Flerkó, B. Control of gonadotropin secretion in the female. In: *Neuroendocrinology*, Vol. 1, edited by L. Martini and W. F. Ganong, pp. 613–668. Academic Press, New York, 1966.
2. Barraclough, C. A. Modifications in reproductive function after exposure to hormones during the prenatal and early postnatal period. In: *Neuroendocrinology*, Vol. II, edited by L. Martini and W. F. Ganong, pp. 61–99. Academic Press, New York, 1967.
3. Everett, J. W. Neuroendocrine aspects of mammalian reproduction. *Ann. Rev. Physiol.*, 31:383–416, 1969.
4. Gorski, R. A., Mennin, S. P., and Kubo, K. The neural and hormonal bases of the reproductive cycle of the rat. In: *Biological Rhythms and Endocrine Function*,

edited by L. Hedlund, J. Franz, and A. Kenny. Plenum Press, New York, 1974 (in press).

5. Gorski, R. A. The neuroendocrine regulation of sexual behavior. In: Advances in Psychobiology, Vol. II, edited by A. H. Riesen. John Wiley, New York, 1974 (in press).

6. Harris, G. W. Sex hormones, brain development and brain function. Endocrinology, 75:627–648, 1964.

7. Gorski, R. A. and Wagner, J. W. Gonadal activity and sexual differentiation of the hypothalamus. Endocrinology, 76:226–239, 1965.

8. Harris, G. W., and Jacobsohn, D. Functional grafts of the anterior pituitary gland. Proc. Royal Soc. B, 139:263–276, 1952.

9. Gorski, R. A. Localization and sexual differentiation of the nervous structures which regulate ovulation. J. Reprod. Fert., Suppl. I:67–88, 1966.

10. Gorski, R. A. Gonadal hormones and the perinatal development of neuroendocrine function. In: Frontiers in Neuroendocrinology, 1971, edited by L. Martini and W. F. Ganong, pp. 237–290. Oxford University Press, New York, 1971.

11. Gorski, R. A. Localization of the neural control of luteinization in the feminine male rat (FALE). Anat. Rec., 157:63–69, 1967.

12. Gorski, R. A., and Barraclough, C. A. The effects of low dosages of androgen on the differentiation of hypothalamic regulatory control of ovulation in the rat. Endocrinology, 73:210–215, 1963.

13. Plapinger, L., McEwen, B. S., and Clemens, L. E. Ontogeny of estradiol-binding sites in rat brain. II. Characteristics of a neonatal binding macromolecule. Endocrinology, 93:1129–1139, 1973.

14. Naftolin, F., Ryan, J. J., and Petro, Z. Aromatization of androstenedione by the anterior hypothalamus of adult male and female rats. Endocrinology, 90:295–298, 1972.

15. Barraclough, C. A., and Gorski, R. A. Studies on mating behavior in the androgen-sterilized rat and their relation to the hypothalamic regulation of sexual behavior in the female rat. J. Endocrinol., 25:175–182, 1962.

16. Harris, G. W., and Levine, S. Sexual differentiation of the brain and its experimental control. J. Physiol., 181:379–400, 1965.

17. Grady, K. L., Phoenix, C. H., and Young, W. C. Role of the developing rat testis in differentiation of the neural tissues mediating mating behavior. J. Comp. Physiol. Psychol., 59:176–182, 1965.

18. Feder, H. H., and Whalen, R. E. Feminine behavior in neonatally castrated and estrogen-treated male rats. Science, 147:306–307, 1964.

19. Goldman, B. D., Quadagno, D. M., Shryne, J., and Gorski, R. A. Modification of phallus development and sexual behavior in rats treated with gonadotropin antiserum neonatally. Endocrinology, 90:1025–1031, 1972.

20. Swanson, H. H. Effects of castration at birth in hamsters of both sexes on luteinization of ovarian implants, oestrous cycles and sexual behavior. J. Reprod. Fertil., 21:183–186, 1970.

21. Goy, R. W., Bridson, W. E., and Young, W. C. Period of maximal susceptibility of the prenatal female guinea pig to masculinizing actions of testosterone propionate. J. Comp. Physiol. Psychol., 57:166–174, 1964.

22. Goy, R. W., and Resko, J. A. Gonadal hormones and behavior of normal and pseudohermaphroditic nonhuman female primates. Recent Progr. Horm. Res., 28:707–733, 1972.

23. Rothchild, I. M. Functional amenorrhea. In: The Neuroendocrinology of Human Reproduction, edited by H. C. Mack and A. I. Sherman, pp. 171–182. Charles C Thomas, Springfield, Illinois, 1971.

24. Money, J., and Ehrhardt, A. A. Man and Woman, Boy and Girl. Johns Hopkins University Press, Baltimore, 1972. 311 pp.

25. Netter, F. H. Endocrine system and selected metabolic diseases. In: The CIBA Collection of Medical Illustrations, Vol. 4, pp. 122–123. CIBA, 1965.

26. Dörner, G., and Hinz, G. Induction and prevention of male homosexuality by androgen. J. Endocrinol., 40:387–388, 1968.

27. Arai, Y., and Gorski, R. A. Protection against the neural organizing effect of

exogenous androgen in the neonatal female rat. *Endocrinology*, 82:1005–1009, 1968.

28. Everett, J. W. The mammalian female reproductive cycle and its controlling mechanisms. In: *Sex and Internal Secretions*, Vol. I, edited by W. C. Young, pp. 497–555. Williams and Wilkins, Baltimore, 1961.

29. Sutherland, S. D., and Gorski, R. A. An evaluation of the inhibition of androgenization of the neonatal female rat brain by barbiturate. *Neuroendocrinology*, 10:94–108, 1972.

30. Arai, Y., and Gorski, R. A. The critical exposure time for androgenization of the developing hypothalamus in the female rat. *Endocrinology*, 82:1010–1014, 1968.

31. Gorski, R. A. Influence of age on the response to paranatal administration of a low dose of androgen. *Endocrinology*, 82:1001–1004, 1968.

32. Neumann, F., and Steinbeck, H. Influence of sexual hormones on the differentiation of neural centers. *Arch. Sex. Behav.*, 2:147–162, 1972.

33. Arai, Y., and Gorski, R. A. Critical exposure time for androgenization of the rat hypothalamus determined by anti-androgen injection. *Proc. Soc. Exp. Biol. Med.*, 127:590–593, 1968.

34. Stern, J. M., and Eisenfeld, A. J. Distribution and metabolism of ^{3}H-testosterone in castrated male rats; Effects of cyproterone, progesterone and unlabeled testosterone. *Endocrinology*, 88:1117–1125, 1971.

35. Shimada, H., and Gorbman, A. Long lasting changes in RNA synthesis in the forebrains of female rats treated with testosterone soon after birth. *Biochem. Biophys. Res. Comm.*, 38:423–430, 1970.

36. Clayton, R. B., Kogura, J., and Kraemer, H. C. Sexual differentiation of the brain: Effects of testosterone on brain RNA metabolism in newborn female rats, *Nature* (Lond.), 226:810–812, 1970.

37. Moguilevsky, J. A., Scacchi, P., and Christot, J. Amino acid incorporation into proteins of anterior pituitary gland and hypothalamus in androgenized and normal female rats. *Proc. Soc. Exp. Biol. Med.*, 137:653–656, 1971.

38. Litteria, M. Inhibitory action of neonatal androgenization on the incorporation of (^{3}H)-lysine in specific hypothalamic nuclei of the adult female rat. *Exp. Neurol.*, 41:395–401, 1973.

39. Moguilevsky, J. A., Libertun, C., Schiaffini, O., and Scacchi, P. Metabolic evidence of the sexual differentiation of the hypothalamus. *Neuroendocrinology*, 4:264–269, 1969.

40. Gorski, R. A., and Shryne, J. Intracerebral antibiotics and androgenization of the neonatal female rat. *Neuroendocrinology*, 10:109–120, 1972.

41. Baserga, R., and Weiss, L. Inhibition of deoxyribonucleic acid synthesis by pentobarbital. *Biochim. Biophys. Acta.*, 145:361–367, 1967.

42. Kuntzman, R. Drugs and enzyme induction. *Ann. Rev. Pharmacol.*, 9:21–36, 1969.

43. Trolle, D. Decrease of total serum-bilirubin concentration in newborn infants after phenobarbitone treatment. *Lancet*, 2:705–708, 1968.

44. Valaes, T., Petmezaki, S., and Doxiadis, S. A. Effect on neonatal hyperbilirubinemia of phenobarbital during pregnancy or after birth: Practical value of the treatment in a population with high risk of unexplained severe neonatal jaundice. In: *Birth Defects: Original Article Series*, Vol. VI, edited by D. Bergsma, pp. 46–54. Williams and Wilkins, Baltimore, 1970.

45. Gorski, R. A. Steroid hormones and brain function: Progress, principles, and problems. In: *Steroid Hormones and Brain Function*, edited by C. H. Sawyer and R. A. Gorski, pp. 1–26. UCLA Forum Med. Sci. No. 15, University of California Press, Los Angeles, 1971.

DISCUSSION

Cushman: Does phenobarbital alone, given in early infancy, modify subsequent sexual development?

Gorski: In our hands, administration of phenobarbital to five-day-old animals did not modify their subsequent ovulatory function.

Ganong: Does injection of barbiturates into the hypothalamus block the response to early androgenization?

Gorski: In fact, it did not. Although we believe that androgen acts on the brain to cause permanent sterilization in the female rat, we are not absolutely sure of this. We did try administering testosterone systemically and administering barbiturates in the hypothalamus, but the barbiturates did not block the action of the androgen.

McCann: Doesn't implantation of testosterone into the preoptic area of young rats produce the syndrome of persistent anovulation?

Gorski: Yes, this has been done and certainly implicates the preoptic area as a site of androgen action. However, we cannot conclude that it is the only site of this action, nor that it is the site at which barbiturates block the response.

Marks: Is this effect specific for barbiturates or does it occur as a result, for example, of anesthesia?

Gorski: We do not know this for sure. What we do know is that progesterone, chlorpromazine, and reserpine can interfere with the response to androgen. However, they are not nearly as effective as the barbiturates.

Way: What is the effect of chloral hydrate, paraldehyde, or alcohol on the effect of androgen? I think it would be important here to rule out a direct drug–drug interaction.

Gorski: We have not studied these agents, and I agree this would be an important possibility to rule out.

Narcotics and the Hypothalamus, edited by
E. Zimmermann and R. George. Raven Press,
New York © 1974

Drug Penetration of the Blood-Brain Barrier

William H. Oldendorf

Research and Neurology Services, Wadsworth Hospital Center, Veterans Administration, Los Angeles, California 90073, and Department of Neurology, Reed Neurological Research Center, UCLA School of Medicine, Los Angeles, California 90024

The restrictive effect of the blood-brain barrier (BBB) can exclude drugs from brain. If a drug is to affect central nervous system (CNS) cells, it must be able to penetrate the BBB and appear in the fluid environment (extracellular fluid, ECF) of these cells.

To arrive ultimately in CNS ECF, a drug must survive in the gut lumen, penetrate the gut wall, resist degradation by blood plasma and other tissue enzymes, remain to some extent unbound to plasma proteins, and finally escape plasma water to enter and penetrate the brain capillary wall.

CNS CAPILLARIES

There is now general agreement that the CNS capillary wall is the anatomic site of the BBB (1–3). In other tissues the walls of capillaries are freely permeable to all molecules having a molecular weight of less than 20,000–40,000 (4, 5). This nearly nonspecific permeability allows the blood plasma to carry out its evident role as a high-velocity mixing subcompartment of the general ECF. This circulation reduces the effective diffusion distance between all body cells to a few microns, even though they may be meters apart in actual distance. Arrest of the circulation increases this effective diffusion path to the distance actually separating various cells. Since the effectiveness of diffusion as a mechanism of molecular transport increases with the square of distance, each cell can no longer contribute its action to other cells and the organism dies.

Whereas non-neural cells are nonspecifically exposed to the chemical output of all other body cells, CNS cells are isolated from the general ECF by the BBB.

The term blood-brain barrier implies an impermeable structure between blood plasma and brain. From our general fund of knowledge we could easily deduce that this cannot be the case. Certain CNS drugs, such as barbiturates, are effective immediately after intravenous injection. The brain is metabolically active so it must obtain a substantial amount of substrate from blood. Accordingly, the BBB must be permeable to some drugs and to at least certain metabolic substrates.

In non-neural capillaries there are several routes by which molecules can move from plasma to the adjacent stationary ECF. Such molecules can pass between adjacent endothelial cells through the intercellular clefts. They can also, in some capillaries, pass through fenestrations in the cell wall. These two routes restrain large molecules. A relatively inefficient pathway for these large molecules (and all others) is pinocytosis (6), in which a portion of the endothelial cell plasma membrane invaginates and forms a vesicle which can now move across to the other side of the cell.

In brain capillaries these relatively nonspecific pathways are absent. The intercellular cleft is sealed shut by a fusion of the adjacent membranes (tight junctions), fenestrations are not present, and there is no pinocytosis (2). Thus all nonspecific routes of transcapillary exchange are blocked.

BBB AND LIPID VERSUS WATER AFFINITY

To penetrate the capillary wall in the CNS, a molecule must pass through the endothelial cell. It must leave the plasma, enter the inner membrane, leave the membranes to enter cytoplasm, leave the cytoplasm, enter the outer membrane, and finally leave this membrane to enter the brain ECF in the pericapillary space. The molecular property governing this sequence is the ability to escape the polar environment of plasma and cytoplasmic water and enter the nonpolar environment of cell plasma membrane lipid. This water–lipid interface constitutes a two-phase compartmental system in which water can be expressed as a lipid/water partition coefficient. For most molecules, this partition coefficient, determined *in vitro*, can predict BBB penetration. Thus, there is a generally recognized rule of thumb that lipid-soluble molecules will also penetrate all other biological membranes and, accordingly, CNS drugs can be absorbed through the gut wall and usually are effective when taken by mouth.

The relationship between lipid/water partition coefficient and BBB penetration can be seen in Fig. 1, where the X coordinate is this partition coefficient and the Y coordinate is the percentage of the ^{14}C-labeled test substances lost to rat brain in a single microcirculatory passage following carotid arterial injection (7–9). This brain uptake percentage is expressed relative to a simultaneously injected, highly diffusible internal standard, ^{3}H-water. This standard is nearly completely lost to brain. Test substances with partition coefficients greater than about 0.02 are largely cleared during a single brain passage, whereas those below about 0.01 are not measurably lost during this brief microcirculatory exposure.

BBB AND MOLECULAR STRUCTURE

By knowing the molecular structure of a compound, an approximate prediction of lipid/water partition coefficient can be made. As diagrammed in

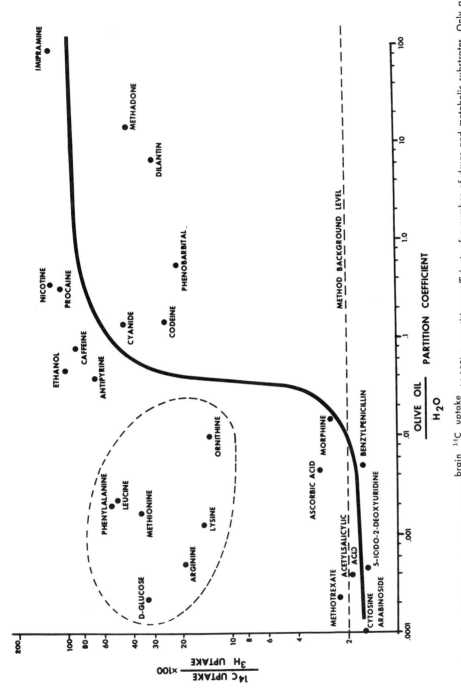

Fig. 1. Relationship of brain uptake index (BUI = $\dfrac{\text{brain }^{14}\text{C uptake}}{\text{brain }^{3}\text{H uptake}}$ $\times$ 100) to partition coefficients of a number of drugs and metabolic substrates. Only a lipid/water partition coefficient greater than about 0.04 is required to permit nearly complete clearance in one pass through brain. The substrates are en-circled at left. They have very low lipid solubility, yet penetrate the BBB because of specific carrier systems.

Fig. 2, two important characteristics determine this relative affinity: ionization and hydrogen bonding. The large charge–dipole interaction between an ionic charge site and adjacent water molecules firmly anchors the molecule into the water, making the achievement of the kinetic level required to overcome this attachment highly unlikely (10). Thus ionization, in general, impedes membrane penetration. With a specific molecule which is partially ionized in solution, it is assumed that it is largely the un-ionized species that penetrates membranes (11).

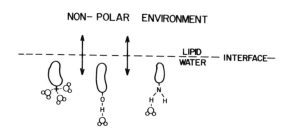

FIG. 2. The lipid-water interface between brain capillary cell plasma membrane lipid and adjacent plasma water is approximated *in vitro* by a two-phase oil-water system. The relative affinities for water and oil strongly favor water for ionized molecules. With these, the ionic charge-dipole interaction anchors the molecule in the water. For un-ionized molecules, hydrogen bonding to water is the most important factor. The strongest hydrogen bonds are formed by —OH and —NH₂ groups. Adding up these and other polar sites of weaker bond formation allows an estimation of the ability of a molecule to penetrate membranes.

With un-ionized molecules, hydrogen bonding largely determines water affinity. The most important groups in most biochemical compounds are $-OH$ and $-NH_2$ groups (11). Other groups form weaker bonds. The water bonding from these groups is about equal, and on the order of 3 to 10 of these groups are equivalent in hydrophilic attachment to a single ionic charge site.

The relationship of hydroxyl groups to permeability can be seen in Fig. 3. The two hydroxyl groups of morphine make it quite soluble in water and its BBB penetration is accordingly quite low. The methylation of one of these reduces the total hydrogen bonding of codeine, and its brain uptake is correspondingly higher. Acetylating both groups causes heroin to be relatively poorly soluble in water and more soluble in lipid. Its brain uptake is accordingly substantially greater than codeine.

The effect of progressive hydroxylation and the lesser effect of methoxylation are indicated in Fig. 4. The uptake of β-phenethylamine is quite high. Adding even one hydroxyl (in addition to the primary amine group already present) reduces the uptake to the background of the method (about 2%). One more hydroxyl in dopamine does not further affect the already unmeasurably low uptake. Adding one, two, and three methoxy groups to the

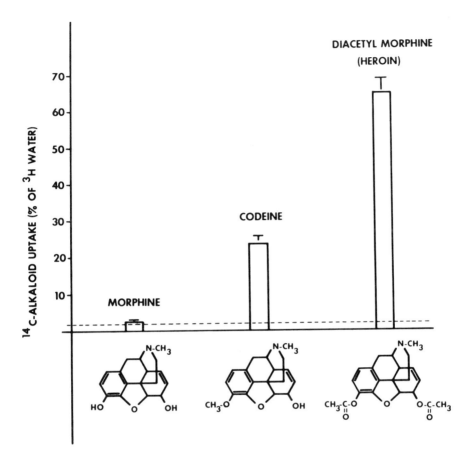

FIG. 3. The methylation of one hydroxyl converting morphine to codeine results in a much greater brain uptake index. Acetylating both hydroxyls produces still more uptake, causing heroin delivery to brain to be nearly flow-limited.

ring shows progressive reduction of uptake but it takes three to bring it down to the background.

CARRIER TRANSPORT SYSTEMS

All BBB penetration is not lipid-mediated. Figure 1 indicates a group of compounds with low partition coefficients which still have appreciable uptakes. These substances are metabolic substrates whose BBB penetration is attributed to the presence of carrier substances which generate specific molecular affinities strong enough to compete with their considerable hydrogen bonding to water. These carrier substances are comparable to hemoglobin in that they greatly increase the pool size of a particular substance or groups of substances in the anatomic compartment they occupy. Hemoglobin increases

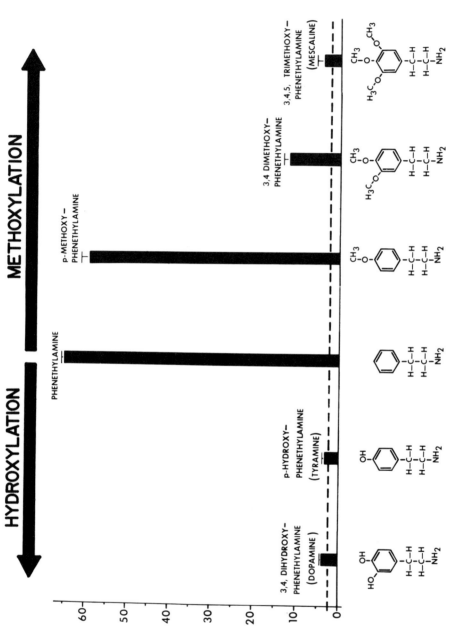

FIG. 4. Comparison of the influence of hydroxylation and methoxylation on the brain uptake index (BUI) of phenethylamine. The hydrogen-bond strength of a methoxy group is much weaker than that of a hydroxyl. Even one hydroxyl reduces the BUI of tyramine to nearly the background of the method (dashed line at 2%). It requires three methoxy groups to bring mescaline down to near-background.

the oxygen pool in blood by perhaps 100 times by virtue of its affinity for and removal of oxygen from free solution in plasma. It provides a finite number of binding sites so its carrying capacity is saturable. Its molecular affinity is not totally specific in that related gases carbon monoxide and carbon dioxide are also removed from free solution.

Membrane carrier proteins can be thought of as analogous to hemoglobin, with the difference that they are studded throughout the membrane lipid. Accordingly, they increase the membrane pool size of their transported molecules much beyond that to be found in their absence. Like hemoglobin, they are saturable and only partially specific in their affinities.

We have demonstrated six such independent BBB carrier systems, each having affinities for a group of related compounds. These carriers are for hexoses (8), short chain monocarboxylic acids (12), neutral amino acids (8, 13), basic amino acids (8, 13), and acidic amino acids (Oldendorf, *unpublished data*). We can also demonstrate still another carrier so far shown to have a saturable affinity for adenine (Oldendorf, *unpublished data*).

Just as carbon monoxide can cause hemoglobin to be bound up by preventing its carriage of oxygen, the high blood levels of phenylalanine present in phenylketonuria can be shown to impede the BBB penetration of all the other large neutral amino acids.

These carrier systems are important to drug penetration in that they could create specific molecular affinities not predictable on the basis of simple lipid versus water affinity.

Our carotid injection studies have shown that many CNS drugs are almost completely lost to brain in a single brain passage (Table 1). These drugs include nicotine, ethanol, caffeine, heroin, and procaine (9). Presumably tetrahydrocannabinol (THC), having a very high partition coefficient ($>$ 1,000), is similarly completely cleared. These drugs, taken for their CNS effects, can accordingly act quickly after administration.

CNS AREAS WITHOUT BBB

There are areas (part of the floor of the hypothalamus and the area postrema at the lower end of the fourth ventricle) in the CNS where there is no BBB and capillaries are nonspecifically permeable. It is possible that CNS responses mediated from these areas could be the basis for obvious central actions of some drugs, such as morphine, exhibiting no appreciable BBB penetration. This speculation is compatible with recent observations (14) of the analgetic effect of microinjections of morphine directly into the posterior hypothalamus, thus circumventing possible BBB restriction. The general BBB penetration of morphine is very low (much less than codeine) (9), and it is possible that its effects are mediated through nonspecific penetration into small, specific regions.

TABLE 1. Brain uptake of drugs following carotid injection and partition coefficient data

Test substance	Concn. injected (mM)	Uptake % of ^{3}HOH		Partition coeff., olive oil/water
^{3}HOH reference		100		
Nicotine	.035	131	± 7	.387
N-Propyl alcohol	.625	131	3	—
Imipramine	.216	128	11	86.6
Procaine	.484	113	8	.341
Isopropanol	.069	110	2	—
Ethanol	.022	104	4	.046
Caffeine	.267	90	3	.084
Antipyrine	.114	68	3	.040
Heroin	.031	68	6	—
L-Methadone	.054	42	3	14.5
Cyanide	1.17	41	4	.148
5,5-Diphenylhydantoin	.269	31	3	6.83
Codeine	.021	26	2	.158
Phenobarbital	.397	22	2	.570
Mescaline	.276	5.62	1.4	—
L-Ascorbic acid	.260	3.0	.2	.0046
Morphine	.022	2.6	.2	.0160
Methotrexate	.020	2.3	.4	.00024
Acetylsalicylic acid	.678	1.8	.4	.00037
Benzylpenicillin	.044	1.7	.2	.0051
Cytosine arabinoside	.00061	1.6	.4	.00010
5-Iodo-2-deoxyuridine	.00036	1.54	.21	.00047
p-Aminohippuric acid	.053	.87	.14	—

For each mean and SD, $n = 3$ except for codeine, $n = 6$. All compounds were carbon-labeled except for methadone, methotrexate, cytosine arabinoside, and iododeoxyuridine, which were tritiated. The pH of all solutions was 7.55 to 7.58. The brain uptake index values for tritiated compounds were based on a ^{14}C-isopropanol diffusible reference and were corrected back to ^{3}HOH reference. Radiochemical purity averaged 98%. Substances were from Amersham/Searle, Chicago; New England Nuclear, Boston; Schwarz/Mann, Orange-burg, N.Y.; and Dhom, Los Angeles.

TAILORING PARTITION COEFFICIENTS

Ethanol probably has the optimal partition coefficient (± 0.04) for a CNS drug. It is high enough to allow rapid BBB penetration but not sufficient to accumulate appreciably in depot fat. It favors the water phase by about 25 times.

In designing CNS drugs, a partition coefficient in this same range should be sought. THC is poor in this respect, having a very great lipid solubility. One of its pharmacologically active hydrogen derivatives with a lower coefficient would seem much more desirable.

Most metabolic processing of nonpolar compounds results in their conversions to more polar compounds. Membranes cannot transport lipid-soluble substances unidirectionally because they "leak" in both directions. When rendered more polar, unidirectionality of transport becomes feasible. In nature, the brain encounters very few significantly lipid-soluble compounds; most notable of these is ethanol (which is not very lipid-soluble). The permeability of the BBB to such substances is, accordingly, not a great handicap.

In the process of "latentiation," a compound is made intentionally lipid-soluble by shielding polar sites by adding, reversibly, nonpolar groups. The resulting compound will then penetrate the BBB and the brain can remove these lipophilic groups, restoring the original structure. This process was first accomplished inadvertently by Wright in 1874 (15), when he first synthesized heroin. The deacetylation of heroin to morphine in brain has been demonstrated by Way (16). Presumably this same ploy can be used to allow penetration into brain of a number of transmitter substances, antibiotics, and other chemotherapeutic agents.

FLOW-LIMITED DRUG DELIVERY

The demonstration that many drugs are completely cleared during one brain passage indicates that their distribution is blood-flow limited; thus, the amount going to various regions of brain is proportional to the fraction of cardiac output going to that region. From this it could be predicted that the fraction of a given dose of drugs such as ethanol, nicotine, THC, or heroin will be a direct function of the fraction of cardiac output distributing to brain (17). Since the absolute blood flow volume to brain is reasonably constant, variable amounts of blood going to adipose tissue, muscle, and skin could significantly affect the fraction of a dose delivered into brain. Thus an obese, hyperventilating heroin addict who gave himself an intravenous dose of heroin immediately after running up several flights of stairs might deliver only perhaps 3 to 5% of this dose to his brain. On a $100-a-day habit this means that only $3–5 worth of the heroin is actually supporting his habit. Were the site of action in brain known, it would perhaps be found that only a few cents worth was actually being used to this end. The remainder is delivered to muscle, fat, skin, and other tissues presumably in no way related to the prevention of withdrawal symptoms. This same individual might deliver several times this amount of drug to brain when administering the same dose if he were completely relaxed in a cool room and generated a hypercapnia and thus an increased brain blood flow at the time of injection of the heroin. Since the distribution to brain and other tissues occurs in the first 30 sec (9) after i.v. injection, such transient patient manipulation at the time of injection might be a practical means to increase the effectiveness of a dose of expensive medication. These same parameters affecting drug distribution may account for some of the variable effects often observed with drugs of abuse.

REFERENCES

1. Brightman, M. The intracerebral movement of proteins injected into blood and cerebrospinal fluid in mice. In: *Progress in Brain Research, Vol. 29: Brain Barrier Systems,* edited by A. Lajtha and D. H. Ford, pp. 19–40. Elsevier, Amsterdam, 1968.
2. Reese, T. S., and Karnovsky, M. J. Fine structural localization of a blood-brain to exogenous peroxidase. *J. Cell Biol.,* 34:207–217, 1967.
3. Crone, C., and Thompson, A. M. Permeability of brain capillaries. In: *Capillary Permeability,* edited by C. Crone and N. Lassen, pp. 447–453. Academic Press, New York, 1970.
4. Landis, E. M., and Pappenheimer, J. R. Exchange of substances through the capillary walls. In: *Handbook of Physiology, Vol. II. Sect. 2, Circulation,* edited by W. F. Hamilton and P. Dow, pp. 935–960. American Physiological Society, Washington, D.C., 1963.
5. Renkin, E M. Transport of large molecules across capillary wall. *Physiologist,* 7:13–28, 1964.
6. Palade, G. E. Fine structure of capillaries. *J. Appl. Physiol.,* 24:1424, 1953.
7. Oldendorf, W. H. Measurement of brain uptake of radiolabeled substances using a tritiated water internal standard. *Brain Res.,* 24:372–376, 1970.
8. Oldendorf, W. H. Brain uptake of radiolabeled amino acids, amines and hexoses after arterial injection. *Am. J. Physiol.,* 221:1629–1639, 1971.
9. Oldendorf, W. H., Hyman, S., Braun, L., and Oldendorf, S. Z. Blood-brain barrier penetration of morphine, codeine, heroin, and methadone after carotid injection. *Science,* 178:984–986, 1971.
10. Stein, W. D. *The Movement of Molecules Across Cell Membranes.* Academic Press, New York, 1971.
11. Goldsworthy, P. D., Aird, R. D., and Becker, R. A. The blood-brain barrier—The effect of acidic dissociation constant on the permeation of certain sulfonamides into brain. *J. Cell Comp. Physiol.,* 44:519–526, 1954.
12. Oldendorf, W. H. Carrier-mediated blood-brain barrier transport of short-chain monocarboxylic organic acids. *Am. J. Physiol.,* 224:1450–1453, 1973.
13. Richter, J. J., and Wainer, A. Evidence for separate systems for the transport of neutral and basic amino acids across the blood-brain barrier. *J. Neurochem.,* 18:612–620, 1971.
14. Jacquet, F. Y., and Lajtha, A. Morphine action at central nervous system sites in rat: Analgesia or hyperalgesia depending on site and dose. *Science,* 182:490–492, 1973.
15. Wright, C. R. A. On the action of organic acids and their anhydrides on natural alkaloids. Part I. *J. Chem. Soc. Lond.,* 24:108–1043, 1874.
16. Way, E. L. Distribution and metabolism of morphine and its surrogates. In: *The Addictive States,* Res. Publ. Assn. Res. Nerv. Ment. Dis., Vol. 46, edited by A. Wikler, pp. 13–31. Williams and Wilkins, Baltimore, 1968.
17. Sapirstein, L. Measurement of the cephalic and cerebral blood flow fractions of the cardiac output in man. *J. Clin. Invest.,* 41:1429–1435, 1962.

DISCUSSION

Kerr: What is the explanation for the increased permeability of a compound following acetylation?

Oldendorf: The reason relates to the fact that the hydroxyl group forms a strong hydrogen bond and when you shield the oxygen with an acetyl group, it forms a much weaker hydrogen bond.

Brazeau: We have very recently obtained evidence that the activity of SRF is greatly increased by acetylation and this could relate to the increased entry into brain as you have described with other compounds.

Way: We must be careful, however, not to generalize on this phenomenon since expression of the activity of a compound may require deacetylation once it enters the brain.

Oldendorf: In fact, your work would indicate that it is necessary to deacetylate heroin in the brain to form morphine, which is presumably the active molecule.

Hayward: What other mechanisms have you thought about regarding entry of substances into brain tissue?—for example, in areas of the brain like the area postrema where there is no blood-brain barrier.

Oldendorf: Well, for one, I think that distribution of a drug within the brain must play an important role. For example, approximately 30 times as much morphine presumably enters the brain when it is administered as heroin than as morphine, yet heroin is only three times as effective as morphine in analgesic potency. Something must explain the missing order of magnitude involved here. One possibility here is that heroin, like nicotine and ethanol, is delivered to the brain regionally in proportion to local blood flow. Thus, these flow-limited substances are delivered to brain in proportion to the amount of the cardiac output which reaches various portions of the brain. Thus, while delivery of morphine as heroin to the brain may be, in fact, much greater than the delivery as morphine, it may, in fact, be reaching for the most part a bunch of useless areas.

Ganong: Is it true that injection of hypertonic solutions into the cerebral circulation results in diminution of blood-brain barrier?

Oldendorf: Yes, it is true. If we inject ordinary contrast medium, which is 1.6 molar in concentration, unilaterally into the carotid artery of dogs, that is, in clinically relevant amounts, that side of the brain will show increased staining with fluorsceine dye administered subsequently for several hours. I must add, however, that we failed to see any evidence of diminished blood-brain barriers in patients following carotid angiography. That is, there is no altered behavior or EEG or anything evident. It is interesting that if the brain gets along so well without a blood-brain barrier, why does it continue to maintain one? At least on a short-term basis, it seems to function well without it.

Mirsky: I think we should remember that any of a wide variety of injuries to the brain can reduce the blood-brain barrier, sometimes for days at a time.

Narcotics and the Hypothalamus, edited by
E. Zimmermann and R. George. Raven Press,
New York © 1974

Maturation of the Blood-Brain and Blood-Cerebrospinal Fluid Barriers and Transport Systems

Dixon M. Woodbury, Conrad Johanson, and Hans Brøndsted

Department of Pharmacology, University of Utah College of Medicine, Salt Lake City, Utah 84132

In considering the effects of drugs of abuse on hypothalamic function, it is important to elucidate the routes and mechanisms by which those drugs that act on the brain enter and leave it. Many factors determine the concentration of drugs in the brain, including the volume of distribution of a drug, its pK_a, the properties of the cerebral capillary endothelial cells that constitute the "blood-brain barrier," the rate of cerebrospinal fluid (CSF) flow, and, the subject of this chapter, the properties of the systems that transport drugs across the choroid plexus, neurons, and glial cells. The developing animal is ideal for studying the blood-brain barrier and brain and choroid plexus transport systems because large changes take place in a short period of time. Thus the maturation of these systems will be stressed. [For discussions of the ontogeny of the blood-brain barrier, see (1) and (2).]

CELL BARRIERS IN BLOOD-CNS TRANSPORT

A diagrammatic representation of the anatomic basis for the "blood-brain" and "blood-CSF" barrier and transport systems in *adult* animals is shown in Fig. 1. In order to enter the brain and CSF, a drug must cross several epithelial cell barriers which are important because transport occurs across these cells. These will be discussed in the order that they are crossed when entering the central nervous system from the cerebral capillaries.

Cerebral Capillaries

The endothelial cells of the cerebral capillaries constitute the site of the so-called blood-brain barrier. The characteristics of these cells have been discussed by Brightman and Reese (3), Pappenheimer (4), and Chrone (5). Large molecules such as albumin, trypan blue (largely bound to plasma protein), horseradish peroxidase, and ferritin do not cross the cerebral capillaries, except possibly very slowly and in small amounts by the process of pinocytosis. This is true even for the capillaries of fetal animals (6, 7). However, molecules as large as inulin (MW 5,000), ouabain, and sucrose do cross these capillaries, albeit slower than capillaries elsewhere in the body.

225

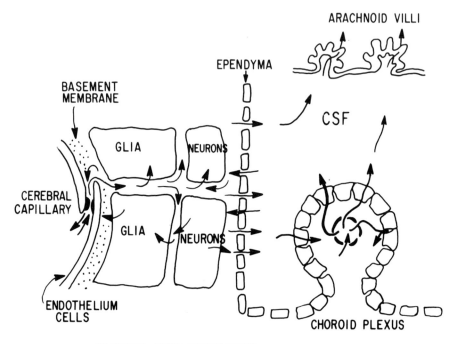

CHANGES WITH MATURATION

1 ↓ PERMEABILITY OF CEREBRAL CAPILLARIES
2 ↓ EXTRACELLULAR SPACE
3 ↑ NUMBER AND VOLUME OF GLIAL CELLS
4 ↑ GROWTH OF NEURONAL PROCESSES
5 ↓ PERMEABILITY OF EPENDYMAL LINING
6 ↑ CSF PRODUCTION AND FLOW
7 ↑ TRANSPORT ACROSS CHOROID PLEXUS

FIG. 1. Schematic representation of the anatomic basis for the "blood-brain" and "blood-CSF" barrier systems in adult animals. The pathways by which various substances can enter and leave the various compartments in the system are also shown. Listed at the bottom are the changes that take place during development of the system. The width of the pathway of substances moving between the endothelial cells of the cerebral capillaries is thought to be about 15 Å. Note also that the capillaries of the choroid plexus are fenestrated.

These data have been interpreted to show that since molecules like inulin (which measures extracellular space) cannot enter cerebral capillary cells, their entrance into the interstitial space of the brain must be by way of intercellular channels between the endothelial cells. The channels are postulated to be approximately 15 Å in diameter, a size just large enough to allow a molecule the size of inulin to pass through slowly, but not large enough for albumin or other large molecules. Channels about 40 to 60 Å in diameter are thought to be present between the endothelial cells of muscle capillaries. This is large enough for albumin to enter. The basement membrane that separates the endothelial cells of the capillaries from the glial endfeet and the interstitial channels of the brain does not appear to be a barrier to movement of large molecules. For example, Brightman and Reese (3) showed that both horseradish peroxidase and ferritin injected into the CSF readily pass through the interstitial space of the brain to the endothelial cell border without being impeded by the basement membrane. However, these substances do not cross the endothelial cells, which are therefore impermeable to large molecules in both directions. Inulin and smaller molecules can leave the brain by this route through the 15-Å pores between the endothelial cells. The permeability of the cerebral capillaries to inulin is greater in fetal and neonatal rats than in adults, and the rate of entrance decreases with increasing age (8, 9). Electron microscopic studies suggest that changes in capillary structure occur with increasing age and that these changes may account for the decrease in the permeability of the capillaries to various molecules that occur (10).

Most drugs are weak electrolytes and as such exist in both the nonionized and ionized form. The extent of ionization depends on the pK_a of the molecule and the pH of the solution. The nonionized form of drugs readily crosses the cell membrane, whereas the ionized form is impermeable or only slowly permeable. The rate of penetration of the nonionized form depends on the lipid:water partition coefficient of the molecule. The greater the lipid solubility, the faster the movement of the nonionized forms of drugs across the endothelial cells of the cerebral capillaries. The rate of movement also depends on the extent of plasma and tissue binding of the drug. These movements are across the endothelial cells, whereas the movement of larger water-soluble molecules (inulin, sucrose, etc.) that cannot cross cell membranes is probably by way of the channels between the endothelial cells.

Ependymal Lining

After crossing the endothelial cells and the basal membrane (which offers no resistance), a drug enters the narrow interstitial channels of the brain that constitute the extracellular space. These are about 150 to 200 Å in diameter and allow free diffusion of all size molecules through them, as Brightman and Reese (3) clearly demonstrated by electron microscopic measurements of the distribution of horseradish peroxidase or ferritin in brain. From the interstitial channels the drugs have access to neurons or their surrounding glial cells or can move into the CSF by crossing the *ependymal* epithelium lining the ventricular cavities. Movement across the ependyma can occur readily except for large protein molecules, because the cells are joined together by gap junctions in many places and this allows ready movement of all molecules between the cells and around the junctions. This movement is mainly dependent on molecular size. For example, in the study by Reed and Woodbury

(11), the rate of movement of various substances across this border was: albumin < inulin < sucrose < iodide.

Glial Endfeet and Glial Cells

Few data are available on the movement of drugs into glial cells or into the glial endfeet bordering on the basal membrane and the capillary endothelial cells (see Fig. 1). Weak electrolytes undoubtedly enter by nonionic diffusion as is the case with all other cells, and their rate, therefore, is dependent on the pH, pK_a and partition coefficient of the nonionized drugs. There is evidence that Na, K, and Cl are actively transported across glial cells and that they are high-K, relatively high-Na and -Cl cells [cf. Kuffler and Nicholls (12) for review]. Active uptake of amino acids and some neurotransmitters also occurs in glial cells. There is evidence that they are sinks for removing neurotransmitters from the synaptic areas after their release following a nerve impulse. Glial cells are also sinks for K and thereby maintain a constant extracellular K concentration under conditions of excessive neuronal activity, a process which would otherwise increase extracellular K concentration as a result of its leakage from the nerve [cf. (13–16)].

The role of the glial endfeet lining the capillaries (see Fig. 1) is not known, but it has been speculated that they function to exchange various metabolic waste products (collected from the neurons they surround and then transported down the glial cell processes to the endfeet) for nutrients and electrolytes such as K and phosphate. Further work in this area is obviously needed.

Neurons

From the interstitial channels, drugs also enter neuronal cells as depicted in Fig. 1. Movement of drugs across neuronal cell membranes appears to occur by the same mechanisms as for other cells, i.e., pH-dependent nonionic diffusion, active transport of ionized molecules, and Na-dependent non-electrolyte transport.

Epithelial Cells of the Choroid Plexus

These cells are the site of formation of most of the CSF. This process involves the active transport of Na across the choroidal epithelial cells and is similar to that which occurs across the epithelial cells of frog skin and toad bladder. The capillaries supplying the choroid plexus differ from the cerebral capillaries in that they are fenestrated between the endothelial cells, and large molecules such as peroxidase and ferritin can readily penetrate them and enter the stromal space. However, the choroid plexus cells are held together by tight junctions, and peroxidase and ferritin as well as inulin and sucrose cannot easily cross them and enter the CSF. Thus these cells are the site of the "blood-CSF" barrier.

Entrance into the CSF via the choroid plexus cells takes place only by substances passing through the cells. Thus, small molecules such as urea, antipyrine, and formamide, can enter the CSF by diffusion across both cell membranes. However, their rate of passage is slower than that of water and this sieving effect can account for CSF/plasma ratios of < 1.0 that often result. Weak electrolytes enter the CSF across the choroid epithelial cells by pH-dependent nonionic diffusion, as is the case for other cells. Electrolytes such as Na^+ and Mg^{++} enter the CSF by active transport across the choroid plexus. Chloride also enters by an active process that appears to involve carbonic anhydrase. Potassium is maintained constant in the CSF, at a value of 0.6 that of plasma, by active transport of this ion out of the CSF across the choroidal epithelial cells into plasma, and possibly by active transport across the endothelial cells or glial endfeet. CSF secretion is inhibited by ouabain, which blocks active Na transport across the choroid plexus cells, and by acetazolamide, which appears to inhibit Cl and HCO_3 transport across these cells by decreasing the activity of carbonic anhydrase. The potential difference across choroid plexus cells is sensitive to acid-base changes in the plasma which, therefore, can alter the distribution of ions between CSF and plasma and thereby affect CSF secretion. The vitamins folic acid and ascorbic acid are also actively transported into the CSF, as is the narcotic analgesic morphine. After the CSF is formed at the choroid plexus the fluid flows through the ventricles, enters the subarachnoid space, and exits into the cerebral venous system via the arachnoid villi as shown in Fig. 1. The exit of CSF via the arachnoid villi is a pressure-dependent filtration process (17, 18).

Substances that enter the CSF, either by way of the cerebral capillary–brain interstitial space–ependymal cell pathway or by crossing the choroid plexus, can exit from the CSF by two routes. One is by bulk flow of the substance in the CSF and exit via the arachnoid villi; nonelectrolyte molecules such as inulin, sucrose, albumin, and even red blood cells exit by this pathway. Small nonelectrolytes and both weak and strong electrolytes can leave by this mechanism and also by the second mechanism, which involves active transport of the substance across the choroid plexus from CSF to blood. This is the predominant system for exit of the anionic and cationic forms of weak and strong organic electrolytes, the inorganic halide anions, and probably K ion.

The anion system transports inorganic anions such as I^-, ClO_4^-, SCN^-, Br^-, and Tc^- out of the CSF into blood. The system is similar to the anion transport system in the thyroid. The choroid plexus cells concentrate these anions, as does the thyroid. This system also transports organic anions and the anionic species of weak acids out of the CSF, and the choroid plexus concentrates them against a concentration gradient. Thus, drugs such as penicillin, probenecid, and p-aminohippuric acid leave the CSF by this route. This is a carrier-mediated, energy-dependent system that obeys saturation kinetics and, therefore, can be blocked by competing anions, e.g., probenecid. This is the route by which many endogenous metabolites leave the brain and CSF, e.g., 5-hydroxyindoleacetic acid, homovanillic acid, and possibly lactate. These substances cross the cerebral capillaries only slowly and can exit at a much faster rate via the choroid plexus anion transport system, although there is some evidence that they also may be transported into plasma from brain across the endothelial cells of the cerebral capillaries.

The cation system transports inorganic cations such as K^+ out of the CSF across the epithelial cells of the choroid plexus. It also transports organic cations and the cationic species of weak bases out of the CSF. Such cations as choline, tetraethylammonium, and N-methyl nicotinamide leave the CSF by this route.

As a result of the rapid exit of substances from the brain and CSF by bulk flow thru the arachnoid villi and/or by active transport across the choroid plexus, and their slow entrance into the brain and CSF via the cerebral capillaries (site of blood-brain barrier), there occurs a low steady-state concentration in the brain and CSF. This has given rise to the concept of the "sink effect," which results from the low permeability of the cerebral capillaries coupled with their rapid exit from the CSF by bulk flow and/or active transport across the choroid plexus. This explains the mechanism of the so-called blood-brain barrier. If CSF secretion is inhibited or active transport of ions out of the CSF blocked, the steady-state levels of substances in the brain and CSF increase because the sink effect is negated. However, substances that enter the CSF by active transport and do not readily cross the cerebral capillary endothelial cells generally enter the brain from the CSF; in this case the brain is the sink for the substance.

CHANGES IN THE BLOOD-CNS TRANSPORT SYSTEM DURING MATURATION

It is now pertinent to discuss the changes in this system that occur during maturation. These are listed in Fig. 1. Changes in transport across the choroid plexus will be discussed first, then alterations in neuronal and glial transport systems.

Changes in Rate of CSF Production and Flow with Age

Figure 2 shows the changes in the rate of CSF production in rats during maturation. The rate of production was determined by ventriculo-cisternal perfusion with ^{14}C-inulin. The production rate increased linearly from a very low rate of about 0.2 μl/min in 3-day-old rats to a value of approximately 0.8 μl/min in 24-day-old rats. Thus, total CSF production increases markedly with age, an effect that is probably due to both increased transport of Na and Cl during early maturation (see below) and increased amounts of choroid

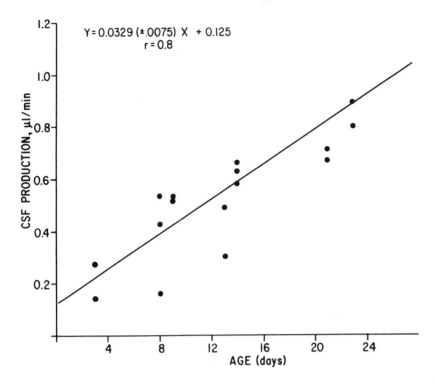

FIG. 2. Relation between cerebrospinal production rate and postnatal age in rats. Ordinate is CSF production rate in μl/min; abscissa is age in days.

plexus tissue during later maturation. The data of Ferguson and Woodbury (9) demonstrate a decrease in the CSF/plasma ratio of inulin with age. Since inulin is not actively transported out of CSF and exits only by bulk flow through the arachnoid villi, it is a measure of CSF flow rate. These results also suggest that immature animals have lower rates of CSF formation than do adult animals. Others have also demonstrated low rates of CSF production in immature animals [e.g., Shaywitz et al., (19).]

That immature animals have lower CSF formation rates than adults is also suggested by the data shown in Fig. 3, which depicts changes in CSF electrolytes with age (9). The concentrations of Na and Cl in CSF increase with age, whereas the concentration of K decreases. At 9 days after birth the CSF electrolyte values, particularly that of K, have leveled out and reached the adult value. These data suggest that the Na-K transport system in the choroid plexus has matured. Prior to this time, CSF-transport of electrolytes has not completely developed; hence, CSF formation is also immature.

The reduced CSF flow rate in immature animals, coupled with increased permeability of the cerebral capillaries to various substances and a larger extracellular volume compared with adult animals, as described below, all

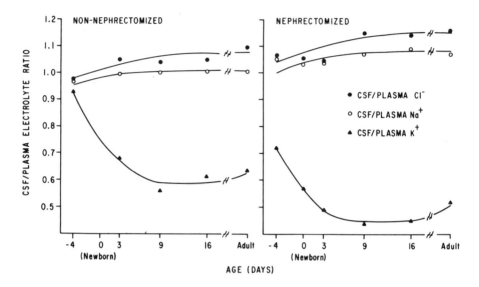

FIG. 3. Plot of CSF/plasma electrolyte concentration ratios for rats of various ages. Graph on left represents changes with age in normal rats and that on the right, changes occurring in nephrectomized rats of various ages. From Ferguson and Woodbury, *Exp. Brain Res.*, 7:181–194, 1969.

result in faster rates of entrance and higher concentrations of drugs and other molecules in brain and CSF. The sink effect is reduced by the lower CSF flow. As the animal matures, CSF flow increases, cerebral capillary permeability decreases, and the extracellular volume decreases. This increases the sink effect, and the rate of entrance of substances into brain and CSF and their concentration in these compartments are reduced.

Changes in Transport of Substances Across the Choroid Plexus with Age
[see (9) and summary by Saunders and Bradbury (2)]

Cation Transport

As indicated from the data presented in Fig. 3 and discussed above, the Na-K choroid plexus transport system does not appear to mature until about 9 days after birth in rats. Magnesium ion is also transported actively from blood to CSF against an electrochemical gradient. This system appears to be immature in fetal animals (but is the first cation system to mature). According to Saunders and Bradbury (2), the specific transport systems for ions mature in the order: Mg first (fetal stage), Na and Cl next, and K last (postnatal). Calcium levels in the CSF reach adult values after birth, but there is no convincing evidence as yet that Ca^{++} is actively transported across the choroid plexus. Thus the transport systems are established at adult values at very different ages for different ions.

Organic cation transport across the choroid plexus also occurs, but the changes with age have not been well documented. However, the accumulation of morphine in the choroid plexus *in vitro* appears to be lower in neonatal than in adult rats. Further work is indicated.

Anion Transport

Mediated transport of Cl from blood into CSF has been described by Bourke et al. (20), and inhibitors of anion transport system in other tissues have been shown to inhibit Cl transport into CSF (21). Changes with age have been little studied, however. As already described and as shown in Fig. 3, Cl levels in the CSF increase with age and reach adult values at about 9 days of age. Whether these changes are a result of development of an active transport system cannot be decided, because the potential difference between CSF and blood at the different age periods studied was not measured. However, the fact that perchlorate ion, which inhibits other inorganic anion transport (e.g., iodide), decreases the movement of Cl ion from blood into CSF suggests that it is an active process and that perchlorate is a competitive inhibitor (Barham and Woodbury, *unpublished observations*). Perchlorate is a less effective inhibitor of Cl movement in neonatal than in mature animals.

The monovalent inorganic anions such as perchlorate, iodide, thiocyanate, and bromide are also transported across the choroid plexus, but in a direction opposite from that of Cl, i.e., from CSF to blood. The changes of this transport system for ^{36}Cl-perchlorate with age are shown in Fig. 4. This figure also

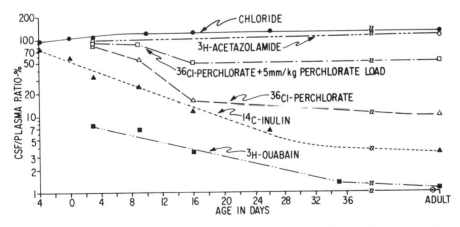

FIG. 4. Changes in CSF/plasma ratio of various radiolabeled ions and drugs during maturation in rats.

shows the changes with age of the CSF/plasma ratio for Cl, which increases and reaches a maximum between 3 and 9 days; acetazolamide, which stays at a value of 1.0 from 3 days to adulthood; inulin, which is used for comparison since it exits from the CSF by bulk flow; and ouabain, which like perchlorate is transported out of the CSF by an active process, but enters the brain and CSF at a slower rate than inulin. It is evident that in neonatal animals little transport of ^{36}Cl-perchlorate from CSF to blood occurs, and that a large load of perchlorate has little effect. The transport system, therefore, has not yet developed. As the animals mature, the ratio of CSF to plasma decreases and a large load of perchlorate has greater and greater effect in inhibiting perchlorate transport and increasing CSF levels. As the CSF levels decrease with age the brain levels also decrease. When the CSF levels increase with perchlorate treatment the brain levels increase. Thus the perchlorate in the CSF appears to determine the levels of perchlorate in the brain.

Iodide transport out of the CSF across the choroid plexus also changes with age (21, 22), as does that of sulfate (22), but at a slower rate. The ability of the isolated choroid plexus of rabbits and cats to accumulate iodide and sulfate at different age periods is shown in Table 1. The tissue to medium

TABLE 1. Uptake of ^{35}S-sulfate and ^{125}I-iodide by isolated choroid plexus of rabbits and cats at different ages of development

| | Tissue/medium ratio | | | |
| | ^{35}S-Sulfate | | ^{125}I-Iodide | |
Age	rabbits	cats	rabbits	cats
Early fetus	1.6	—	39	—
Late fetus	1.7	2.1	60	45
1–3 days	2.9	3.3	30	25
10 days	3.2	2.7	31	25
Adult	2.5	2.4	26	26

From Robinson, Cutler, Lorenzo, and Barlow, J. Neurochem., 15:455–458, 1968.

ratio (T/M) for iodide increases from the early fetal stage value of about 40 to the late fetal stage value of 60, decreases thereafter until a few days after birth, and then levels out into the adult stage (ca. 25). Even in the early fetal stage, however, the T/M is higher than that of the neonatal and adult animals, and, although there is a transient rise in the accumulative ability, there is an overall decrease with age. However, since iodide levels in the CSF decrease with age, the concentration in the choroid plexus may not reflect the rate of removal from CSF. Further work is indicated. The T/M for sulfate is about 1.5 in the early fetal stage, increases thereafter to about 3 in the late fetal and early postnatal stages, and then decreases to the adult value of 2. Thus sulfate is actively transported out of the CSF across the choroid plexus and the transport ability increases with age, but it appears to be an independent system from that of Cl.

Changes in *organic anion transport* with age have been noted, and the results indicate the transport properties of these anions develop early in some cases and late in others. For example, Tissari (23) showed that the rate of active transport of 5-HIAA, a metabolite of 5-hydroxytryptamine (5-HT), out of brain is very low in newborn rats and increases with age; adult values are reached at about 21 days of age. Probenecid blocks the transport, which probably occurs at the choroid plexus and possibly at the cerebral capillaries. On the other hand, Bass and Lundborg (24) studied the elimination of *p*-aminohippuric acid (PAH) from the CSF in rats of different ages by the technique of subarachnoid infusion. CSF bulk flow rate as measured by inulin elimination was considerably slower in 5-day-old rats than in 30-day-old rats, but PAH was rapidly eliminated by an active transport mechanism across the choroid plexus which was inhibited by 5-HIAA and probenecid. However, rats younger than 5 days of age were not tested, and it is likely that this system matures either in the late prenatal stage or in the immediate postnatal period. The complexity of the situation is indicated by the fact that active transport out of the CSF had disappeared in 30-day-old rats and the efflux of PAH from CSF could be accounted for by the increased bulk flow; however, a system for transport of PAH out of the brain across the cerebral capillaries that was inhibited by 5-HIAA and probenecid had developed. This system was absent in the 5-day-old rats, although an equally rapid efflux of PAH from the brain occurred through the highly permeable cerebral capillaries. Thus, an early-developing transport system across the choroid plexus was replaced by a late-developing transport system across the brain capillaries. These interesting observations of Bass and Lundborg (24) should be confirmed by other workers.

Capillary Permeability Changes During Development

The histologic and ultrastructural changes in cerebral cortex and in cerebral capillaries with age have been described by Donahue and Pappas (10) and Caley and Maxwell (25, 26), and are summarized in Table 2. The basement membrane progresses from a thin band of variable thickness and density to a thicker structure of more or less uniform width and density above any given capillary. The endothelial cells in the immature animals are relatively thick. These cells become attenuated in the adult. The rather complete glial investment of the cerebral capillaries in the adult is absent in the immature animals. Cell bodies rather than cell processes (as in the adult brain) are in close proximity to the capillaries in the immature brain. It would appear that the decreased ability of various substances to enter the brain from the plasma in the mature animal is related to the anatomic changes in the cerebral capillaries and extracellular space and to the glial investment of the capillaries.

TABLE 2. *Ultrastructural changes during maturation of the cerebral cortex*

Age	Changes
Birth to 7 days	Increased cortical thickness to adult value due to proliferation of dendritic tree of pyramidal neurons and invasion of axons Large extracellular space Few blood vessels Presumptive synapses
8–14 days	Transition period Blood vessel lamina open; extracellular space reduced nearly to adult size Astrocytic processes replace the extracellular spaces around the blood vessels and developing synapses Myelination begins
15–21 days	Establishment of the mature neuropil of tightly packed axons, dendrites, synapses, and glial processes

From Caley and Maxwell, in: *Brain Development and Behavior*, pp. 91–107, Academic Press, New York, 1971.

As already described, the permeability of the cerebral capillaries to large molecules such as albumin and trypan blue is absent in the immature as well as the adult animal. However, molecules such as inulin, sucrose, sodium, potassium, chloride, iodide, perchlorate, ouabain and other drugs, glutamic acid, lysine and other amino acids, phosphate, and cholesterol enter brain and CSF more rapidly or have higher steady-state concentrations relative to plasma in fetal and neonatal animals as compared with adults (8, 9, 21, 27–33).

The rate of uptake of these materials might be even faster, but there are fewer arterioles per square centimeter of brain surface in young than in older animals. The number of vessels per square centimeter increases sharply with age in both man and rats and then levels out; in the rat this occurs at 21 days (25, 34). Thus the rate of uptake of substances in the young animals may be blood flow-limited.

An example of the change in rate of entrance of substances into the brain with age is the observation of Luciano (32) that the half time for the uptake of ^{22}Na by newborn rat brain was 40 min, whereas it was 75 min in the adult. Even correcting for the larger volume of distribution of Na in the younger animals, the rate constant was faster than that of adult rats. The same is true for ^{36}Cl uptake in neonatal as compared with adult rats (8) and for ^{14}C-inulin. The rate of entry of the latter into the brain was seven times faster in −4-day-old (17 days of gestation) rats than in 16-day-old rats and about 25 times faster than the uptake into the brain of adult rats (9).

Changes in Brain Extracellular Volume During Development

Figure 5 summarizes the changes in K concentration, Na and Cl spaces, and extra- and intracellular volume of brain during development of the rat.

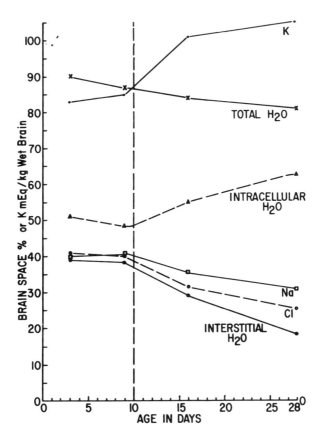

FIG. 5. Changes in K concentration, Na and Cl spaces, and extra- and intracellular volume of brain during maturation in the rat. The ordinate is changes in brain concentration or space of the various parameters; the abscissa is age in days after birth.

The extracellular fluid (ECF) volume was measured by the brain/CSF ratio of ^{14}C-inulin in rats of different ages (-6 days old to adult) (9). The values are in agreement with the extracellular spaces determined from the second component of brain ^{36}Cl uptake curves in animals of the same age (8). In animals -6 days old the CSF/plasma ratio of inulin was about 1.0 and in the adults it was 0.01. The corresponding brain spaces of inulin measured simultaneously with the CSF values are 50% and 1%. The brain/CSF ratio measures the ECF volume up to 16 days of age in rats since CSF and brain interstitial fluid appear to be in rapid equilibrium during this period of time. The second component of the brain ^{36}Cl uptake curve measures the extracellular space into the adult stage.

It is evident, therefore, that the volume of the extracellular space of the brain as measured by the marker technique decreases with age. A decrease in ECF volume with age has also been noted with anatomic studies of the brain utilizing the electron microscope [see, for example, (35) and (25)].

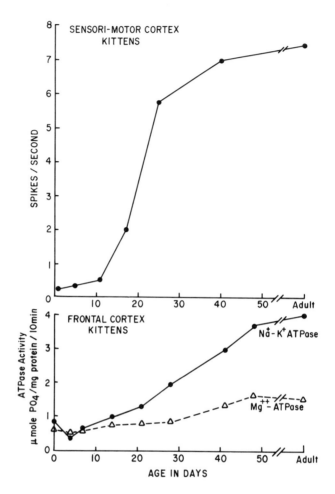

FIG. 6. Changes with age in kittens of electrical activity of the sensorimotor cortex (upper graph) and Na⁺,K⁺-ATPase and Mg⁺⁺-ATPase activity in the frontal cortex (lower graph). Ordinate in upper graph is number of spikes/sec and in lower graph, ATPase activity in μmoles phosphate/mg protein/10 min. Abscissa is age in days after birth. From Huttenlocher and Rawson, *Exp. Neurol.,* 22:118–129, 1968, with permission of the publisher.

Figure 5 also shows that the Na and Cl spaces of brain decrease with age, intracellular water increases (despite a decrease in total water, because the ECF volume decreases to a greater extent than total water decreases), and K concentration increases (36, 8). The increase in K concentration and decrease in Na and Cl concentrations with age are indicative of the increase in number of neuronal cell processes and glial cells and the decrease in the extracellular space with age, as indicated by electron microscopic studies.

Changes in Neuronal Cell Volume and Transport Ability with Age

Electron microscopic and neurophysiologic evidence demonstrates that there is marked proliferation of neuronal processes (axons and dendrites) and synapses during maturation of the brain. As they proliferate, these processes and the glial cells fill in the large extracellular space of the neonatal animal and account for its decrease with age. This is evident from the increase in brain K concentration and decrease in Na and Cl concentration in the brain that occurs with age (see Fig. 5). Very few data are available on the changes in the permeability of neuronal membranes to drugs and other substances with age.

However, the development of transport systems concerned with electrical activity of the brain does seem to correlate with maturation. As shown in Fig. 6, taken from the work of Huttenlocher and Rawson (37), there is a correlation between the development of spikes induced by stimulation of the sensorimotor cortex of different aged kittens and the Na^+,K^+-ATPase activity in the same area. Thus, electrical activity of the brain appears to develop *pari passu* with development of the transport system for Na and K. Similar findings were observed in the rat (38).

Since ouabain is a selective inhibitor of Na^+,K^+-ATPase, it was of interest to study its distribution in brain and CSF during maturation. ^3H-Ouabain was used and the concentrations of the free and bound forms of the drug were measured. Ouabain binds to Na^+,K^+-ATPase; therefore the amount in this form represents the amount of this enzyme present. The amount of bound ouabain increased with age and paralleled the increase in activity of Na^+,K^+-ATPase with age as described by Abdel-Latif et al. (38). An interesting finding, however, was the result shown in Table 3, taken from Brøndsted and Woodbury (33), that the ratio of the free concentration of ^3H-ouabain in brain cells to that in extracellular fluid (CSF) was zero (extracellularly distributed) in 3- and 9-day-old rats and increased with age thereafter. It was greater than 1.0 after 16 days of age. Thus ouabain is actively transported into brain cells (also muscle, heart, and liver cells) as well as out of CSF. That this is carrier-mediated transport is indicated by the fact that loading the animals with ouabain decreased the transport of the drug into brain, muscle,

TABLE 3. ^3H-Ouabain distribution in rat brain
and CSF during maturation

Age (days)	Brain cell ^3H-ouabain/ extracellular ^3H-ouabain	CSF ^3H-ouabain/ plasma ^3H-ouabain
3	0	0.076
9	0	0.067
16	1.0	0.034
35	2.1	0.013

heart, and liver cells. Increase in plasma K^+ also inhibited the active transport of ouabain into these cells. It appears that, since ouabain competes with K for the inward (K) arm of the Na-K transport system, its active transport may involve binding to the same carrier as K^+. Whether the active uptake of ouabain is into neurons, glial cells, or both has not yet been assessed. It is clear, however, that the system does mature with age.

The permeability of the cerebral capillaries to ouabain also decreases with age, as indicated by the fact that the levels of the drug in the brain decrease with age. This is reflected in the LD_{50} and CD_{50} values of the drug in different aged rats as shown in Fig. 7 (Brøndsted and Woodbury, *unpublished observa-*

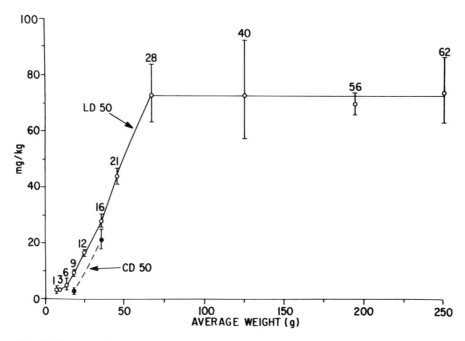

FIG. 7. Changes in the CD_{50} and LD_{50} for ouabain during maturation of rats. Vertical bracketed lines are 95% fiducial limits. Ordinate is CD_{50} or LD_{50} in mg/kg; abscissa is age in days after birth.

tions). The LD_{50} is very low in neonatal animals and increases markedly with age until 28 days when it reaches a plateau. Thus, low doses of the drug readily produce seizures and death in infant rats but large doses are required to kill adult rats and seizures do not result. Ouabain levels in brain and CSF of adult animals are therefore very low because of low permeability of the cerebral capillaries to the drug and because active transport and bulk flow out of CSF rapidly remove the small amount that enters.

Further evidence for change in the properties of nerve membranes during

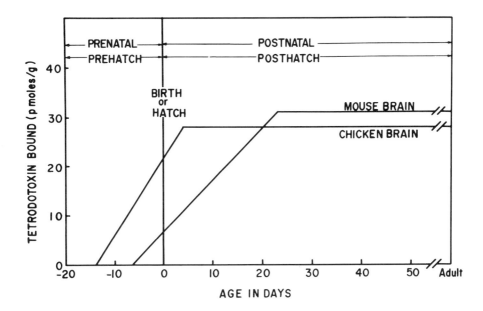

FIG. 8. Changes with age in ^{3}H-tetrodotoxin binding sites in brain from mice and chickens. Ordinate is amount of tetrodotoxin bound in pmoles/g brain; abscissa is prenatal or postnatal age in days. From Hafemann and Unsworth, *J. Neurochem;* 20:613–616, 1973, with permission of the publisher.

maturation is derived from the ^{3}H-tetrodotoxin experiments of Hafemann and Unsworth (39) shown in Fig. 8. Tetrodotoxin binds tightly to nerve cell membranes and blocks the Na channels. Thus electrical activity is inhibited. Figure 8 indicates the amount of tetrodotoxin bound to the mouse and chicken brain at different age periods. The amount found, which is a measure of the number of Na channels in the brain, increased with age until 1 to 4 days after hatch in the chick, and until 23 days in the mouse, times in both animals when the brain is functionally mature. Thus the number of Na channels correlates, as would be expected, with the development of electrical activity and function.

Changes in Glial Cell Numbers, Volume, and Transport Ability with Age

Figure 9 shows the changes in weight, carbonic anhydrase activity, and total CO_2 of the brain with age. The brain weight has reached about half its maximal value by 10 days but neither the carbonic anhydrase activity, which is very low in the first 10 days of life, nor the total CO_2, which is very high, has changed during this period. However, from 10 to 21 days the brain carbonic anhydrase activity increases rapidly and then levels out somewhat, although it continues to increase for the rest of the life of the rats. Total CO_2 decreases rapidly from 10 to 21 days and then levels out and also tends to decrease more slowly thereafter. Since carbonic anhydrase is localized to glial

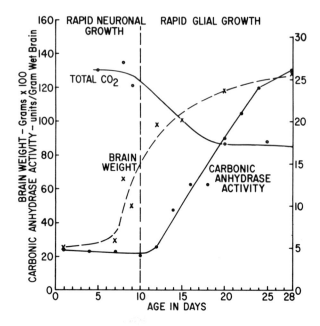

FIG. 9. Changes in weight and carbonic anhydrase activity (left ordinate) and total CO_2 (right ordinate) of the brain with age in days (abscissa). The period of rapid neuronal growth is separated from the period of rapid glial growth by a vertical dashed line at 10 days of age. From Woodbury, Discussion, in *Ion Homeostasis of the Brain*, Munksgaard, Copenhagen, pp. 337–339.

cells (40) and it is assumed that the activity per cell does not change, then the increase in carbonic anhydrase activity during development indicates increased glial cell growth with age. This is in line with observations of Brizzee and Jacobs (41) that the glial-neuron index (number of glial cells per number of neurons per unit area) increases with age; electron microscopic evidence [see, for example, (42) and (43)] and evidence from tissue fractionation studies in which glial cells and neurons are separated also demonstrate increased number and volume of glial cells with maturation of the brain.

Acetazolamide is a selective inhibitor of carbonic anhydrase, and as such binds avidly to this enzyme. If ^{3}H-acetazolamide is given, the activity of the drug present in tissues at 24 hr after administration represents the amount bound to carbonic anhydrase in a well-perfused tissue in which blood has been removed. Figure 10 shows the distribution with time of ^{3}H-acetazolamide in 3-day-old versus adult rats. The amount of drug present is considerably lower in blood and brain (related to both CSF and plasma) in 3-day-old as compared with adult rats. Other data show that the brain/CSF ratio follows the same time course of increase with maturation as does the carbonic anhydrase curve shown in Fig. 9. Thus this index of carbonic anhydrase activity also indicates that glial cell growth increases with age.

Experiments in our laboratory (*unpublished*) and by others (44, 45) have

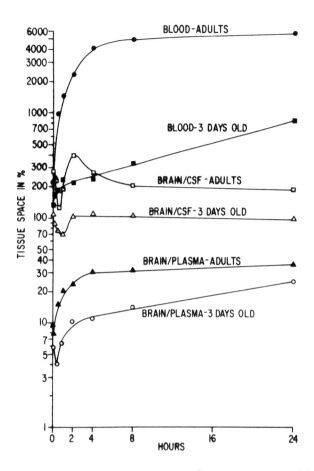

FIG. 10. Tissue/plasma, tissue/CSF ratios in percent of ^{3}H-acetazolamide in adult as compared with 3-day-old rats. The ordinate is tissue space in percent; the abscissa is time in hours. From Woodbury, in *Antiepileptic Drugs*, Raven Press, New York, pp. 465–475.

demonstrated that Cl is transported into glial cells by a K-dependent, carrier-mediated system that is inhibited by thiocyanate and perchlorate. This system also appears to actively transport perchlorate anion, and shows saturation kinetics as the perchlorate load is increased. A schematic representation of this process is illustrated in Fig. 11 and is based on data from ^{36}ClO$_4$ uptake curves. The control situation is shown in the upper portion of the figure. The cells represent both neurons and glia, although the system probably involves only glial cells since perchlorate transport is not blocked by perchlorate loads in animals younger than 10 days of age, a time when glial cells are not developed. The ratio of extracellular to intracellular perchlorate is such as to indicate that it is not distributed passively according to the membrane potential and that active transport into the cells is involved. Transport of perchlorate

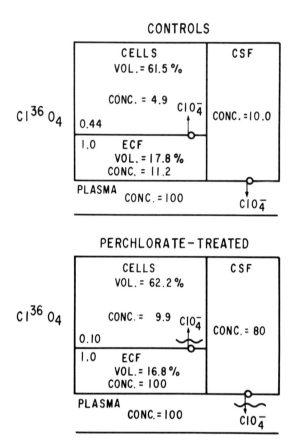

FIG. 11. Schematic drawing of the plasma-brain-CSF system showing the distribution of ^{36}Cl-perchlorate (^{36}ClO$^-_4$) in the various compartments of the brain in control and perchlorate-loaded rats. Two pumps are shown, one for transporting ^{36}ClO$^-_4$ out of the CSF across the choroid plexus to the blood and one for transporting it into brain cells. The wavy line crossing the arrow on the two pumps in the perchlorate-loaded group (lower diagram) indicates inhibition of the pumps by perchlorate. The brain extracellular space values were derived from the second component of the brain and CSF ^{36}Cl$^-$ uptake curve measured at the same time in control and perchlorate-loaded rats. The concentrations of ^{36}ClO$^-_4$ in the various compartments are relative to a plasma concentration of 100. Extracellular concentrations are based on the CSF levels and also on the second component of the ^{36}ClO$^-_4$ uptake curves. The intracellular values were derived from the total brain ^{36}ClO$^-_4$, water content, extracellular volume, and extracellular ^{36}ClO$^-_4$ concentration.

out of the CSF across the choroid plexus is also present, as already described. When a large load of perchlorate is given (lower portion of figure), the concentration of perchlorate in the CSF and correspondingly in the brain interstitial space is increased as a result of inhibition of the active transport across the choroid plexus. The perchlorate load also results in inhibition of the cellular transport of perchlorate, since, despite the increase in the total amount in the cell, the ratio of extracellular to intracellular perchlorate increases and approaches the ratio that would be predicted for passive distribution.

Measurement of ^{36}Cl-perchlorate uptake in maturing animals has shown that this transport system matures with age in parallel with the development of the glial cells, maturation of brain carbonic anhydrase, and maturation of the glial Cl transport system. Thus the perchlorate anion transport probably uses the same system as Cl and appears to involve carbonic anhydrase.

Changes in Permeability of the Ependymal Lining with Age

As maturation proceeds, the ability of drugs or other substances to cross the ependymal lining decreases. This layer of cells possesses gap junctions, and small molecules can cross freely. However, large molecules such as albumin and to some extent even the smaller inulin molecule are restricted in their movements. The increase in the brain/CSF ratio for inulin that occurs after 16 days in the study by Ferguson and Woodbury (9) can be explained by a decrease in the ability of inulin to cross the ependymal border as the animal matures.

SUMMARY

It is apparent from this discussion that the entrance of drugs into brain and CSF with age and their exit therefrom depend upon a number of properties of the blood-brain–CSF system: permeability of the brain capillaries; rate of flow of CSF; active transport across the choroid plexus, cerebral capillaries, neurons, and glia; and volume of the ECF. Other factors such as protein binding affinity of the drug, lipid solubility, and pK_a are also important. Many of these factors change with age and, therefore, in order to define the changes in distribution of drugs with age, each of these properties has to be identified. The dose of a drug is also important in affecting its own distribution or that of another drug. For example, probenecid competes with many organic anions for transport across choroid plexus cells. It thus blocks the exit of penicillin, 5-HIAA, homovanillic acid, etc., but if given in large doses can also block its own transport out of the CSF. Many drugs may act on the brain by inhibiting transport of other drugs or endogenous metabolites out of the brain and CSF. This would result in an increase in their level in CSF and in brain, and if this level is sufficiently elevated, can cause pharmacologic effects on the brain. Effects of drugs on transport processes in glial and neuronal cells occur and also appear to be age-dependent.

ACKNOWLEDGMENTS

Unpublished data presented in this paper were supported by a grant (5–P01–NS–04553) from the National Institute of Neurological Diseases and Stroke. D.M.W. is the recipient of U.S. Public Health Service Research Career Award 5-K6-NB-13,838 from the National Institute of Neurological Diseases and Blindness, National Institutes of Health.

REFERENCES

1. Davson, H. Ontogeny of the blood-brain barrier. In: *Fetal Pharmacology*, edited by L. O. Boréus, pp. 75–88. Raven Press, New York, 1973.
2. Saunders, N. R., and Bradbury, M. W. B. The development of the internal environment of the brain. In: *Fetal Pharmacology*, edited by L. O. Boréus, pp. 93–109. Raven Press, New York, 1973.
3. Brightman, M. W., and Reese, T. S. Junctions between intimately apposed cell membranes in the vertebrate brain. *J. Cell Biol.*, 40:648–677, 1969.
4. Pappenheimer, J. R. On the location of the blood-brain barrier. In: *Proceedings of a Symposium on the Blood-Brain Barrier*, edited by R. V. Coxon, pp. 66–84. Truex Press, Oxford, 1970. (See also discussion by M. R. Brightman on pp. 237–238 of this same symposium, and figure opposite p. 240.)
5. Chrone, C. The blood-brain barrier facts and questions. In: *Ion Homeostasis of the Brain*, Alfred Benzon Symposium III, edited by B. K. Siesjo and S. C. Sorensen, pp. 52–66. Munksgaard, Copenhagen, 1971.
6. Grazer, F. M., and Clemente, C. D. Developing blood brain barrier to trypan blue. *Proc. Soc. Exp. Biol. Med.*, 94:758–760, 1957.
7. Olsson, Y. Blood-brain barrier to albumin in embryonic, new born and adult rats. *Acta Neuropath.*, 10:117–122, 1968.
8. Vernadakis, A., and Woodbury, D. M. Cellular and extracellular spaces in developing rat brain. *Arch. Neurol.*, 12:284–293, 1965.
9. Ferguson, R. K., and Woodbury, D. M. Penetration of ^{14}C-inulin and ^{14}C-sucrose into brain, cerebrospinal fluid, and skeletal muscle of developing rats. *Exp. Brain Res.*, 7:181–194, 1969.
10. Donahue, S., and Pappas, G. D. The fine structure of capillaries in the cerebral cortex of the rat at various stages of development. *Am. J. Anat.*, 108:331–347, 1961.
11. Reed, D. J., and Woodbury, D. M. Kinetics of movement of iodide, sucrose, inulin and radioiodinated serum albumin in central nervous system and cerebrospinal fluid of rat. *J. Physiol.* (Lond.), 169:816–850, 1963.
12. Kuffler, S. W., and Nicholls, J. G. The physiology of neuroglial cells. *Ergebn. Physiol.*, 57:1–90, 1966.
13. Orkand, R. K. Neuroglial-neuronal interactions. In: *Basic Mechanisms of the Epilepsies*, edited by H. H. Jasper, A. A. Ward, and A. Pope, pp. 737–746. Little, Brown, Boston, 1969.
14. Pollen, D. A., and Trachtenberg, M. C. Neuroglia: Gliosis and focal epilepsy. *Science*, 167:1252–1253, 1970.
15. Trachtenberg, M. C., and Pollen, D. A. Neuroglia: Biophysical properties and physiologic function. *Science*, 167:1248–1252, 1970.
16. Henn, F. A., Haljamäe, H., and Hamberger, A. Glial cell function: Active control of extracellular K^+ concentration. *Brain Res.*, 43:437–443, 1972.
17. Shabo, A. L., and Maxwell, D. S. The morphology of the arachnoid villi: A light and electron microscopic study in the monkey. *J. Neurosurg.*, 29:451–463, 1968.
18. Shabo, A. L., and Maxwell, D. S Electron microscopic observations on the fate of particulate matter in the cerebrospinal fluid. *J. Neurosurg.*, 29:464–474, 1968.
19. Shaywitz, B. A., Katzman, R., and Escriva, A. CSF formation and ^{24}Na clearance in normal and hydrocephalic kittens during ventriculocisternal perfusion. *Neurology*, 19:1159–1168, 1969.
20. Bourke, R. S., Gabelnick, H. L., and Young, O. Mediated transport of chloride from blood into cerebrospinal fluid. *Exp. Brain Res.*, 10:17–38, 1970.
21. Woodbury, D. M. Distribution of nonelectrolytes and electrolytes in the brain as affected by alterations in cerebrospinal fluid secretion. In: *Progress in Brain Research*, Vol. 29, edited by A. Lajtha and D. Ford, pp. 297–313. Elsevier, Amsterdam, 1968.
22. Robinson, R. J., Cutler, R. W P., Lorenzo, A. V., and Barlow, C. F. Development of transport mechanisms for sulphate and iodide in immature choroid plexus. *J. Neurochem.*, 15:455–458, 1968.
23. Tissari, A. H. Serotoninergic mechanisms in ontogenesis. In: *Fetal Pharmacology*, L. O. Boréus, pp. 237–257. Raven Press, New York, 1973.

24. Bass, N. H., and Lundborg, P. Postnatal development of mechanisms for the elimination of organic acids from the brain and cerebrospinal fluid system of the rat: Rapid efflux of [³H] para-aminohippuric acid following intrathecal infusion. *Brain Res.,* 56:285–298, 1973.
25. Caley, D. W., and Maxwell, D. S. Development of the blood vessels and extracellular spaces during postnatal maturation of rat cerebral cortex. *J. Comp. Neurol.,* 138:31–48, 1970.
26. Caley, D. W., and Maxwell, D. S. Ultrastructure of the developing cerebral cortex in the rat. In: *Brain Development and Behavior,* edited by M. B. Sterman, D. J. McGinty, and A. M. Adinolfi, pp. 91–107. Academic Press, New York, 1971.
27. Bakay, L. Studies on BBB with radioactive phosphorus. III. Embryonic development of the barrier. *Arch. Neurol. Psychiat.,* 70:30–39, 1953.
28. Katzman, R., and Leiderman, P. H. Brain potassium exchange in normal adult and immature rats. *Am. J. Physiol.,* 175:263–270, 1953.
29. Himwich, H. E., and Himwich, W A. The permeability of the blood-brain barrier to glutamic acid in the developing rat. In: *Biochemistry of the Developing Nervous System,* edited by H. Waelsch, p. 202. Academic Press, New York, 1955.
30. Lajtha, A. Amino acid and protein metabolism of the brain II. The uptake of L-lysine by brain and other organs of the mouse at different ages. *J. Neurochem.,* 2:209–215, 1958.
31. Dobbing, J., and Sands, J. A. The entry of cholesterol into rat brain during development. *J. Physiol.* (Lond.), 166:45P, 1963.
32. Luciano, D. S. Sodium movement across the blood-brain barrier in newborn and adult rats and autoradiographic-localization. *Brain Res.,* 9:334–350, 1968.
33. Brøndsted, H. E., and Woodbury, D. M. Uptake and distribution of ³H-ouabain in brain and other tissues of developing rats. In: *Fetal Pharmacology,* edited by L. O. Boréus, pp. 89–92. Raven Press, New York, 1973.
34. Rhodes, A. J., and Hyde, J. B. Postnatal growth of arterioles in the human cerebral cortex. *Growth,* 29:173–182, 1965.
35. Pysh, J. J. The development of the extracellular space in neonatal rat inferior colliculus: An electron microscopic study. *Am. J. Anat.,* 124:411–430, 1969.
36. Vernadakis, A., and Woodbury, D. M. Electrolyte and amino acid changes in rat brain during maturation. *Am. J. Physiol.,* 203:748–752, 1962.
37. Huttenlocher, P. R., and Rawson, M. D. Neuronal activity and adenosine triphosphatase in immature cerebral cortex. *Exp. Neurol.,* 22:118–129, 1968.
38. Abdel-Latif, A. A., Brody, J., and Ramahi, H. Studies on sodium-potassium adenosine triphosphatase of the nerve endings and appearance of electrical activity in developing rat brain, *J. Neurochem.,* 14:1133–1141, 1967.
39. Hafemann, D. R., and Unsworth, B. R. Appearance of binding sites for radioactive tetrodotoxin during the development of mouse and chick brain. *J. Neurochem.,* 20:613–616, 1973.
40. Giacobini, E. A cytochemical study of the localization of carbonic anhydrase in the nervous system. *J. Neurochem.,* 9:169–177, 1962.
41. Brizzee, K. R., and Jacobs, L. A. The glial-neuron index in the submolecular layers of the motor cortex in the cat. *Anat. Rec.,* 134:97–105, 1959.
42. Caley, D. W., and Maxwell, D. S. An electron microscopic study of the neuroglia during postnatal development of the rat cerebrum. *J. Comp. Neurol.,* 133:45–70, 1968.
43. Vaughn, J. E., and Peters, A. Electron microscopy of the early postnatal development of fibrous astrocytes. *Am. J. Anat.,* 121:131–152, 1967
44. Bourke, R. S. Evidence for mediated transport of chloride in cat cortex *in vitro. Exp. Brain Res.,* 8:219–231, 1969.
45. Bourke, R. S., and Nelson, K. M. Further studies on the K⁺-dependent swelling of primate cerebral cortex *in vivo:* The enzymatic basis of the K⁺-dependent transport of chloride. *J. Neurochem.,* 19:663–685, 1972.
46. Woodbury, D. M. Discussion. In: *Ion Homeostasis of the Brain,* Alfred Benzon Symposium III, edited by B. K. Siesjo and S. C. Sorensen, pp. 337–339. Munksgaard, Copenhagen, 1971.
47. Woodbury, D. M. Acetazolamide. In: *Antiepileptic Drugs,* edited by D. M. Woodbury, J. K. Penry, and R. P. Schmidt, pp. 465–475. Raven Press, New York, 1972.

DISCUSSION

Mirsky: I would like to apologize, first, for referring to work which was done back in 1938 and 1939, but the results of those studies, based on relatively crude methods, agree closely with results we've seen here this morning. We found that injection of acid fuchsin into the ventricular system of the immature rat caused convulsions up until approximately 16 to 18 days of age. Thereafter, the incidence of this response dropped tremendously. Likewise, injection of bilirubin into the CSF prior to 18 days of age was followed by significant amounts of bilirubin-staining of brain tissue, but after this time the amount measurable in brain decreased. Thus, we concluded that a blood-brain barrier to these two macromolecular substances developed somewhere in the neighborhood of 16 to 18 days of age in the rat.

Woodbury: That is very interesting. In general, we find that the brain permeability to a number of different drugs decreases dramatically between 10 and 20 days of age.

Ford: I wonder to what extent the changes we are talking about here may relate to something other than a blood-brain barrier. Might they relate to the rather sudden plateau and then cessation of growth of nerve cells during this time? At this time the cells pass from a period of very active growth to one of extremely slow increase in size.

Kerr: From time to time we hear of a CSF-brain barrier, and I am wondering if it is the same thing to inject a compound into CSF as it is to implant it directly into brain. Could you comment on this?

Woodbury: Generally, if you inject a compound into CSF it rapidly gets into brain. However, we find that the rate at which it enters the brain depends upon the size of the molecule. For example, injection of radioactive albumin into CSF shows that it enters brain more slowly than inulin, and inulin enters more slowly than glucose, and glucose enters more slowly than mannitol. Of course, in addition to the size of the molecule, its charge, its solubility in fat, and certain regional considerations are also known to be important.

Weiner: Regional differences can be very important. For example, in the floor and lateral recess of the third ventricle, the ependymal cells have tight junctions. These cells also have microvilli and might function as barriers to some substances and, at the same time, as a point of transport of other materials out of the CSF into direct apposition to the primary plexus of the portal system. These functions may be selective and specific.

Woodbury: It is also possible that the capillaries of the choroid plexus differ from capillaries elsewhere in the brain and these differences might also be important.

Gorsky: I'm wondering if drugs of abuse modify the blood-brain barrier; this being one of the older ideas regarding the development of tolerance to these drugs.

Woodbury: There is evidence that the cells or capillaries of the choroid plexus do concentrate morphine *in vitro*.

Oldendorf: I'm somewhat suspicious of this type of *in vitro* work with choroid plexus cells since we find that they concentrate so many diverse and different agents.

Kerr: We have some recent evidence *in vivo* in the rat which suggests that tolerance to morphine is accompanied by a change in permeability of the blood-brain barrier. These findings are reported in the *Federation Proceedings* and suggest that tolerance to morphine is mediated by the blood-brain barrier.

Narcotics and the Hypothalamus, edited by
E. Zimmermann and R. George. Raven Press,
New York © 1974

Narcotic Analgesics and the Neuroendocrine Control of Anterior Pituitary Function

David de Wied, Jan M. van Ree, and Wybren de Jong

Rudolf Magnus Institute for Pharmacology, Medical Faculty, University of Utrecht, Utrecht, The Netherlands

INTRODUCTION

This chapter surveys recent data on the influence of narcotic analgesics on hypothalamic-pituitary function. The concept that the releasing factor cells operate as neuroendocrine transducers, converting a neuronal input into a humoral output (1, 2), suggests that narcotic analgesics affect pituitary function through modification of hypothalamic transmission. Although the influence of morphine and related drugs on transmission in the central nervous system (CNS) is not well established (3–7), an attempt is made to relate neuropharmacologic data with neuroendocrine effects elicited by the acute and chronic administration of these drugs. The effect of the morphinomimetics on endocrine function has been competently reviewed recently (8–10). George and Lomax (10) stated that the effects on endocrine function of drugs which induce physical and/or psychic dependence have scarcely been studied. In fact, the subject needs more attention and accurate measurements of pituitary activity. With the availability of radioimmunologic techniques it is now possible to assess the influence of acute and chronic administration of morphine and related drugs and of withdrawal effects on anterior pituitary activity. Recent data from studies begun only within the last decade on the influence of morphine on brain transmitter activity are also reviewed here, and again one has to conclude that a detailed study of the influence of the narcotic analgesics on biogenic amine and acetylcholine activity in the brain is needed.

PITUITARY-ADRENAL ACTIVITY

The effect of morphine and related drugs on pituitary-adrenal function has been studied more extensively than for other pituitary functions. A single injection stimulates pituitary-adrenal activity in the conscious rat, mouse, and dog, but not in guinea pigs and man (8–11). Acute administration of morphine blocks vasopressin-induced release of ACTH and prevents the early morning rise in plasma cortisol in pentobarbital-sedated man (12). In fact, morphine in the presence of pentobarbital in rats also inhibits stress-induced

ACTH release (10, 11). Munson (11) argued that pentobarbital serves to prevent the pain and alarm of the injection, but this seems too simple an explanation. Morphine injection elicits a more marked and a much longer lasting pituitary-adrenal activation than placebo injection, and in the rat this effect increases with the dose (13, 14). Pentobarbital itself brings pituitary-adrenal activity back to very low (basal) levels and it may be that the narcotic analgesics potentiate the blocking action of pentobarbital as they potentiate its anesthetic effects (15). This potentiation may therefore be responsible for inhibition of stress-induced pituitary-adrenal activity.

From studies with hypothalamic lesions and intrahypothalamic microinjection (10, 16–18), it is evident that the stimulatory effect of morphine on ACTH release is located in the CNS. Hypothalamic lesions, in particular in the median eminence, block morphine-induced ACTH release, indicating that the effect of morphine is not on the pituitary directly. Application of microgram quantities of morphine in the mid-hypothalamus has the reverse effect. Microinjection of morphine in or close to the nucleus arcuatus elicits a long-lasting release of ACTH (18).

Chronic administration induces tolerance to the stimulatory effect of morphine in the rat within a few days (10, 11, 14) and depresses the pituitary-adrenal response to stress in various species (8–11). During morphine addiction in man, plasma and urinary 17-hydroxycorticosteroids were reported low, with an unchanged hydrocortisone half-life (19, 20). Withdrawal of morphine, however, rapidly results in a large increase in adrenocortical activity in these addicts as well as in rats on chronic morphine (9, 10, 14, 19, 20). Abstinence elicited by the injection of nalorphine or naloxone in rats has the same effect (9, 14). Generally, an unimpaired response of the adrenal cortex to exogenous ACTH is found after acute and chronic morphine treatment (8–12, 14, 19–21). Nalorphine and naloxone in relatively low doses antagonize the stimulatory effect of morphine as well as its inhibitory action on pituitary-adrenal activity (8–11, 14).

In summary, ACTH release in some species is stimulated by a single injection of morphine, while chronic morphine administration reduces ACTH release in animals and man. Both effects are mediated through a CNS action of morphine (8–10).

PITUITARY-THYROID ACTIVITY

In general, morphinomimetics depress basal pituitary-thyroid activity in different species, as reflected by various parameters of thyroid function (8, 10, 22). However, a single injection of various morphine derivatives, except codeine, stimulated thyroidal ^{131}I release in mice (23). Chronic injection of these compounds inhibits release of thyroid-stimulating hormone (TSH). Adrenalectomy does not block the depressing effect of morphine on TSH release and TSH still activates the thyroid in morphine-treated rats (22). Lomax and

George (24) studied the locus of the depressing action of morphine on TSH release in the CNS. Lesions in the caudal region of the hypothalamus block morphine-induced thyroid inhibition. Microinjection of morphine reduces thyroid activity when injected into the rostral and caudal parts of the hypothalamus but not into the mid-hypothalamus, from which ACTH release can be elicited (17, 25). The effect on thyroid activity in the caudal area was maintained throughout the period of administration, while some tolerance seems to develop to the injection into rostral sites. Lomax et al. (25) suggested that morphine stimulates inhibitory neurons in the caudal hypothalamus which depress pituitary-thyroid function. The pituitary-thyroid axis responds normally to thyrotropin-releasing factor in patients on chronic methadone therapy (26). Similar studies in animals treated chronically with the narcotic analgesics are lacking.

PITUITARY-GONAD ACTIVITY

After either a single or chronic injection, morphine affects the secretion of gonadotropins (10, 27). Barraclough and Sawyer (27) found that administration of morphine between 12 and 2 P.M. on the day of proestrus in rats prevents ovulation. Chronically injected morphine daily between 12 and 2 P.M. inhibits ovulation for a considerable period of time. Tolerance to the drug results in the recurrence of ovulation, although cycles remain irregular. The site of the morphine effect is near the median eminence. Electrical stimulation in the median eminence, but not in the posterior tuberal region, overcomes the morphine blockade of ovulation (28). Addicts have irregular menstrual cycles and decreased gonadotropin secretion as reflected by a diminished urinary excretion of 17-ketosteroids, while the response to exogenous gonadotropins is enhanced (20, 21, 29). These and other data suggest that the release of luteinizing hormone (LH), and possibly of follicle-stimulating hormone (FSH), is reduced by morphine (8, 10).

The effect of morphine and related compounds on prolactin release has not been studied extensively. Several years ago, Meites (30a) reported that acute administration of morphine stimulates lactation in the rat, indicating an increase in the discharge of prolactin. Recently, increased circulating levels of prolactin have been observed in rats following systemic (30b) or intraventricular (30c) administration of morphine.

PITUITARY GROWTH HORMONE RELEASE

The narcotic analgesics have an interesting effect on growth hormone (GH) secretion in the rat. Whereas stress causes inhibition of GH release in this species (31, 32), the acute administration of morphine and related compounds causes an increase in both radioimmunoassayable circulating GH and plasma corticosterone (14, 31). The release of GH by morphine and related compounds occurs in doses lower than those necessary for pituitary-adrenal activation. Thus, stress-induced inhibition of GH release seems to interfere with the effect of the narcotic analgesics (14). Naloxone, which has no narcotic properties, does not affect GH release and only slightly stimulates pituitary-adrenal activity. In fact, naloxone inhibits morphine-induced ACTH release but not GH release. Thus, these two pituitary hormones are secreted under different control mechanisms (14). Chronic treatment with morphine produces tolerance to pituitary-adrenal activation (10, 11, 14). In contrast, the release of GH is enhanced during repeated administration of morphine (14).

In summary, a single injection of morphine and related compounds in rats stimulates the release of ACTH, GH, and possibly TSH and prolactin, and blocks FSH/LH release. Chronic administration in the same species reduces the release of ACTH, TSH, and FSH/LH while the release of GH is enhanced (Table 1).

TABLE 1. *Effect of the narcotic analgesics on anterior pituitary function in rats*

Treatment	ACTH	TSH	FSH/LH	GH	Prolactin
Acute	+	±	−	+	+
Chronic	±	−	−	++	?

+, Stimulation; −, reduction.

MORPHINE AND BRAIN TRANSMITTER ACTIVITY

Studies specially devoted to the relationship between anterior pituitary function and altered brain neurotransmitter activity after administration of morphine are scarce. The majority of studies on the effect of narcotic analgesics on brain transmission have concerned the involvement of norepinephrine (NE), dopamine (DA), serotonin (5-hydroxytryptamine, 5-HT), and acetylcholine (ACh) activity in analgesic mechanism, tolerance, and dependence. No uniform conclusion has emerged from these studies (3–7). The present data mainly concern recent observations in the rat, in particular hypothalamic changes.

Catecholamines

Reviews of earlier work (3, 4, 7) indicate that single doses of morphine mainly decrease brain NE content in various species, whereas tolerance to this effect develops after repeated administration. Data on brain DA content are less consistent. Accumulation studies with ^{14}C-tyrosine indicate a possible increased catecholamine synthesis rate, particularly of DA. Considerable variation in the results obtained by different authors may, at least in part, be explained by species and strain differences, inadequate doses, and differences in time interval after administration of morphine. Moreover, considerable regional variation in the effects of morphine on brain DA and NE exists in various species.

In the rat, single high doses of morphine decrease brain NE content (4, 33–35). Hypothalamic NE was found decreased in rats and cats (18, 35, 36). Whole rat brain and striatal DA content have been reported unaltered or slightly increased after acute morphine treatment (18, 34, 37, 38). We observed an increase in hypothalamic DA content (Table 2).

TABLE 2. *Effect of a single injection of morphine HCl (80 mg/kg) on hypothalamic catecholamine content and pituitary adrenal-activity in rats, assessed 30 min after administration*

	Corticosteroid production in vitro μg/100 mg adrenal/hr	Norepinephrine concentration % of controls	Dopamine concentration % of controls
Saline	12.2 ± 1.2[a]	100 ± 4	100 ± 6
Morphine HCl	23.5 ± 1.3[b]	90 ± 4[c]	115 ± 5[d]

[a] Mean ± SEM of 19 to 21 rats.
[b] $p < 0.001$.
[c] $p < 0.1$.
[d] $p = 0.05$.

A single dose of morphine increases the accumulation of labeled NE and DA in mouse brain after administration of radioactive tyrosine (39, 40). A similar increased accumulation of labeled brain DA occurs in various parts of rat brain (35, 37, 41). The turnover rate of DA as estimated by synthesis inhibition by α-methyl-p-tyrosine increases in rat striatum (38, 42), while the homovanillic acid content of rat and mouse brain also increases after acute morphine administration (43, 44). However, the accumulation of labeled NE in rat brain is not increased (35, 45), and has even been found decreased in the hypothalamus and striatum (35). The changes in synthesis rates of NE and DA apparently cannot be explained by altered tyrosine hydroxylase activity, since the activity of this enzyme was unchanged after acute morphine treatment in whole brain as well as in hypothalamus and other brain parts (41, 46).

Chronic treatment with morphine causes an increase in rat brain NE level, in particular in cortical areas (3, 4, 18, 33). No data concerning DA level in rats chronically treated with morphine are available. We found an elevation in the rat mesencephalon only (18). During chronic morphine treatment, tolerance develops to the increased accumulation of labeled NE and DA in mouse brain (40). Under these conditions the DA synthesis rate in several brain areas remains elevated in the rat (35, 45). Chronic treatment did not change rat brain tyrosine hydroxylase activity (46).

The decrease in NE content after a single injection of morphine, together with the increase in DA content and turnover of DA in the rat hypothalamus (35), may possibly be explained by an inhibitory effect of the analgesic on dopamine-β-hydroxylase activity. This would induce NE depletion and DA accumulation. Evidence for an influence of the narcotic analgesics on this enzyme, however, is lacking.

5-Hydroxytryptamine

Way (4, 47) reviewed the available data on the effect of acute and chronic administration of morphine on brain 5-HT. The bulk of evidence suggests that in various species single doses of morphine hardly alter 5-HT levels of the brain, but may increase 5-HT synthesis (4, 7, 47). In the rat an increased 5-HT turnover was found in the brain after a single injection of morphine (48–50).

Repeated administration of morphine also does not materially affect the concentration of brain 5-HT in various species (4, 47, 50, 51). The 5-HT turnover rate may be increased or unchanged in chronic morphinized animals (4, 47, 48, 50–52). No significant alteration of tryptophan hydroxylase activity has been found after acute and chronic morphine administration (50, 53).

Acetylcholine

ACh concentration of whole brain increases following an acute injection of a high dose of morphine (5, 7, 54–57). This increase is not caused by an accelerated synthesis or a diminished enzymatic destruction (5, 7, 58) but is probably due to prevention of release, since the narcotic analgesics reduce the release from peripheral and central cholinergic neurons (5, 7, 57). Chronic administration of morphine induces tolerance to these effects (5, 7, 54, 57).

MORPHINE AND THE NEUROENDOCRINE CONTROL OF ANTERIOR PITUITARY FUNCTION

The acute effect of morphine on hypothalamic NE and DA may have a bearing on its influence on anterior pituitary activity. The increased release of ACTH, GH, and possibly TSH and prolactin and the reduction in FSH/LH release as a result of acute morphine administration may be related to NE depletion and/or DA accumulation in the rat hypothalamus. Indeed, it has been suggested that the release of ACTH is under a central inhibitory noradrenergic control mechanism (32, 59). For example, stimulation of α-adrenoreceptor activity in the brain inhibits stress-induced ACTH release, while a decrease in hypothalamic NE elicits an increased pituitary-adrenal activity (60, 61). In particular, the NE-depleting effect of a single injection of morphine may be causally related to the reported increased release of ACTH. It was therefore of interest to study the effect of morphine on both hypothalamic catecholamine concentration and on ACTH release. Morphine HCl in a dose of 80 mg/kg was administered intraperitoneally to female Wistar rats weighing between 120 and 150 g. Half an hour after the injection of the morphine, pituitary-adrenal activity was determined by the rate of corticosteroid production of excised adrenal glands *in vitro* (62). Hypothalamic catecholamine concentration was determined fluorometrically according to Laverty and Taylor (63).

Morphine caused a marked increase in the rate of corticosteroid production *in vitro* while hypothalamic NE content declined and DA content increased significantly (Table 2). A significant negative correlation ($p < 0.01$) between corticosteroid production rate *in vitro* and the hypothalamic NE content appeared to exist. No significant correlation was found between steroid production rate and the hypothalamic DA content (Fig. 1). These results may suggest that morphine stimulates pituitary ACTH release by removing a central

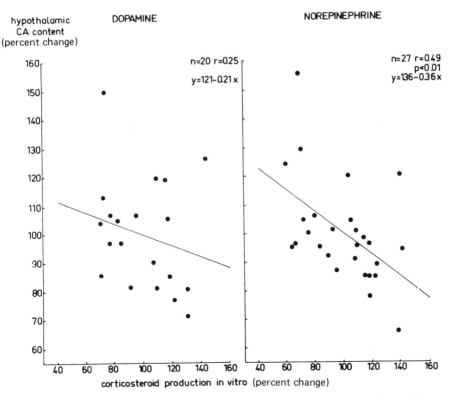

FIG. 1. Relation between corticosteroid production rate of rat adrenal glands *in vitro* and hypothalamic dopamine and norepinephrine content half an hour after i.p. administration of morphine HCl (80 mg/kg). The data were obtained in experiments carried out on different days and individual values were calculated as the percent deviation of the mean of each experiment.

inhibitory noradrenergic control on the cells in the median eminence producing corticotropin-releasing factor (32, 59).

Removal of the adrenal glands potentiates morphine-induced hypothalamic NE depletion. Adrenalectomized rats were maintained on a "low" (1 mg/kg per day) or a "high" (10 mg/kg per day) corticosterone regimen for 3 days. Morphine injected on the 4th day, again in a dose of 80 mg/kg, caused a NE depletion to $74 \pm 5\%$ in the "low" corticosterone-substituted rats compared with $88 \pm 4\%$ in sham-operated control rats. Interestingly, no depletion was found in the "high" corticosterone-substituted animals, suggesting a steroid feedback control on hypothalamic NE neurons. This corroborates findings reported by Dallman and Yates (64) and Ganong (65) that the monoamine oxidase inhibitor iproniazide potentiates dexamethasone in blocking stress-induced ACTH release, and those by Ganong (65) that monoamine oxidase inhibitors prevent reserpine-induced ACTH release. However, the same corticosterone treatment which in adrenalectomized rats blocked morphine-induced NE depletion was ineffective in intact rats, although the pituitary-adrenal response was reduced. Thus, other transmitter systems may be involved. For example, p-chlorophenylalanine (p-CPA), which inhibits brain 5-HT synthesis, reduces the feedback action of prednisolone while tryptophan administration abolishes stress-induced ACTH release in adrenalectomized rats (66). Cortisol (67) or betamethasone (68) decreases brain 5-HT levels, although an initial increase followed by a decrease in rat brain after betamethasone treatment has also been reported (69). However, Vermes et al. (70), who found an increase in hypothalamic 5-HT following corticosterone administration, argued that the discrepancy in the literature is caused by the different time intervals used in the various experiments and the uneven distribution of the serotonergic system in the brain, in addition to independent changes in 5-HT content in different parts of the brain. These authors also found that 5-HT administered intraventricularly or implanted in the medial hypothalamus blocks stress-induced pituitary-adrenal activation (71) and compensatory adrenal hypertrophy (72). Thus, 5-HT may be involved in the feedback action of adrenocortical steroids, since these steroids may restore hypothalamic 5-HT concentration. In this respect it is noteworthy that dexamethasone is a more potent inhibitor of morphine-induced ACTH release than of ether stress-induced release (73). However, the findings of Vermes et al. (70–72) argue against the participation of serotonergic pathways in pituitary ACTH release elicited by the acute administration of morphine.

Hypothalamic DA is implicated in the release of FSH/LH, prolactin, and GH (32). DA releases luteinizing hormone-releasing factor from rat hypothalamic fragments (74) and, when injected intraventricularly, stimulates LH release (75). Other studies suggest a stimulatory dopaminergic control of ovulation (32). The tubero-infundibular DA neurons are held responsible for a tonic inhibitory effect on the release of prolactin and GH in the rat (32, 75, 76). The accumulation of hypothalamic DA, together with an increase in the turnover rate of this amine as elicited by morphine, should therefore be consistent with an increase in FSH/LH release and a decrease in the release of prolactin and GH. Since the release of these pituitary hormones is affected in a reverse way by acute morphine treatment, it follows that the alteration in hypothalamic DA may not be related to the secretion of prolactin, GH, and FSH/LH under these conditions. However, the findings of Hökfelt and Fuxe (77) on the tubero-infundibular DA neurons in relation to LH release partly disagree with these considerations.

Morphine has been shown to affect 5-HT synthesis, and several reports (48–50) point to an increase in the turnover of this amine in rat brain. Interestingly, intraventricularly or systemically administered 5-hydroxytryptophan (5-HTP) stimulates prolactin release (75) and intraventricularly injected 5-HT inhibits the release of FSH and LH, as does the systemic administration of 5-HTP (75). Although Müller et al. (78) failed to demonstrate bioassayable GH release following intraventricular 5-HT, Collu et al. (76) reported a marked stimulatory effect of 5-HT on GH release. Thus, the inhibitory effect of morphine on the release of FSH/LH and its stimulatory influence on the release of prolactin and GH release might be the result of an increased activity of 5-HT neurons in the CNS as induced by the analgesic. 5-Hydroxytryptamine depletion in rat brain is associated with a marked depression of serum TSH (79). The enhanced activity of brain serotonergic neurons following morphine might therefore be involved in the release of TSH. However, the evidence that morphine increases the release of TSH is derived from one study in mice only (23), and chronic morphine depresses TSH release in the presence of a possible enhanced 5-HT synthesis (10, 47–50).

Finally, the reduced release of ACh found after a single injection of morphine (5, 7, 57) and the well-known inhibitory effect of atropine on ovulation (80–82) and on ACTH release (83, 84) suggest the possibility of a cholinergic participation in morphine-induced alterations in anterior pituitary function.

CONCLUDING REMARKS

It is clear that the available data do not allow a conclusion as to the nature of the influence of the narcotic analgesics on the neuroendocrine control of the anterior pituitary. We lack adequate information not only about transmitter activity in the brain, in particular in the hypothalamus, under acute and chronic treatment with morphinomimetics, but also about the simultaneous measurement of hypothalamic transmitter activity and the release of anterior pituitary hormones. In addition, the interpretation of the effects of morphine and related compounds on brain neurotransmitters should take into account the influence of releasing factors and anterior pituitary- and target gland hormones on brain neurotransmitter activity. For example, thyrotropin-releasing factor potentiates L-DOPA activity in intact and hypophysectomized rats

(85). ACTH and corticosteroids increase the turnover of brain catechol-amines (32, 86) and the concentration of hypothalamic 5-HT (70). Estrogens and testosterone may increase DA turnover in the tubero-infundibular neurons in the median eminence (77), and progesterone affects 5-HT concentration in the brain (1). Prolactin stimulates DA turnover in the median eminence of intact, castrated, and hypophysectomized rats (77). Finally, the diurnal varia-tion in pituitary activity relates to variation in brain transmitter activity, and the circadian variation in pituitary-adrenal activity disappears in rats whose brains are depleted of 5-HT (87–89).

Admittedly, the impact of the effects of these hormones on brain transmitter activity should not be exaggerated, since pharmacologic rather than physio-logic amounts were used in most of the studies. Nevertheless, alterations in pituitary function by narcotic analgesics may interfere with brain transmitter activity, thereby obscuring the initial effects of these drugs. Thus, morphine effects should be explored in intact rats as well as in animals in which the pitui-tary gland and/or the various target glands are removed, preferably at a time when brain neurotransmitter activity has not materially changed due to hor-mone deficiency. In addition, in order to evaluate the effect of drugs on the neuroendocrine control of anterior pituitary function, their influence should be assessed on the respective transmitter systems to the·releasing factor cells rather than in whole brain, hypothalamus, or parts of these structures.

SUMMARY

The recent literature concerning the influence of morphine on neuroendo-crine control of anterior pituitary activity is briefly reviewed. In particular the effect of narcotic analgesics on the release of anterior pituitary hormones and on hypothalamic neurotransmitters is surveyed. Data are presented on the re-lationship between changes in hypothalamic catecholamine levels and pitui-tary-adrenal activity following single administration of morphine in rats.

REFERENCES

1. Wurtman, R. J. Brain monoamines and endocrine function. *Neurosci. Res. Progr. Bull.,* 9, No. 2, 1971.
2. Wurtman, R. J. Biogenic amines and endocrine function. *Fed. Proc.,* 32:1769–1771, 1973.
3. Dole, V. P. Biochemistry of addiction. *Ann. Rev. Biochem.,* 39:821–840, 1970.
4. Way, E. L., and Shen, F.-Hs. Catecholamines and 5-hydroxytryptamine. In: *Narcotic Drugs, Biochemical Pharmacology,* edited by D. H. Clouet, pp. 229–253. Plenum Press, New York, 1971.
5. Weinstock, M. Acetylcholine and cholinesterase. In: *Narcotic Drugs, Biochemical Pharmacology,* edited by D. H. Clouet, pp. 254–261. Plenum Press, New York, 1971.
6. Clouet, D. H. Theoretical biochemical mechanisms for drug dependence. In: *Chemical and Biological Aspects of Drug Dependence,* edited by S. J. Mulé and H. Brill, pp. 545–561. CRC Press, Cleveland, Ohio, 1972.

7. Smith, C. B. Neurotransmitters and the narcotic analgesics. In: *Chemical and Biological Aspects of Drug Dependence*, edited by S. J. Mulé and H. Brill, pp. 495–504. CRC Press, Cleveland, Ohio, 1972.
8. George, R. Hypothalamus: Anterior Pituitary Gland. In: *Narcotic Drugs, Biochemical Pharmacology*, edited by D. H. Clouet, pp. 283–299. Plenum Press, New York, 1971.
9. Sloan, J. W. Corticosteroid hormones. In: *Narcotic Drugs, Biochemical Pharmacology*, edited by D. H. Clouet, pp. 262–282. Plenum Press, New York, 1971.
10. George, R., and Lomax, P. Hormones. In: *Chemical and Biological Aspects of Drug Dependence*, edited by S. J. Mulé and H. Brill, pp. 523–543. CRC Press, Cleveland, Ohio, 1972.
11. Munson, P. L. Effects of morphine and related drugs on the corticotrophin (ACTH)-stress reaction. *Progr. Brain Res.*, 39:361–372, 1973.
12. McDonald, R. K., Evans, F. T., Weise, V. K., and Patrick, R. W. Effect of morphine and nalorphine on plasma hydrocortisone levels in man. *J. Pharmacol. Exp. Ther.*, 125:241–247, 1959.
13. Nikodijevic, O., and Maickel, R. P. Some effects of morphine on pituitary-adrenocortical function in the rat. *Biochem. Pharmacol.*, 16:2137–2142, 1967.
14. Kokka, N., Garcia, J. F., and Elliott, H. W. Effects of acute and chronic administration of narcotic analgesics on growth hormone and corticotrophin (ACTH) secretion in rats. *Progr. Brain Res.*, 39:347–360, 1973.
15. Briggs, F. N., and Munson, P. L. Studies on the mechanism of stimulation of ACTH secretion with the aid of morphine as a blocking agent. *Endocrinology*, 57:205–219, 1955.
16. George, R., and Way, E. L. The role of the hypothalamus in pituitary-adrenal activation and antidiuresis by morphine. *J. Pharmacol. Exp. Ther.*, 125:111–115, 1959.
17. Lotti, V. J., Kokka, N., and George, R. Pituitary-adrenal activation following intrahypothalamic microinjection of morphine. *Neuroendocrinology*, 4:326–332, 1969.
18. van Ree, J. M. *Unpublished data.*
19. Eisenman, A. J., Fraser, H. F., and Brooks, J. W. Urinary excretion and plasma levels of 17-hydroxycorticosteroids during a cycle of addiction to morphine. *J. Pharmacol. Exp. Ther.*, 132:226–231, 1961.
20. Eisenman, A. J., Fraser, H. F., Sloan, J., and Isbell, H. Urinary 17-ketosteroid excretion during a cycle of addiction to morphine. *J. Pharmacol. Exp. Ther.*, 124:305–311, 1958.
21. Hollister, L. E. Human pharmacology of drugs of abuse with emphasis on neuroendocrine effects. *Progr. Brain Res.*, 39:373–381, 1973.
22. George, R. Effects of narcotic analgesics on hypothalamo-pituitary-thyroid function. *Progr. Brain Res.*, 39:339–345, 1973.
23. Redding, T. W., Bowers, C. Y., and Schally, A. V. The effects of morphine and other narcotics on thyroid function in mice. *Acta Endocrinol. (Kbh.)*, 51:391–399, 1966.
24. Lomax, P., and George, R. Thyroid activity following administration of morphine in rats with hypothalamic lesions. *Brain Res.*, 2:361:367, 1966.
25. Lomax, P., Kokka, N., and George, R. Thyroid activity following intracerebral injection of morphine in the rat. *Neuroendocrinology*, 6:146–152, 1970.
26. Shenkman, L., Massie, B., Mitsuma, T., and Hollander, C. S. Effects of chronic methadone administration on the hypothalamic-pituitary-thyroid axis. *J. Clin. Endocr. Metab.*, 35:169–170, 1972.
27. Barraclough, C. A., and Sawyer, C. H. Inhibition of the release of pituitary ovulatory hormone in the rat by morphine. *Endocrinology*, 57:329–337, 1955.
28. Sawyer, C. H. Neuroendocrine blocking agents: Discussion. In: *Advances in Neuroendocrinology*, edited by A. V. Nalbandov, pp. 444–457. University Illinois Press, Urbana, 1963.
29. Stoffer, S. S. A gynecologic study of drug addicts. *Am. J. Obst. Gynec.*, 101:779–783, 1968.

30a. Meites, J. Control of mammary growth and lactation. In: *Neuroendocrinology,* Vol. 1, edited by L. Martini and W. F. Ganong, pp. 669–707. Academic Press, New York, 1966.

30b. Zimmermann, E., Pang, C. N., and Sawyer, C. H. Morphine-induced prolactin release and its suppression by dexamethasone in male rats. *Endocr. Soc. Abstr.,* 1974.

30c. McCann, S. M., Ojeda, S. R., Libertun, C., Harms, P. G., and Krulich, L. Drug-induced alterations in gonadotropin and prolactin release in the rat. *This volume.*

31. Kokka, N., Garcia, J. F., George, R., and Elliott, H. W. Growth hormone and ACTH secretion: Evidence for an inverse relationship in rats. *Endocrinology,* 90:735–743, 1972.

23. de Wied, D., and de Jong, W. Drug effects and hypothalamic-anterior pituitary function. *Ann. Rev. Pharmacol.,* 14:389–412, 1974.

33. Gunne, L.-M. Catecholamines and 5-hydroxytryptamine in morphine tolerance and withdrawal. *Acta Physiol. Scand.,* 58, suppl. 204:1–91, 1963.

34. Holtzman, S. G., and Jewett, R. E. Some actions of pentazocine on behaviour and brain monoamines in the rat. *J. Pharmacol. Exp. Ther.,* 181:346–356, 1972.

35. Johnson, J. C., and Clouet, D. H. Studies on the effect of acute and chronic morphine treatment on catecholamine levels and turnover in discrete brain areas of rats. *Fed. Proc.,* 32:757 (Abs. 3062), 1973.

36. Reis, D. J., Rifkin, M. and Corvelli, A. Effects of morphine on cat brain norepinephrine in regions with daily monoamine rhythms. *Europ. J. Pharmacol.,* 9:149–152, 1969.

37. Gauchy, C., Agid, Y., Glowinski, J., and Cheramy, A. Acute effects of morphine on dopamine synthesis and release and tyrosine metabolism in the rat stratium. *Europ. J. Pharmacol.,* 22:311–319, 1973.

38. Sugrue, M. F. Effects of morphine and pentazocine on the turnover of noradrenaline and dopamine in various regions of the rat brain. *Brit. J. Pharmacol.,* 47:644P, 1973.

39. Loh, H. H., Hitzemann, R. J., and Way, E. L. Effect of acute morphine administration on the metabolism of brain catecholamines. *Life Sci.,* Part I, 12:33–41, 1973.

40. Smith, C. B., Sheldon, M. I., Bednarczyk, J. H., and Villarreal, J. E. Morphine-induced increases in the incorporation of ^{14}C-tyrosine into ^{14}C-dopamine and ^{14}C-norepinephrine in the mouse brain: Antagonism by naloxone and tolerance. *J. Pharmacol. Exp. Ther.,* 180:547–557, 1972.

41. Costa, E., Carenzi, A., Guidotti, A., and Revuelta. A. Narcotic analgesics and the regulation of neuronal catecholamine stores. *Life Sci.,* 13:xxi–xxii, 1973.

42. Puri, S. K., and Lal, H. Effect of morphine, haloperidol, apomorphine and benztropine on dopamine turnover in rat corpus striatum: Evidence showing morphine-induced reduction in CNS dopaminergic activity. *Fed. Proc.,* 32:758 (Abs. 3065), 1973.

43. Fukui, K., and Takagi, H. Effect of morphine on the cerebral contents of metabolites of dopamine in normal and tolerant mice: Its possible relation to analgesic action. *Brit. J. Pharmacol.,* 44:45–51, 1972.

44. Gessa, G. L. Effect of methadone and other narcotic analgesics on brain dopamine metabolism. *Life Sci.,* 13:xlv, 1973.

45. Clouet, D. H., and Ratner, M. Catecholamine biosynthesis in brains of rats treated with morphine. *Science,* 168:854–856, 1970.

46. Cicero, T. J., Wilcox, C. E., Smithloff, B. R., Meyer, E. R., and Sharpe, L. G. Effects of morphine, *in vitro* and *in vivo*, on tyrosine hydroxylase activity in rat brain. *Biochem. Pharmacol.,* 22:3237–3246, 1973.

47. Way, E. L. Role of serotonin in morphine effects. *Fed. Proc.,* 31:113–120, 1972.

48. Haubrich, D. R., and Blake, D. E. Modification of serotonin metabolism in rat brain after acute or chronic administration of morphine. *Biochem. Pharmacol.,* 22:2753–2759, 1973.

49. Yarbrough, G. G., Buxbaum, D. M., and Sanders-Bush, E. Increased serotonin turnover in the acutely morphine treated rat. *Life Sci.,* Part I, 10:977–983, 1971.

50. Yarbrough, G. G., Buxbaum, D. M., and Sanders-Bush, E. Biogenic amines and narcotic effects. II. Serotonin turnover in the rat after acute and chronic morphine administration. *J. Pharmacol. Exp. Ther.*, 185:328–335, 1973.

51. Ho, I. K., Lu, S. E., Stolman, S., Loh, H. H., and Way, E. L. Influence of p-chlorophenylalanine on morphine tolerance and physical dependence and regional brain serotonin turnover studies in morphine tolerant-dependent mice. *J. Pharmacol. Exp. Ther.*, 182:155–165, 1972.

52. Cheney, D. L., Goldstein, A., Algeri, S., and Costa, E. Narcotic tolerance and dependence: Lack of relationship with serotonin turnover in the brain. *Science*, 171:1169–1170, 1971.

53. Schechter, P. J., Lovenberg, W., and Sjoerdsma, A. Dissociation of morphine tolerance and dependence from brain serotonin synthesis rate in mice. *Biochem. Pharmacol.*, 21:751–753, 1972.

54. Large, W. A., and Milton, A. S. The effect of acute and chronic morphine administration on brain acetylcholine levels in the rat. *Brit. J. Pharmacol.*, 38:452P, 1970.

55. Richter, J. A., and Goldstein, A. Effects of morphine and levorphanol on brain acetylcholine content in mice. *J. Pharmacol. Exp. Ther.*, 175:685–691, 1970.

56. Grossland, J., and Slater, P. The effect of some drugs on the "free" and "bound" acetylcholine content of rat brain. *Brit. J. Pharmacol.*, 33:42–47, 1968.

57. Domino, E. F., and Wilson, A. Effects of narcotic analgesic agonists and antagonists on rat brain acetylcholine. *J. Pharmacol. Exp. Ther.*, 184:18–32, 1973.

58. Sharkawi, M. Effects of morphine and pentobarbitone on acetylcholine synthesis by rat cerebral cortex. *Brit. J. Pharmacol.*, 40:86–91, 1970.

59. Ganong, W. F. Brain mechanisms regulating the secretion of the pituitary gland. In: *The Neurosciences, Third Study Program*, edited by F. O. Schmitt and F. G. Worden, pp. 549–563. MIT Press, Cambridge, 1974.

60. van Loon, G. R., Scapagnini, U., Moberg, G. P., and Ganong, W. F. Evidence for central adrenergic neural inhibition of ACTH secretion in the rat. *Endocrinology*, 89:1464–1469, 1971.

61. Scapagnini, U. Pharmacological studies of brain control over ACTH secretion. In: *The Neurosciences, Third Study Program*, edited by F. O. Schmitt and F. G. Worden, pp. 565–569. MIT Press, Cambridge, 1974.

62. van der Vies, J., Bakker, R. F. M., and de Wied, D. Correlated studies on plasma free corticosterone and on adrenal steroid formation rate in vitro. *Acta Endocrinol. (Kbh)*, 34:513–523, 1960.

63. Laverty, R., and Taylor, K. M. The fluorometric assay of catecholamines and related compounds: Improvements and extensions to the hydroxyindole technique. *Anal. Biochem.*, 22:269–279, 1968.

64. Dallman, M. F., and Yates, F. E. Anatomical and functional mapping of central neural input and feedback pathways of the adrenocortical system. In: *Memoirs of the Society for Endocrinology, 17*, edited by V. H. T. James and J. Landon, pp. 39–72. Cambridge University Press, Cambridge, England, 1968.

65. Ganong, W. F. Evidence for a central noradrenergic system that inhibits ACTH secretion. In: *Brain-Endocrine Interaction Median Eminence: Structure and Function*, edited by K. M. Knigge, D. E. Scott, and A. Weindl, pp. 254–266. S. Karger, Basel, 1972.

66. Vernikos-Danellis, J., Berger, P., and Barchas, J. D. Brain serotonin and pituitary-adrenal function. *Progr. Brain Res.*, 39:301–309, 1973.

67. Curzon, G. Effect of adrenal hormones and stress on brain serotonin. *Amer. J. Clin. Nutr.*, 24:830–834, 1971.

68. Scapagnini, U., Preziosi, P., and de Schaepdryver, A. Influence of restraint stress, corticosterone and betamethasone on brain amine levels. *Pharmacol. Res. Comm.*, 1:63–66, 1969.

69. de Schaepdryver, A., Preziosi, P., and Scapagnini, U. Brain monoamines and adrenocortical activation. *Brit. J. Pharmacol.*, 35:460–467, 1969.

70. Vermes, I., Telegdy, G., and Lissák, K. Correlation between hypothalamic serotonin content and adrenal function during acute stress. Effect of adrenal corticosteroids

on hypothalamic serotonin content. *Acta Physiol. Acad. Sci. Hung.*, 43:33–42, 1973.

71. Vermes, I., and Telegdy, G. Effect of intraventricular injection and intrahypothalamic implantation of serotonin on the hypothalamo-hypophyseal-adrenal system in the rat. *Acta Physiol. Acad. Sci. Hung.*, 42:49–59, 1972.

72. Vermes, I., Molnár, D., and Telegdy, G. The effect of hypothalamic serotonin on compensatory adrenal function. *Acta Physiol. Acad. Sci. Hung.*, 43:27–32, 1973.

73. Zimmermann, E., and Critchlow, V. Inhibition of morphine-induced pituitary-adrenal activation by dexamethasone in the female rat. *Proc. Soc. Exp. Biol. Med.*, 143:1224–1226, 1973.

74. Schneider, H. P. G., and McCann, S. M. Possible role of dopamine as transmitter to promote discharge of LH-releasing factor. *Endocrinology*, 85:121–132, 1969.

75. Kamberi, I. A. The role of brain monoamines and pineal indoles in the secretion of gonadotrophins and gonadotrophin-releasing factors. *Progr. Brain Res.*, 39:261–278, 1973.

76. Collu, R., Fraschini, F., and Martini, L. Role of indoleamines and catecholamines in the control of gonadotrophin and growth hormone secretion. *Progr. Brain Res.*, 39:289–299, 1973.

77. Hökfelt, T., and Fuxe, K. On the morphology and the neuroendocrine role of the hypothalamic catecholamine neurons. In: *Brain-Endocrine Interaction Median Eminence: Structure and Function*, edited by K. M. Knigge, D. E. Scott, and A. Weindl, pp. 181–223. S. Karger, Basel, 1972.

78. Müller, E. E., Cocchi, D., Jalanbo, H., and Udeschini, G. Antagonistic role for norepinephrine (NE) and dopamine (DA) in the control of growth hormone (GH) secretion in the rat. Ineffectiveness of serotonin (5-HT). *Endocrinology, Suppl.* 92, A-248, 1973.

79. Shenkman, L., Sanghvi, I., Shopsin, B., Kataoka, K., Imai, Y., Gershon, S., and Hollander, C. S. T3, T4, TSH and prolactin response to *p*-chlorophenylalanine (PCPA): A role for serotonin in thyro-pituitary function. *Endocrinology, Suppl.* 92, A-138, 1973.

80. Everett, J. W., Sawyer, C. H., and Markee, J. E. A neurogenic timing factor in control of the ovulatory discharge of luteinizing hormone in the cyclic rat. *Endocrinology*, 44:234–250, 1949.

81. Sawyer, C. H., Critchlow, B. V., and Barraclough, C. A. Mechanism of blockade of pituitary activation in the rat by morphine, atropine and barbiturates. *Endocrinology*, 57:345–354, 1955.

82. Kamberi, I. A., and Bacleon, E. S. Cholinergic pathways and gonadotropin releasing factors. *Fed. Proc.*, 32:240 Abs, 1973.

83. Hedge, G. A., and Smelik, P. G Corticotrophin release: Inhibition by intrahypothalamic implantation of atropine. *Science*, 159:891–892, 1968.

84. Kaplanski, J., and Smelik, P. G. Analysis of the inhibition of the ACTH release by hypothalamic implants of atropine. *Acta Endocrinol. (Kbh).*, 73:651–659, 1973.

85. Plotnikoff, N. P., Brange, A. J., Jr., Breese, G. R., Anderson, M. S., and Wilson, I. C. Thyrotropin releasing hormone: Enhancement of Dopa activity by a hypothalamic hormone. *Science*, 178:417–418, 1972.

86. Versteeg, D. H. G. *Personal communication.*

87. Scapagnini, U., Moberg, G. P., van Loon, G. R., de Groot, J., and Ganong, W. F. Relation of brain 5-hydroxytryptamine content to the diurnal variation in plasma corticosterone in the rat. *Neuroendocrinology*, 7:90–96, 1971.

88. van Delft, A. M. L., Kaplanski, J., and Smelik, P. G. Circadian periodicity of pituitary-adrenal function after *p*-chlorophenylalanine administration in the rat. *J. Endocr.*, 59:465–474, 1973.

89. Krieger, D. T., and Rizzo, F. Serotonin mediation of circadian periodicity of plasma 17-hydroxycorticosteroids. *Amer. J. Physiol.*, 217:1703–1707, 1969.

DISCUSSION

Way: With respect to effects of narcotics on serotonin turnover in brain, I would like to point out that although we were unable to find any difference in turnover rate, others have observed an increase in serotonin turnover following administration of morphine.

De Wied: I agree that there is no consistent effect reported in the literature. It seems to depend largely upon the species and there is a great difference between the responses of rats and of mice. I have the feeling that 5-HT may be very important in mediating the effects of morphine on the pituitary. I think more work should be done in this area.

Ganong: How good is the evidence that serotonin is involved in growth hormone secretion?

De Wied: It is difficult to clearly implicate serotonin in growth hormone secretion and the available evidence is not clear-cut. One of the complicating factors is that many of the available studies have been performed in anesthetized animals.

Weiner: The evidence you've reviewed would indicate that serotonin is involved in the stimulation of prolactin secretion by morphine. On the other hand, morphine causes increased turnover and brain content of dopamine which itself inhibits prolactin secretion. It is possible that dopamine would also act to inhibit prolactin in the presence of stimulation by serotonin. Would you care to comment on this potential conflict?

De Wied: From the available evidence it is difficult, if not impossible, to say that dopamine is released under these conditions. The only consistent finding we have is that dopamine content in brain increases. This may indicate an increased synthesis without increased release of dopamine. Another problem is that most of the available evidence is based on dopamine concentrations in whole brain tissue. To really get at the question, it is necessary to look specifically at hypothalamus and probably at medial hypothalamic tissue in particular.

Gorski: I would like to pose a very difficult question. Is there a relationship between changes in neuroendocrine function produced by drugs of abuse and drug addiction?

De Wied: Perhaps Dr. Zimmermann would like to respond to this question. There has been a dialogue on this question between our laboratories now for several years.

Zimmermann: You have raised a fundamental question for which there is, at the present time, no satisfactory answer. I think it is safe to say that all that is known about the phenomenon of addiction, or tolerance and physical dependence, cannot be accounted for simply on the basis of changes in production, storage, or removal a single endogenous neural chemical substance, be it a neurotransmitter or hormone. We have obtained evidence that hormones can antagonize certain specific actions of narcotics *in vivo* or on isolated spinal cord preparations, but it is not yet possible to generalize upon these findings and say that they therefore explain addiction. Nevertheless, I think hormonal changes should be looked at more diligently in relation to the causes of tolerance and physical dependence.

INDEX

A